Rethra

I0028582

Mark Campbell and Viktor Harsch

Hubertus Strughold

Life and Work in the Fields of Space Medicine

2013

RETHRA VERLAG NEUBRANDENBURG

Rethra Verlag GbR, Neubrandenburg, www.rethra-verlag.de
23 Aalstrasse, Neubrandenburg, 17033, Germany
First edition

Copyright © 2013 Rethra Verlag ™
All rights reserved

Printed by Books on Demand, Norderstedt, Germany.

No part of this publication may be reproduced, stored in a retrieval system or transmitted in any form or by any means electronic, mechanical, photocopying, recording or otherwise without the prior written permission of the publisher

Permissions may be sought directly from Rethra Verlag Rights Department in Germany: fax (+49) 395 5667564;
For information on all Rethra publications
visit our website at www.rethra-publishing.de

Die verwendeten Abbildungen, sofern nicht explizit ange-
führt, befinden sich aufgrund ihres Alters in der public do-
main bzw. im Verfügungsstand der Autoren. Gleichwohl
unterliegt die etwaige Weiterverteilung den engen Grenzen des Urheberrechtes.

Das Werk einschließlich aller seiner Teile ist urheberrechtlich geschützt.
Jede Verwertung außerhalb der Grenzen des Urheberrechtes ist
ohne Zustimmung des Verlages unzulässig. Das gilt insbesondere für
Vervielfältigungen, Übersetzungen, Mikroverfilmungen und die
Einspeicherung und Verarbeitung in elektronischen Systemen.

Die Beiträge geben ausschließlich die Meinung der Autoren wieder.

ISBN 978-3-937394-47-3

Contents

Hubertus Strughold, The Father of Space Medicine

Introduction

Man mag vielleicht sagen, daß Raumfahrtphysiologie in das Reich der Phantasie gehört. Wir sollten jedoch immer wissen, daß in zahlreichen Fällen die Phantasie von gestern die Wirklichkeit von morgen ist.

Some will say that aerospace physiology belongs to the kingdom of fantasy. However, we should always remember that in many cases the fantasies of yesterday will become reality tomorrow.

Strughold 1951 (1)

Dr. Hubertus Strughold (1898-1986) is known as the "Father of Space Medicine". The Space Medicine Branch of the Aerospace Medical Association initiated the "Hubertus Strughold Award" in 1963, given to the person each year for the greatest achievement in space medicine. Dr. Strughold has become extremely controversial since his death based upon alleged, but unsubstantiated links, to war atrocities in Nazi Germany during World War II. However, he was never a member of the Nazi party and no evidence of his involvement in any war crimes has ever been found. Despite many outstanding contributions in aerospace medicine, several books and many internet sites describe him in derogatory terms and most of his honors have been removed. A review of all available evidence, including examination of his files from the U.S. Dept. of Justice obtained under the Freedom of Information Act, shows no direct involvement, direction or participation by Dr. Strughold in any war crimes.

The commandant of the School of Aviation Medicine, Col. Harry G. Armstrong, organized the first Department of Space Medicine in the world on February 9, 1949. Dr. Hubertus Strughold became the first and only Professor of Space Medicine in 1958. Under his leadership, the school became a major center for basic and clinical investigations into the physiological and behavioral effects of spaceflight and the space environment.

In November 1948, Dr. Armstrong organized a panel discussion on the "Aeromedical Problems of Space Travel." Strughold resolved the contradiction inherent in the title of the symposium during his presentations by emphatically using the term "space medicine" for the first time. Dr. Strughold estimated that the main medical problems of space flight could be formulated, the majority of the questions fully answered within 10 to 15 years, and that the first manned space flights would become feasible between 1964 and 1969. In March of 1950, another symposium, "The Biological Aspects of Manned Space Flight", featured Dr. Strughold as one of the main presenters. This conference led to discussions to form a permanent space medicine organization. On May 31, 1950, Dr. Strughold and 17 other aerospace medical experts founded the Space Medicine Branch of the Aerospace Medical Association.

In November 1951, Dr. Strughold organized a symposium discreetly entitled "Physics and Medicine of the Upper Atmosphere." A good portion of the material presented covered the nature of space, the mechanics of space flight, and the medical difficulties of sending a man beyond the sensible and breathable atmosphere. Two other space medicine symposiums were later organized by Dr. Strughold and conducted in 1960 and 1965.

In 1951, Dr. Strughold published this seminal paper in the Journal of Aviation Medicine (the forerunner of Aviation, Space and Environmental Medicine) in which he proposed a dramatic thesis concerning the human potential for space exploration. Dr. Strughold addressed the central problem of where space began and proposed that space was present in small gradations as altitude levels increased rather than existing in the remote regions of the atmosphere.

At the urging of Hubertus Strughold, the Air Force funded the construction of a space cabin simulator. In 1958, an Air Force airman spent seven days in the chamber performing a number of tasks for psychological monitoring and wearing biological instrumentation. Strughold had a long career at the School of Aviation Medicine. Among the fundamental studies initiated were those in acceleration, noise and vibration, atmospheric control, and nutrition. He contributed enormously to such space-travel problems as weightlessness, visual disturbances, and disruption of normal time cycles. He was particularly interested in the aspects of the space medical problems related to Mars.

Dr. Strughold's World War II record did not become a public issue until 1958, when a magazine article charged that he used prisoners in his German research. This charge was disproved by a Justice Department investigation. This 1958 investigation was dropped when the Air Force stated that Strughold already had been "appropriately investigated". The allegations resurfaced in 1974, when the Immigration and Naturalization Service (INS) investigated him for allegations of Nazi war crimes and considered possible deportation. The investigation was terminated several months later due to lack of evidence. The INS Director Leonard Chapman reported that inquiries to the military and other federal agencies had disclosed "no derogatory information" and therefore the INS considered the case closed. The Department of Justice – Office of Special Investigations reopened the investigation again in 1983, but this was terminated upon Dr. Strughold's death in 1986.

Several popular books have been published that have commented on the Strughold controversy. In "The Paperclip Conspiracy, The Hunt for Nazi Scientists" (1987), Dr. Strughold is not accused of any direct involvement in any war crimes, but of knowing about medical experiments that occurred at Dachau and trying to cover-up for his colleagues

The statement was made, "The Office of Special Investigation had an open investigation file on him (Dr. Strughold) since the early 1980's, with abundant evidence of his knowledge of and complicity in the Dachau experiments.

In the "Secret Agenda: The United States Government, Nazi Scientists and Project Paperclip, 1944-1990" (1991), it was stated, "Strughold was not arrested, interrogated, or even called as a witness at the trial, despite the derogatory information against him. It was a glaring example of how far the military went to protect him."

Mark L. Kornbluh, an assistant professor of history at Washington University in St. Louis, Missouri stated in 1992, "American scientific recruiting teams ignored the inhumane basis of much of their work and treated Nazi scientists as both colleagues and friends. The records of the Nazi activities of these scientists were altered, hidden, expunged, or classified. U.S. officials not only ignored the fact that many of these men were Nazis; they actively concealed that information in order to shield the Nazi scientists from prosecution. They then relocated them to new homes in America, with the understanding that the recruits would then share their technology with the U.S. government. The American space program became a veritable haven of ex-Nazis. Dr. Strughold pioneered aviation medicine through gruesome experiments conducted on prisoners in Dachau".

Brooks AFB Aeromedical Library was named after him in honor of his accomplishments in aerospace medicine in 1977. In 1995, the U.S. Air Force removed Strughold's name after the Jewish Anti-Defamation League (ADL) protested. "Paying tribute to Dr. Strughold was an obscene mockery of the pain and death suffered by his victims," commented ADL National Chairman Richard Strassler. The basis of the claim was his presence at the October 1942 meeting in Nuremburg where Dachau experiments were presented. The letter from the Air Force Chief of Staff to the ADL stated, "We are not in a position to draw any specific conclusions beyond this (his presence at the meeting) regarding the possibility of his complicity in or responsibility for the torture of concentration camp inmates in the guise of medical research. Although available information lends some support to those, including your organization, who maintain that Dr. Strughold was aware of and in some way aided such experiments, his death and the cessation of any formal investigation or proceedings concerning him make it unlikely that this question will ever be resolved conclusively. Nevertheless, and as you suggest, the evidence of Dr. Strughold's wartime activities is sufficient to cause concern about retaining his name in an honored place on the library."

In 1993, his portrait was also removed from a mural of medical heroes in a display of the "The World History of Medicine" at Ohio State University at the request of the World Jewish Congress. The German Society of Aviation and Space Medicine (DGLRM) had an award named after Dr. Strughold but canceled it due to the controversy. Dr. Strughold was inducted into the New Mexico Museum of Space History Hall of Fame in 1978. The museum removed him from the hall of fame in May 2006 after protests from the ADL.

At the time of his removal from the museum, the Institute of Ethics at the University of New Mexico released the following statement: "Surely recognition in a "Hall of Fame" should be reserved for those who represent widely held values of tolerances and respect for human dignity, and surely Hubertus Strughold, whatever his scientific contributions, should not be given a place of honor when his conduct failed to uphold those basic human values."

A careful review of Internet links using standard search techniques for "Strughold" reveals many obvious distortions. Some of these are minor and others outrageous. The most prevalent (all apparently from the same original source and simply repeated or magnified) state with confidence that Dr. Strughold was a Nazi, in charge of the Dachau experiments, was protected at the Nuremburg Trials, and involved in mind control experiments with psychoactive drugs at both Dachau and later in the U.S. under the C.I.A. In other web links, he is described as the examining physician when the aliens landed in Roswell, N.M. in 1947.

Dr. Stan Mohler tells the story of attending a lecture when he was a medical student in 1955 (this was two years before Sputnik brought space to the public's conciousness) where Dr. Strughold presented a talk on the "Medical Aspects of Space Travel". Halfway through the talk, a professor of physiology turned to Dr. Mohler and said in a loud voice, "This man is crazy!" This was loud enough to be heard by everyone in the room, including Dr. Strughold, who continued his talk without hesitation. I think that it serves as a good example of Dr. Strughold's life. Frequently misunderstood and a decade ahead of everyone else, but pressing forward with what he knew to be true and important; unwavering in his principles, beliefs, and ideas. As an example, Dr. Strughold never joined the Nazi party or allowed his staff to do so at a time when it would not only be advantageous to his career, but actually dangerous to not do so. He was as anti-Nazi as you could possibly be in his position without being arrested or executed. He specialized in aviation medicine at such an early time that he was discredited by his colleagues for his expansive ideas on future aeronautical possibilities. He then was a pioneer in the advancement of space medicine when the only activity was short unmanned suborbital flights using captured V-2s. He was pivotal in developing this discipline to such an extent that the U.S. was well prepared for the Mercury program in 1959. Finally, he was an advocate of the possibility of life on Mars and kept a "Mars jar" on his desk during the 1950s. This jar was growing lichen in an atmosphere of extremely dry, low pressure CO_2. In 1964, when Mariner 4 showed Mars to be more Moon-like, everyone dropped the idea of finding any life on Mars, except for Dr. Strughold. Now that there are hints of atmospheric methane and flowing salt water on Mars, exobiologists are becoming more confident that we will eventually discover some form of life on Mars.

It is important that future debate of Dr. Strughold's World War II activities be carried on with documented and well referenced facts and not with blatantly false information or politically inspired revisionist history. Everyone is entitled to their own opinion, but they are not entitled to their own facts. The Internet and several books criticizing Dr. Stughold have multiple distortions, misrepresentations, and assumed guilt by even casual association. It is highly unlikely that new information will become available in the future concerning Dr. Strughold as the true facts are either already known or will never be known. It is recognized that this issue will continue to be debated and will always be controversial. The Holocaust and the Nazi regime were horrific and any ties to that part of German history, whether real or remote, will always follow Dr. Strughold. Hubertus Strughold is still known (and will always be known) as the "Father of Space Medicine".

Chapter 1. Childhood and Adolescence (1898-1918)

In 1898, Ferdinand and Anna Strughold from Westphalian Westtuennen looked forward to the birth of their third child. On June 15, a son was born whom they baptized four days later as Hubert Joseph Heinrich Strughold at the Catholic church, St. Regina, in the neighboring community of Rhynern (1). Anna Strughold had already delivered two sons: Ferdinand was born in 1895, but died at the age of two. Joseph Strughold followed in 1896. Hubertus's sister, Mathilda, was finally born in 1899. All the births took place at the home of the Strughold family (2). Hubertus' father, Ferdinand Strughold, came from an agricultural family located in the Lippstadt area. His mother, Anna Strughold, whose maiden name was Tillmann, also came from an old farming family from the Sauerland area. They were married in the summer of 1894 in Elspe (3). Ferdinand Strughold began his career as a school official candidate at the primary school in Halberbracht, which is close to Olpe in 1887. The next year he was offered a teaching post at the Catholic primary school of Eckmannshausen, in the Siegen area. On December 1, 1893 he finally took over at the school office of the Catholic school Westtuennen in the Hamm area (4).

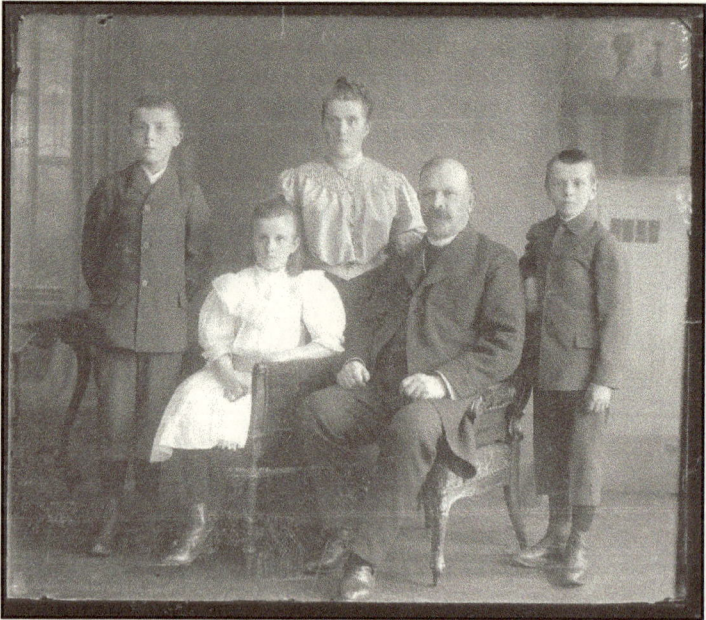

Fig. 1 The Strughold family in the early 20th century: Hubertus is on the right.
From left to right: Joseph, Mathilda, Anna, Ferdinand, Hubertus.
Photo archive Dr. Harsch, Neubrandenburg (Nbdbg.)

Hubert Strughold's childhood was marked by a very rural lifestyle with close relationships (Fig. 1) (5). His schooling began in 1904 at the primary school of Westtuennen, where he attended the first four grades (Fig. 2) (6). At that time there was not a local church, so a church in Rhynern had to be visited, which was a walk several kilometers away. Strughold's astronomical interest was pioneered by the observation of the comet Johannesburg in February of 1910 (this was later named after its South African discoverer, Brooks). Three months later Strughold's astronomical impressions were further peaked by his observation of "Halley's Comet" (7). The astronomical observations were performed from a tree house that was built by his father. These direct experiences were significant for Strughold as they developed a later passion to deal with phenomena that was beyond the ordinary (8). In that same year Strughold was injured while viewing a solar eclipse with a poorly tinted glass and the resulting retinal burn on his right eye was permanent (9).

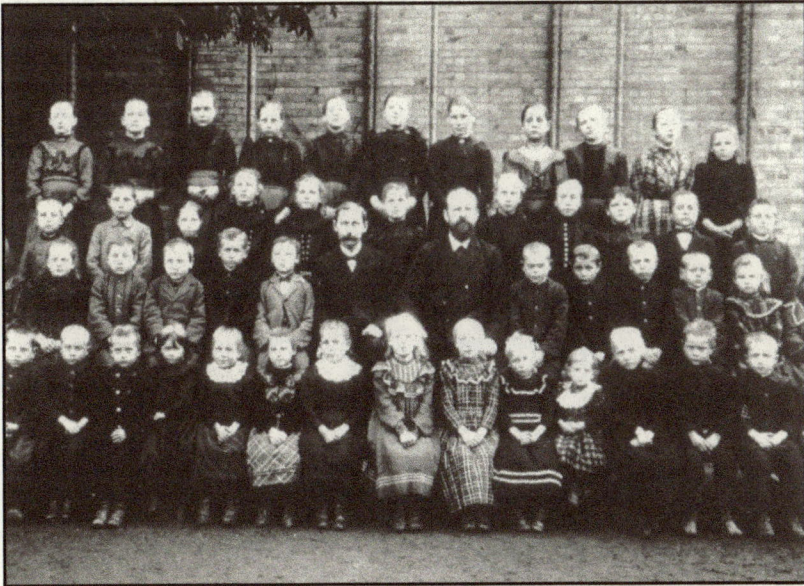

Fig. 2 The class of Hubertus Strughold 1905/06. He is immediately to the left of the teachers Buhsmann and F. Strughold with the typical school dress of the times, but only one with a bow tie. Photo archive Dr. Harsch, Nbdbg.

The Strughold household had a formative influence on his development. While his mother sparked his interest in astronomy and art, his father brought him closer to the natural sciences. Strughold's father died on July 19, 1912 at the age of 45 due to heart and kidney disease (10). Strughold would write later about his father: "[He] never instilled in me a special knowledge of my direction, but he inspired me to study botany and zoology. Of course, he considered it important that I enjoyed a well-rounded education. I perceived all of this and was always conscious of it, to observe and to explore nature. I still remember the many wonderful hikes through the woods, when I would shower him with questions. Most, of course, were silly. But my father was always patient and persistent. He had a touching concern for my older brother, my little sister, and me. It was, therefore, a very painful loss when he died so early - I was only 13 years old. "

Strughold's youth was overshadowed by the untimely death of his father, who was only recently appointed to be one of the "first teachers" of the school (11). The education of the children was now in the hands of his mother. Strughold characterized her as strict and competent. Despite their rural origins, his mother enjoyed a high level of education. Her most important traits that he considered unique were her curiosity and the ability to deal with unconventional new questions. She was interested in poetry and encouraged her youngest (Struggi), to "express unusual and colorful art" and to write minor poems. Despite limited financial capabilities, Hubert Strughold attended the Catholic church school in Hamm (1908-1911) and the grammar school "Hammonense" (Fig. 3). Strughold's mother died on June 28, 1931 at the age of 70 (12).

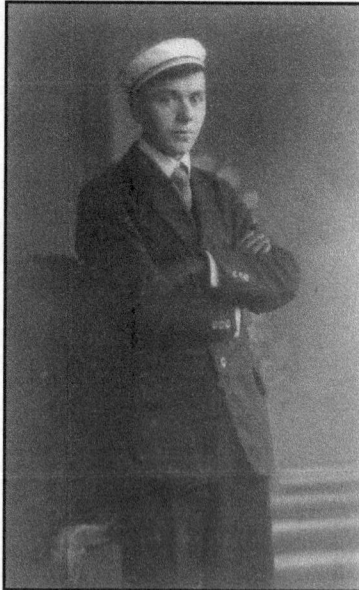

Fig. 3 Hubertus Strughold in his school uniform at the Hammonense school in 1917. Photo archive Dr. Harsch, Nbdbg.

With the outbreak of World War I, the entire upper class (*Oberprima*) of the Royal Grammar School "Hammonense" reported for the preliminary exam (*Notreifepruefung*) that was available for the patriotic and expected military service (13). When the church organist of Westtuennen was appointed to the front, Hubert Strughold had the opportunity to close the gap and played the church organ every sunday. His musical performance was graded by himself as rather unorthodox, but that seemed to please the audience. So he took courage and ventured further, even trying pieces by Wagner (14). His passion for music - which began with his father - went with him into his old age. In his adopted home in Texas an organ was always a permanent fixture (15). In the years 1917 and 1918 younger recruits, including 17-year-olds, were called up for military service (16). In 1916, Strughold was indeed issued a permit for "one year's voluntary service" by the Examination Commission (Doc. 2), but he was deferred from military service (17). His older brother Joseph, however, was conscripted and in the service of Infantry Regiment No. 94 in the late summer of 1918 and was eventually wounded (18). Hubertus Strughold, meanwhile, continued his education, and was identified as one of five graduates of the "Hammonense" on February 15, 1918. Interestingly enough for a future scientist, the final exam only shows sufficient performance in handwriting, mathematics, and physics. He received good grades in english, geography and history (19).

Chapter 2. Years of Study (1918-1924)

After his graduation in February 1918, Hubertus Strughold was enrolled on April 25, 1918 in the philosophical-scientific faculty of the Westfaelische-Wilhelms-Universitaet (WWU) in Muenster to study medicine (1). On May 1, 1918, he joined the Association of German Catholics under the student fraternity "CV Cheruskia-Muenster", with which he remained connected to for life (Fig. 4). This sectarian-oriented fraternity was one of the largest in Muenster and was close to the democratic Center Party (2). The ongoing military actions of World War I had an impact on Strughold's study: From June 1918 until February 1919, he was formally in the employ of Infantry Regiment No. 13 in Muenster (3). However, according to the University book voucher, he took part in four courses during the summer term and in five courses during the winter term (4). Further study was then continued without interruption, but his *Physikum* (the first major exam in medicine after two years of pre-clinical medical education) was delayed. After five terms in the summer of 1920 he completed his preclinical education with an overall grade of "Two" (subjectively good) (5).

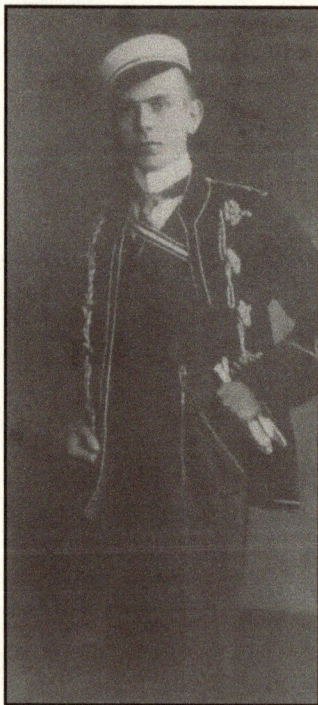

Fig. 4 Hubertus Strughold in the uniform of the catholic fraternity "CV Cheruskia-Muenster". Photo archive Dr. Harsch, Nbdbg.

By Strughold's own admission, his years of study were punctuated by parsimony and privation. Traditionally, students in Germany changed the course of their training and the location of their study. Strughold justified this by saying that a student who would remain for the duration of his studies at only one university, would not appear to be well rounded. For example, a physician would have more confidence when he had studied patients at several universities under several different professors. Therefore, he preferred to go through his training at several different universities (6). After Muenster, Strughold chose the Georg-August-University in Goettingen, which he entered on October 29, 1920 and where he completed his matriculation (7). During the same years at the Goettingen University, Hermann Oberth was studying physics. Oberth would later be known as the "Father of Space Travel" (8). While Oberth had already dealt intensively for many years with the idea of space, Strughold's interest in astronomy was still much more conservative. The later "Father of Space Medicine" wrote his first space medical paper in 1949. Sometimes, Strughold in his free time walked the 200 km long route home, and he was always known throughout his life to be a passionate hiker (8).

Strughold's medical curriculum allowed him to go for six months to Munich, where he enrolled for the summer term in 1921 at the Ludwig-Maximilians-University. Here he was educated by the renowned surgeon, Sauerbruch (9). This carefree time in Munich was used to expand his horizons, because he wanted, in addition to his books and lectures, to experience many new influences. Munich's international atmosphere captivated the medical student. Here he joined the Catholic fraternity "KDStV Rheno-Franconia to Munich" and sometimes relaxed with friends at the "*Hofbräuhaus*" (Royal brewery house). He also had time to study painting and to attend a dance course – initiating several life-long passions. Beginning in high school he had studied art and was especially interested in Egyptian, Greek, Italian and Dutch painters. His own paintings were mostly landscapes and with a preference on the Munich river Isar (10).

At the Julius-Maximilians-University in Wuerzburg, he was enrolled for the winter term 1921-22, and then for four complete semesters. On May 26, 1923, he took the medical final examination and received a grade of "Good" (11). Up to this point, it appeared that Strughold's life was mapped out to be similar to any other clinically active physician. At the Institute of Physiology, however, he found a subject that increasingly captivated him. Here Strughold met the renowned Salzburg physiologist, Max von Frey (1852-1932), who influenced his future scientific life in a crucial way. Since 1899 Frey had been the Head of the Physiological Institute at Wuerzburg and specialized in the field of sensory physiology and cardiovascular research and was also the Associate Editor of the "Journal of Biology" (12). Later, during the mid 1930s, Strughold would publish numerous groundbreaking works in sensory physiology. On June 13, 1923 Strughold concluded the medical state examination in philosophy from his earlier studies begun in Muenster (a preliminary step to a Ph.D.). Supervised by the work of Frey, "The Effect of the Agents Diphenylarsinchlorid (Blue Cross Agent) and Aethylarsindichlorid (Yellow Cross Agent) on the Skin of People" was evaluated by the physiologist Professor Rosemann and classified as "cum laude" (13). Strughold dedicated the medical theses (*Dissertation*) to his father. It was the strong effect of eliciting pain by exposure to this gas during World War I that the substances Blue Cross and Yellow Cross had first become known. This substance was then used in small doses by Strughold for the investigation of pain sense. Other sensations on the skin (pressure, heat and cold sense) were also investigated (14). This work was first published in 1923 in J.F. Lehmann's Verlag in Munich and later in that same year published in the "Journal of Biology".

In his medical thesis which Strughold submitted while in Wuerzburg there was also a dedicated section on other neuro-physiological problems. The doctoral thesis on the distribution of pain receptors in the skin was evaluated in 1923 with "summa cum laude" (15). For this outstanding performance he was rewarded by the refund of his examination fee. This benefit, however, during these times of high inflation, was mostly of a symbolic value. Of the 50,000,000.- Mark, that Strughold had to pay to the university for the examination fee, he could have bought at least a new pair of shoes. Six weeks later, when the fee was refunded, the amount was only equivalent to a pack of cigarettes (16). The doctor's degree (similar to an Ph.D. and called a "Dr. med et phil") was awarded on October 18, 1923. However, it was not until November 24, 1926 that this was formally approved. This delay was caused due to the necessity to distribute 60 copies of the medical theses in times of the the financial crisis in Germany. This severe inflationary period with its peak in 1923 was remembered later by Strughold as extreme privation (17):

"Sometimes I spent three days in bed, only in this way I could reduce my energy consumption, since I had nothing to eat. (...) I only ate bread, margarine and spinach. Until this day I hate spinach! Sometimes, I was so hungry that if I had enough money I would go eat horse meat at a local restaurant. "

During his internship year, he attended the medical clinic and continued to conduct research at the Physiological Institute. In June 1924, he fulfilled the requirements for the practical year and a month later became an assistant at the Physiological Institute. He received a license to practice as a physician in Wuerzburg on November 6, 1925 from the Bavarian State Ministry of the Interior and of Education and Culture (18).

Chapter 3. The Wuerzburg Years (1924-1935)

During his internship Strughold became an assistant at the Physiological Institute in Wuerzburg, beginning on July 1, 1924 (1). During this period he realized that he had a complete lack of interest in a clinical medical practise (2). His scientific activity at the Physiological Institute secured only a meager living during difficult economic times. His income of 320, - Mark he described as being adequate, and at times he could even afford a pitcher of beer (3). It is essential to note that Strughold was further channeled into his professional and scientific career in physiology while in Wuerzburg. Dr. Frey enabled him to quickly become involved at the Freiburg Institute of Physiology (4):

"The licensed physician, Dr. phil. et med. Hubert Strughold started his work as an assistant in the Physiological Institute on 1 July 1924 after he was already there in his ninth and tenth terms in 1922/23 as well as a medical practitioner (*Medizinalpraktikant*) with scientific studies mainly engaged in the field of sensory physiology. Various publications are partly his own, and sometimes in association with Dr. Rein & the undersigned (Dr. Frey), which he intends to continue even further. The same is distinguished by a purely scientific approach, careful execution, skill and tenacity in overcoming experimental difficulties and through critical self-control. To give him the opportunity for a broader training in physiology, the undersigned is willing to allow Dr. Strughold for the period 1 October 1925 to 31 March 1926 to become a full research scientist for Dr. H. Rein at the Physiological Institute in Freiburg. "

At the Ludovica Albertina University in Freiburg, Strughold continued his physiological research for the next six months (5). The head of the Freiburg institute, Dr. Paul Hoffmann, was a former assistant to Frey and still had close connections to the Wuerzburg institute as well. Strughold concentrated his research on the field of tendon reflexes. His work, "Contributions to the Knowledge of the Refractory Period of the Human Spinal Cord", was completed during the spring of 1927 at the Wuerzburg University as a postdoctoral medical thesis. For his habilitation lecture (followed by his thesis-defense in order to obtain the "*venia legendi*") he was invited to personally appear at the auditorium of the Physiological Institute in Wuerzburg on February 27, 1927. After Strughold mastered this academic hurdle (termed habilitation or "Dr. med habil", which is similar to a Ph.D. and qualifies the person to be able to teach at an university) he became an assistant professor of physiology at 29 years of age. From now on he was devoted to research on sensory physiology and performed experimental work while also in the classroom. Focal points were on the field of somatovisceral sensitivity of the mechanoreceptors in the skin (surface sensitivity), the sensitivity of tissue receptors (muscle, joint and tendon receptors) and the reflexes in general (6). In the summer term of 1927 Strughold lectured on

"General physiology" and the "Physiology of reproduction, growth, and the restitution of the people in the light of the doctrine of internal secretion." In the winter term of 1927-28 Strughold taught "Physiology of the central nervous system and sensory organs of the people" along with "Neurophysiological work in the laboratory" (7).

In 1927 Strughold's interest turned to a new direction initiated by Charles Lindbergh's Atlantic crossing. Just days before Lindbergh's flight, he spoke in a visionary presentation to his students that thousands would cross the Atlantic in aircraft in the near future (8). His interest in aviation went back to his youth (9):

"I have always been interested in balloons and airships. I eagerly watched all of that since 1910, when I was a child, watching them rising in the air. I was watching very carefully the development of aviation in Germany and the epochal flight of Lindbergh crystallized my thoughts. I had the certainty that there dawned a new era - the era of general aviation. "

Strughold discussed with his teacher, Max von Frey, about how physiology could make a decisive contribution in this field. Consequently, during the following summer term of 1928 he presented the lecture, "Flight of human physiology for medical practitioners, scientists and aviators". It was, according to him, a one-hour lecture presented in the small auditorium of the Physiological Institute and about 60 interested people attended (10). This event was the first documented aviation physiology lecture in Germany and probably the first worldwide (11). Strughold used as his preparatory reading the work of the physiologist Sir Joseph Barcroft and of Dr. Edward Christian Schneider. Both worked with laboratory chambers at the atmospheric level equivalent to the summit of Pike's Peak in Colorado (12). Later these experiment were supplemented by practical tests in flight by Strughold (Fig. 05) (13). The Wuerzburg newspaper "*General Anzeiger*" wrote about a "scientific demonstration flight" at the airport given to students (14):

"On Wednesday afternoon Dr. Strughold visited with his students at the Wuerzburg Flight School for the practical part of his aeromedical course. Here flying demonstrations were offered. WW I ace Knight [Ritter] von Greim and Dr. Strughold took a Udet-Flamingo plane for the following physiological test flight to test the behavior of the musculoskeletal system through the so-called balance test of Baranni during the different phases of looping (´Barannische´ or ´Bárány Zeigerversuch´ which is associated with the finger nose test) (15). The fast changes between positive and negative acceleration enable the physiologist to perfectly study the functions of the organs of balance. It was flown by a series of loops and after a quick roll, the descent was established through a tailspin."

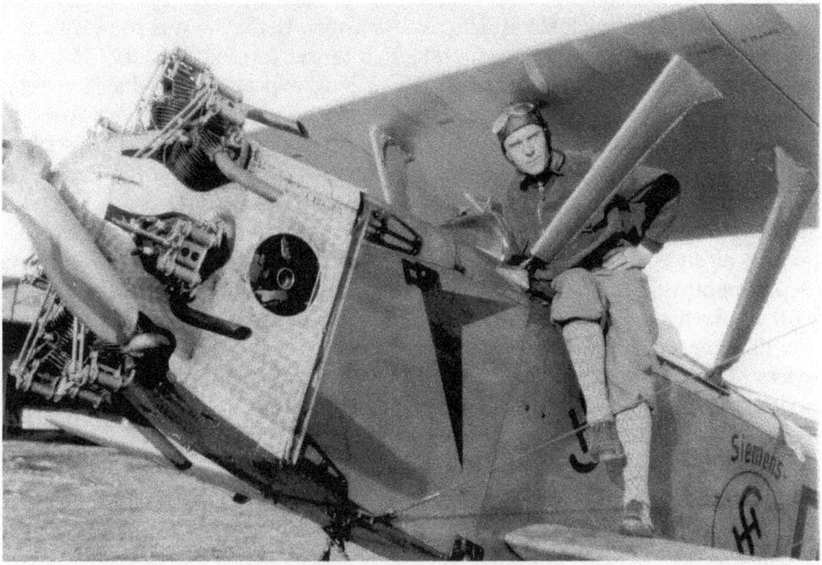

21

Fig. 5 Hubertus Strughold as a flight student in the Siemens Flamingo aircraft in Wuerzburg. Photo archive Dr. Harsch, Nbdbg.

During his presentations, the audience followed his topic with exceptional interest, but according to his predominantly conservative group of colleagues it seemed that the lectures of this unconventional, enthusiastic teacher were really only a product of his own dreams (16). Strughold, however, was not giving up and continued to work in the field of aviation medicine (17):

"At that time my colleagues ridiculed me about my crazy course on aviation physiology with the practical demonstrations. I have since learned that when I take something that others will make fun of, then I'm almost always on a really good track. One must have the courage to walk new paths, if you really want to do pioneering work."

Strughold's lectures benefited from his practical aero-medical interests and his understanding of neurosensory and cardiovascular physiology. He carried out laboratory investigations at altitude in a hot air balloon, a small airship, and also in airplanes. Since no altitude chamber was available in Wuerzburg, Strughold took advantage of a metabolic chamber at the Wuerzburg hospital for his hypoxia experiments (18). By increasing the nitrogen content of the breathing gas mixture equivalent to that of the oxygen that was reduced in content he was able to investigate many aspects of high altitude hypoxia. At an equivalent hypoxic altitude of 2,300 meters, he performed sensorimotoric tests on himself for three hours, while an assistant during this interval took blood samples. A chronic headache was the result and his performance was degraded enough that he labeled this the "disorder threshold" (*Stoerschwelle*). The effects of long exposure to reduced oxygen content in the air above this threshold disorder range from paralysis to unconsciousness and death. The time to onset of paralysis was first described by Strughold as the "reserve time". Together with the dentist Anton Poppe, he took a balloon trip from Wuerzburg up to the Czech border (Lochau). He used a dynamometer to measure and record the arm force strength in relationship to the altitude up to 4,000 meters. Strughold had to pay for this private experiment with 300, - Mark out of his own finances (19). For further studies and to take flying lessons for himself, he developed a personal relationship with the director of the only flying school in Bavaria which was in Wuerzburg. The pilots Marga von Etzdorf and Heinzinger also took experimental subjects with recording instruments on their experimental flights (20). For flight lessons with Robert Ritter von Greim, a former member of the "Richthofen Squadron," Strughold paid the equivalence of a six-months salary (21). His flying lessons had to be terminated because of his later trips to the USA. Interestingly, Strughold was later known to take every opportunity to not have to travel by airplane. A significant physiological neuro-sensory self-experiment was performed sometime during this period. By injecting a local anesthetic into his "bottom", Strughold switched off his sense of position ("seat of his pants" flying) and flew multiple aerobatic maneuvers, which led to severe spatial disorientation. The movements of the horizon, which he could still visually acquire, appeared to follow him "senseless, unmotivated and confused." After the aerobatic flight in the flamingo biplane, Strughold had the feeling that he was sitting "beside the chair." These "neural therapeutic" interventions were surely some of the world's first aviation experiments in sensory physiology. He was very happy to feel solid ground under his feet after these experiments (22).

In 1928 Strughold obtained a one-year U.S. research position with a Rockefeller Foundation Fellowship. This was the beginning of a lifelong connection to the New World (23). Under the internationally recognized circulatory physiologist, Carl John Wiggers at Western Reserve University in Cleveland, Ohio he studied the effects of hypoxia on the heart (Fig. 6). During an evening symposium Strughold presented his results based upon his Wuerzburg experiments. The topic was the effect of oxygen deficiency on the sensorimotor function of pilots, which was of particularly keen interest to the expert panel that was present. Concerning the question of his motivations for studying abroad, Strughold answered in a letter to Dr. Wiggers on the occasion of his retirement in 1952 (24):

"As I recall, it was during the year 1925 when I played with the idea of studying in the U.S. Shortly after, you made a trip to Europe and visited my former director, Professor Max von Frey, the Director of the Physiological Institute of the University of Wuerzburg. After only a brief conversation with you, my decision was clear, and here in the U.S. to go first to you in Cleveland. I did never regret this decision, on the other hand, it would be a great loss to my career if I wouldn´t have worked even for a short time as a research assistant in your department. After seeing a large number of other Physiological Institutes, I am convinced that this was the most suitable place in the world to study the full range of circulation physiology. What I have learned from you was later on valuable for my physiology lectures, also for scientific aeronautics and medical lectures. I found in you a personality and a professor of the classical type. (...) Please accept my deep gratitude for the shown kindness and for the privilege of working in your department. "

For another six months in 1929 Strughold was at the University of Chicago (Illinois) at the department of the physiologist, Professor Anton Carlson (25). After his return from the U.S. Strughold continued his work at the Physiological Institute in Wuerzburg beginning on October 16, 1929 (26). On July 7, 1930, he was installed as a "private teacher for special flight physiology", the first one so designated in Germany (27).

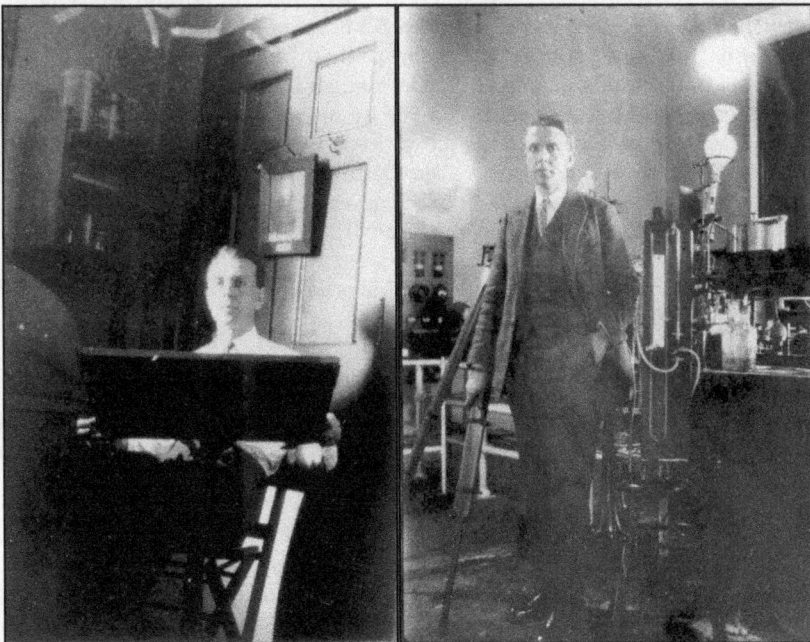

Fig. 6 a/b Strughold at the physiological laboratory in Cleveland, OH in 1929.
Photo archive Dr. Harsch, Nbdbg.

At this point it should be noted that there was not any state funding for aviation medical research. Secret military aeromedical research was present to a small extent, but civil aviation was without any significant capital resources. Aviation medicine experts in Germany at that time included Strughold (Wuerzburg), Brauer (Hamburg), Gillert (DVL in Berlin), and Koschel (Luft-Hansa Airline Base in Braunschweig) as well as several temporarily-paid aviation doctors. The Scientific Society for Aeronautics (WGL) in the late 1920s tried to support the creation of an aeromedical institution and tried to install a full Professor for Aviation Medicne (28). In Wuerzburg, there was a discussion by the city and the university to install a full professorship during the "crisis year" of 1931. A lively exchange of letters documented this difficult task as additional funding would be necessary. In a letter to the "Ministry of State for Education and Culture" from April 1, 1931, Strughold was proposed to become a full Professor of Aviation Medicine. The Wuerzburg city council and the head of the Physiological Institute (Professor Max von Frey) were supporting Strughold. They justified their proposal because the University of Wuerzburg in Germany held the leading role in the aerophysiological field. It seemed to them that it was necessary to strongly advocate for this support for Wuerzburg since the competition was so strong. Berlin had an advantage as it was the capital, Braunschweig was the center of the German commercial pilot school, and Hamburg had closer proximity to the capital. Strughold's position within the WGL (which he had joined in 1927) would be advantageous for the negotiations with the "Bavarian State Ministry of Foreign Affairs" and the "Ministry of Transportation" with respect to funding questions. Beside Strughold's outstanding scientific achievements it was felt that procurring for him a corresponding post at the university would be advantageous. Further-more, this would interfere with the present monopoly of experts that were transferring into this field to Dr. Brauer in Hamburg (29). The Wuerzburg flight school would also benefit from the advancement of flight physiology. The Faculty of Medicine supported the establishment of a professorship in the Physiology of Airship Travel in its statement dated June 1, 1931 (30). Emphasis was placed on the increasing importance of air traffic and it seemed to be important to promote aeromedical research (31):

"Since Dr. Strughold has dealt with these problems successfully and is renown in the circles of the WGL, it seems to this faculty that it would be wise to establish a Professorship for Flight Physiology to ensure the continuation of these important investigations. This would promote the work of ´aspiring young scholars´ on this new and important branch of science" (32).

The difficult economic situation in Germany during the global recession was demonstrated in the letter from the city mayor Loeffler to the University Rector on July 8, 1931. He stated that neither the city nor the country had the financial ability to support the University in those days. Expectations for possible support by the industry were also limited (33):

"But the support by the aviation industry is currently beyond any discussion. The German aerospace industry is at a standstill. Most plants are decommissioned. The few works that are still supported transmit from the Imperial (government) and can hardly be maintained. There are not any significant contracts by the German Lufthansa due to the steady decline in air travel. Sales to private entities is minimal in the difficult economic situation that is in Germany. With the general intensification of the global economic crisis, the possibilities of export are very limited. The only existing aircraft industry company in Bavaria, to which we can address ourselves, is the Bavarian Aircraft Works at Augsburg which, incidentally, went bankrupt a month ago. Even if it successfully recovers, which will be very difficult, this company will initially have other worries than to make donations to a German university. According to my knowledge of the situation at this time, the procurement of funds for the construction of a professorate in aviation medicine seems not possible."

Strughold was not a supporter of the totalitarian regime, for personal, political, scientific, and religious reasons. Raised in a conservative christian environment, he was politically close to the German Center Party. In the 1932 and 1933 elections he chose "Center" party (34). In 1934, he feared an arrest for this reason as the party was by then banned. Because of his U.S. contacts he was one of an exposed group of people controlled by the secret service (*Gestapo*). He was repeatedly interrogated by the secret service, so that he always had the fear of being arrested and, therefore, lived at three different places in Wuerzburg (35). As a former Catholic Fraternity student he supported their work against the Nazi regime after their ban and even when they were in the underground by political, moral and religious motivation (36).

Further efforts by Dr. Strughold to become involved in aviation research were not successful throughout the rest of the early 1930s (37). On March 13, 1933, however, he became a Honorary Associate Professor of Physiology (*außerordentliche Professur der Physiologie mit besonderem Lehrauftrag für Flugphysiologie, "Titular"-Professor*) by the "old Bavarian government," (as Strughold called it later) (38). Strughold was voting for the German Center Party, which was representative of catholic Germany until the end of the Weimar Republic in 1933. He was a strong supporter of Heinrich Bruening, who was a German politician of the Center Party and Chancellor of Germany from March 30, 1930 until May 30, 1932. Bruening had been active in the campaign for the reelection of Hindenburg. In May 1932, Hindenburg (in a move to the right to appease the National Socialists) dropped Chancellor Bruening. In the following period, Strughold was excluded for political reasons from becoming a full professor. In 1935 he became a civilian employee at the military Aero Medical Research Institute (AMRI) in Berlin (39):

"Since I was not a Nationalist Socialist party member and, in fact, was an outspoken opponent of the National Socialists Movement (which was partly due to my long stay in the U.S.), no prospect of obtaining a teaching chair at a German university was possible. On the basis of me being arrested as a supporter of Bruening's policy in 1934, I did not feel safe, and so I took an offer in 1935 by the Chief of the Medical Inspectorate of the Army Surgeon General, Dr. Waldman, to be the head of the newly created military Aero Medical Research Institute in Berlin." (Fig. 7).

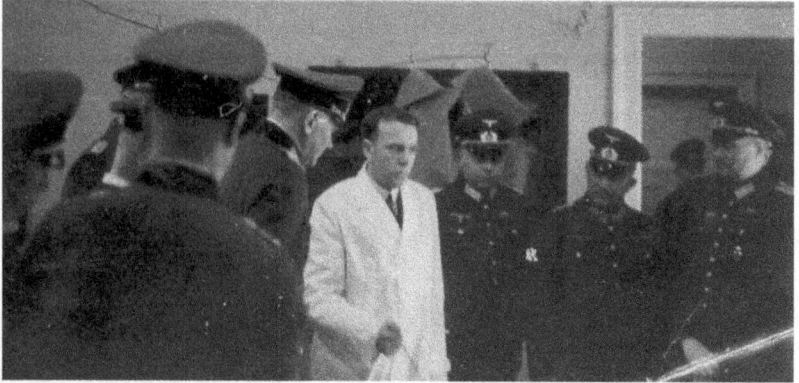

Fig. 7 Strughold during a presentation at the Aeromedical Research Institute (AMRI) in Berlin. To his right is General Waldmann. Photo archive Dr. Harsch, Nbdbg.

Strughold finished his activity at the Physiological Institute in Wuerzburg on March 31, 1935. Just before his move to Berlin, Strughold became an Aviation Medical Examiner (February 15, 1935) with the intent of examining glider pilots and free balloon pilots for the Bavarian Aviation Office in Nuremberg (40).

Chapter 4. The Berlin Years (1935-1945)

As a result of the Nazi takeover in 1933 and the subsequent transformation of Germany into a totalitarian state there occurred an intensification of military power. The German Air Force (Luftwaffe) was secretly expanded and became an independent military branch separate from the Army and Navy. This resulted in a drive for the further development of aviation medicine, whose main contributions until that time had been mainly basic scientific research. Following the outbreak of World War II, research was devoted to an increasing extent on operational issues. The leading aviation medicine institutions in 1934 before the establishment of the Luftwaffe are shown in Table 1 (1):

Table 1: Principle institutions involved in aviation medicine research in 1933:

Medical department of the DVL in Berlin-Adlershof (**S. Ruff**)
Aviation Medical Laboratory at the Military Medical Academy, Berlin
(**H. von Diringshofen**)
Aviation Medical Laboratory in Rechlin (**T. Benzinger**)
Institute for Aviation Medicine and Air Research at University of Hamburg-Eppendorf (**L. Brauer**)
Institute of Physiology at University Wuerzburg (**H. Strughold**)

Strughold's professional career in Berlin (1935-1945) began with Strughold replacing Heinz von Diringshofen as the head of the aeromedical laboratory at the Military Medical Academy (2). This was also known as the Aero Medical Research Institute (AMRI). The "Ministry of State for Education and Culture," announced that Strughold was changing his position as an Associate Professor of Physiology from Wuerzburg to Berlin (3). From the winter term of 1935-36 he was commissioned to give additional lectures in aviation medicine (4). On October 20, 1939 he was appointed as a full Professor (5). He previously had not become a full Professor in the Third Reich presuambly because he was not adequate "politically reliable" (6). (Fig. 8)

When Strughold was transferred to Berlin in 1934-1935, he was investigated as a routine security check by the *Gestapo*. It states that he was regarded to be one of a "German national group of university professors to be more oriented towards the old German (monarchistic) state". There were no entries about his political orientation before the Nazi-takeover (7).

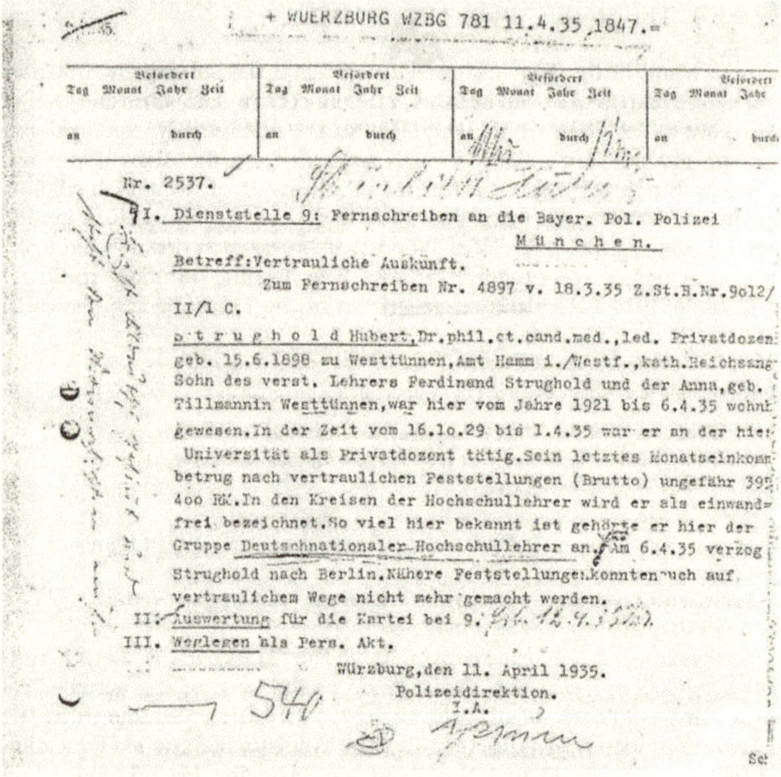

+ WUERZBURG WZBG 781 11.4.35 1847. =

Befördert		Befördert		Befördert		Befördert	
Tag Monat Jahr Zeit		Tag Monat Jahr Zeit		Tag Monat Jahr Zeit		Tag Monat Jahr	
an	durch	an	durch	an	durch	an	durch

Nr. 2537.

I. Dienststelle 9: Fernschreiben an die Bayer. Pol. Polizei
M ü n c h e n.

Betreff:Vertrauliche Auskunft.

Zum Fernschreiben Nr. 4897 v. 18.3.35 Z.St.B.Nr.9o12/

II/1 c.

S t r u g h o l d Hubert,Dr.phil.et.cand.med.,led. Privatdozent
geb. 15.6.1898 zu Westtünnen,Amt Hamm i./Westf.,kath.Reichsang
Sohn des verst. Lehrers Ferdinand Strughold und der Anna,geb.
Tillmannin Westtünnen,war hier vom Jahre 1921 bis 6.4.35 wohnt
gewesen.In der Zeit vom 16.1o.29 bis 1.4.35 war er an der hie:
Universität als Privatdozent tätig.Sein letztes Monatseinkomm
betrug nach vertraulichen Feststellungen (Brutto) ungefähr 39:
4oo RM.In den Kreisen der Hochschullehrer wird er als einwand-
frei bezeichnet.So viel hier bekannt ist gehörte er hier der
Gruppe Deutschnationaler Hochschullehrer an. Am 6.4.35 verzog
Strughold nach Berlin.Nähere Feststellungen konnten auch auf
vertraulichem Wege nicht mehr gemacht werden.

II. Auswertung für die Kartei bei 9.

III. Weglegen als Pers. Akt.

Würzburg,den 11. April 1935.
Polizeidirektion.
I.A.

Fig. 8 Strughold´s GeStaPo-File No. 15720 (English translation in Ref. 6).
Photo archive Dr. Harsch, Nbdbg.

The tremendous technical developments that resulted in advanced aircraft performance in the 1930s made it necessary to perform additional research in acceleration physiology. Operationally oriented research was performed at the Luftwaffe Medical test center in Jueterbog, while basic research was performed using the AMRI-centrifuge. The Ph.D. student U. Fischer (1938) studied the effects of acceleration in animals with experiments using the AMRI-centrifuge. Physiology was investigated by using contrast medium with x-ray techniques, studying the visible changes in heart filling with different changes in the direction of centrifugal force (8). Research in high altitude physiology was the most important project in the aeromedical community during those years. The mountaineer and aviator Hans Hartmann, located at the AMRI since 1934, was involved with the German Nanga Parbat expedition to carry out physiological studies in the western Himalayas (Karakorum) in 1937. He was accompanied by Ulrich C. Luft (9). Of practical aerospace medical relevance was the problem of increasing the level of hypoxia tolerance. The knowledge that altitude sickness resistance could be achieved by altitude acclimatization was of significant importance. Further research was performed on the possibility of preservation of these acclimatization effects by physical training, medicine, regular training in the altitude chamber or breathing oxygen-reduced gas mixtures (10). At a St. Johann (Tyrol) meeting held on mountain physiology during 1943, it was significant that 10 of the 16 speakers were from the scientific centers of Berlin (11).

By the late 1930s, aircrafts were already equipped with pressurized cabins, which caused additional medical problems if rapid decompression from a sudden loss of cabin pressure occurred (12). Animal experiments on decompression were performed first, followed by some validation experiments on humans. This scientific research was years ahead of the practical applications (13). At the AMRI, experiments were conducted in 1939 by Clamann with rapid depressurization trials on humans up to altitudes of 15,000 meters. With the outbreak of war in 1939 flight crews took part in a high-altitude training program in a vacuum chamber in Rechlin. The rapid decompression was first tested in 1937 and again in 1941 with extended self-tests up to an altitude of 17,000 m where a relative pressure loss of 60,000 m / sec was performed. Response times at these heights were examined and were included in the "Technical guidelines for the development and testing of aircraft with pressurized cabins (14). Benzinger (Rechlin) and Lutz (Munich), also examined issues of rapid and explosive decompression (15). They performed experiments with gas mixtures at pressure altitudes corresponding to 7,500 m, which was equivalent to hypoxia as high as 12,000 m in the vacuum chambers when performing a *"Blitzaufstieg"* profile (rapid ascent followed by decompression). Air crews were exposed in altitude chambers to both hypoxia and rapid decompression: The subjects had to act quickly, as the remaining time (reserve time) for consciousness to be able to perform a safe descent was short (16). An outline of the effect of altitude was introduced by Strughold based upon his tendon reflex studies. In human experiments at AMRI, it was the standard to perform these experiments on themselves or on voluntary colleagues and members of aviation personnel (17). The objectives of these studies were to determine the tolerance times to hypoxia (reserve time), resistance level to hypoxia, and further advanced research which served to increase the understanding of the altitude effects. Strughold divided the reaction zones into the following different phases: ground up to 2.000 m altitude showing no physiological changes, a reaction threshold above that with physiological changes to compensate for the changes, an interference threshold (*Stoerungsschwelle*) beginning at 4000 m altitude with the occurance of physiological deficiencies, and a critical threshold beginning at 7000 m altitude where prolonged exposition leads to death. The concept of reserve time was of operational relevance, and was introduced by Strughold in 1938. It demonstrated the necessity for oxygen supplementation or immediate descent to lower altitudes (18). The breathing of 100% oxygen raised these altitude thresholds, and the use of positive pressure breathing, pressure suits, and pressurized cabins were proposed for further higher altitude ascents. Since oxygen breathing was regarded as dangerous in aeronautical circles, Strughold's assistants, Becker-Freyseng and Clamann, performed prolonged self-investigations using 100% oxygen breathing in the altitude chamber (19).

Through the centralized control of aerospace medical research by the Reich´s Air Ministry (RLM), the gap in the international aviation medicine field was successfully closed within a few years in many areas and this contributed decisively to further research development (20). Meetings between the various institutes were organized to share experiences and to improve the coordination of research activities. Initially these meetings took place with international participation (1937). The central research facility in Germany in 1935 and over the next few years was at the AMRI in Berlin headed by Strughold. This Luftwaffe controlled AMRI institute was also responsible for directing the Aviation Medical Institute in Hamburg, the Institute for Aviation Medical Pathology in Freiburg, the Aeromedical Test Center of the Air Force in Jueterbog, as well as the Institute of Hygiene in Pfaffenrode. In addition, the AMRI was coordinating with the DVL Institute of Aviation Medicine in Berlin-Adlershof e.V., the Medical Department of the Flight Test Center at Rechlin, and the Munich Medical Institute of Aviation Research (21). The Luftwaffe´s medical headquarters sponsored all of the aeromedical research and funded the contracts. In this way a central coordination agency for research activities was established by the Luftwaffe (Fig. 9). Aviation medicine was also represented in the "German Academy of Aviation Research" and in the "*Lilienthal-Gesellschaft*". Lecturers in Aviation Medicine were appointed at several universities and technical colleges by the Reich Ministry of Education with the participation of the RLM (22).

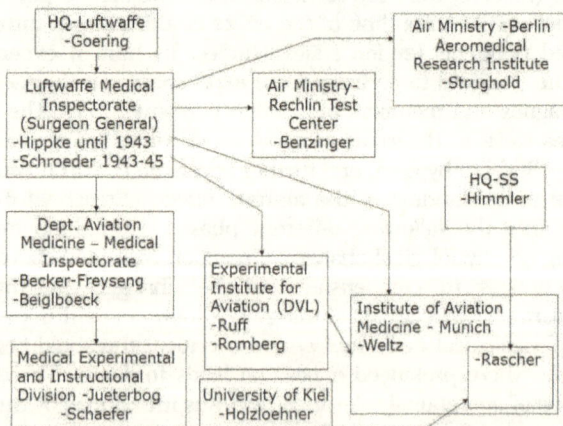

Fig 9 Organizational chart of the German aviation medical research centers during WW II.

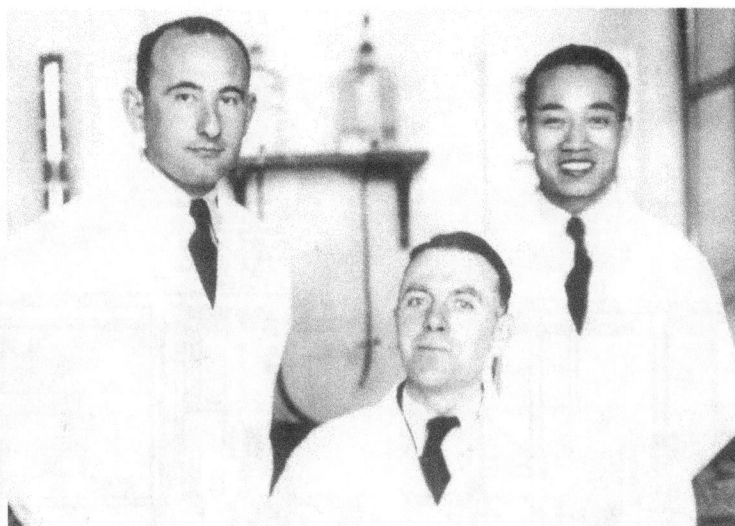

Fig. 10 Strughold with the Chinese scientist Chang and another Yugoslavian researcher.
Photo archive Dr. Harsch, Nbdbg.

The Luftwaffe´s Aeromedical Research Institute AMRI (also called
LMFI of the RLM) in Berlin was composed of the chief and nine research
departments. Since April 1, 1935, Hubertus Strughold was its head (*Leiter*),
and on January 15, 1942 his official title and position changed to Director
(23). The institute's reputation was also expanded by the involvement and
activities of several foreign scholars (Fig. 10). Numerous international awards
bear witness to the excellent scientific reputation of Strughold and his group.
The former deputy to the Luftwaffe Surgeon General, Erich Hippke, was E. A.
Lauschner. He described in 1984 Strughold as being young and enthusiastic.
The ideas of these researchers could be developed, in a rather liberal academic
atmosphere, without insurmountable external constraints. According to
Lauschner, this rather academic freedom was made possible by Strughold's
farsighted leadership, his organizational skills, his eye for detailed observation,
and by keeping politics out of the research efforts. The research focus of AMRI
was in the aerophysiological field, primarily on the effects of high altitude and
acceleration (Fig. 11 and 12). The AMRI organizational chart from the 1940´s
is shown in Table 2 with the nine separate departments, their managers,
significant employees, and the main working areas of reponsibility (24):

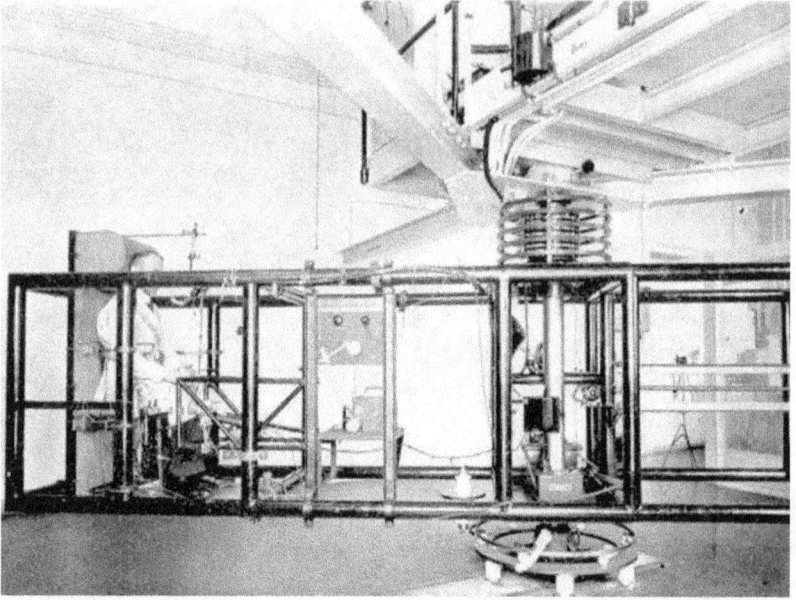

Fig. 11 AMRI centrifuge, Berlin (Strughold as test object, Atlas of Aviation Medicine 1942).

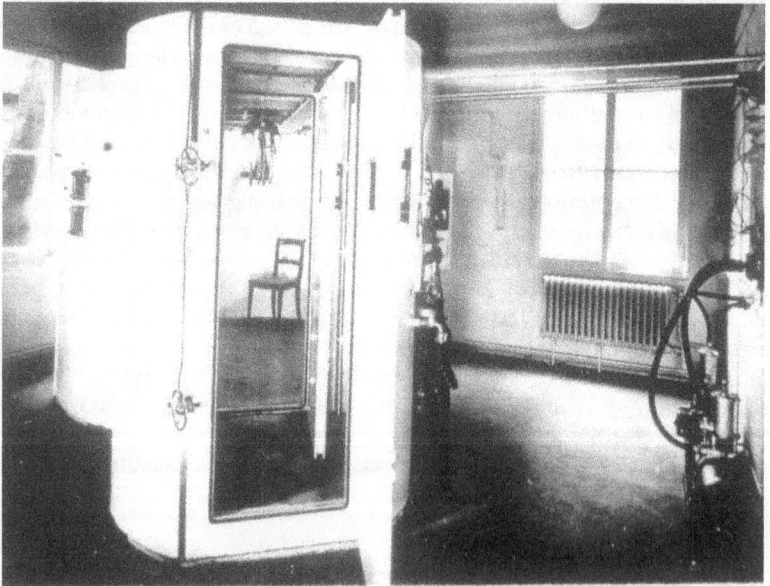

Fig. 12 AMRI altitude chamber in Berlin. Photo archive Dr. Harsch, Nbdbg.

Table 2 Departments and personnel of the Aeromedical Research Institute (AMRI) in WW2:

Chief of the department:

Maj. Prof. Dr. **Schuetz** (Dir. Physiol. Instit. Univ. Muenster)	altitude effects, sensory physiology, optics, elektrokardiography, bibliographie of aviation medicine, comperative
Dr. Ingeborg **Schmidt**	physiology, biological isotope research,
Doz. Dr. phil. Hansjochem **Autrum**	experimental animal breeding, colour and
Dr. phil **Denzer**	night vision
Capt. Dr. Heinrich **Rose**	
Dr. phil. **Suchalla**	

1. Dept. of high altitude research

Doz. Dr. Ulrich Cameron **Luft**	altitude adaptation
Dr. Friedrich **Noltenius** (died 1936)	
Dr. Hans **Hartmann** (died 1937)	

2. Dept. of histophysiology

Doz. Dr. Erich **Opitz**	oxygen supply to the tissues, respiratory
Dr. Franz **Palme**	control, height strenght (Höhenfestigkeit), elektroenzephalography

3. Dept. of respiratory and circulatory physiology

ORegMedRat Dr. Hans Georg **Clamann** (deputy direktor of AMRI)	metrology, rapid decompression research, hypoxia, oxygen toxicity, electrical and Sensory physiology, stress, stratosphere

4. Dept. for acceleration research

Prof. Dr. Otto F. **Ranke**	acceleration
Capt. Doz. Dr. Otto **Gauer**	

5. Dept. for experimental and practical issues

Capt. Doz. Dr. **Hermann** **Becker-Freyseng**	oxygen poisoning, altitude associated accidents, thurst and thirst control in
AssArzt Dr. Konrad **Schaefer**	maritime distress

6. Dept. for nutritional physiology

Capt. Doz. Dr. Horst **Hanson**	special flyers diet, general troops
Cadet Dr. **Habild**	nutritional issues

7. External Dept. for brain research, Berlin-Buch

LtCol. Prof. Dr. Hugo **Spatz**	physiology and pathology of the
OArzt Doz. Dr. **Werner K. Noell**	central nerval systems
Capt. Dr. Hugo **Noetzel**	
Capt. Dr. Eduard **Welte**	

8. External Dept. for aviation physiology, Goettingen

LtCol. Prof. Dr. Friedrich Hermann **Rein**	physiology of breathing and circulation,
Capt. Prof. Dr. Wolfgang **Schoedel**	oxygen deficiency, hypothermia
Capt. Doz. Dr. F. **Grosse-Brockhoff**	
Capt. Dr. Otto **Mertens** (also AMRI)	
OArzt Doz. Dr. Hans Hermann **Loeschcke**	
Dr. Max **Schneider**	
Cadet Dr. Juergen **Aschoff** (also Helmholtz institute)	
Erich **Opitz** (also AMRI)	

9. External Dept. at the Helmholtz institute for vibration research, Brandenburg/Inn

Capt. Dr. **Desaga**	experimental air protection research,
Capt. Dr. **Pichotka**	detonation effects (air blast),
Capt. Dr. **Reismann**	dust effect
Cadet Dr. Juergen **Aschoff** (also Goettingen)	

10. External Dept. for Aviation Medicine, Hamburg

In aeromedical meetings, mutual exchange of research experience occurred and demonstrated the scientific status of the various laboratories and professional groups. The Surgeon General of the Luftwaffe Medical Corps (E. Hippke) organized an aeromedical symposium in the post-olympic year on October 25-28, 1937. This was attended by representatives of several European countries. Other symposiums dealt with oxygen deficiency (in Goettingen in Febuary of 1941), altitude resistance (Hamburg in April of 1942), and "Medical questions in water and winter distress" (Nuremberg) (25). Keynote addresses dealt with altitude and acceleration research as well as aviation accident research. Strughold delivered the lecture "Altitude effect on the neurophysiological examination." Before this 1937 symposium Strughold attended the 9th scientific annual meeting of the Aero Medical Association, where he was elected as an honorary member (26). Strughold presented a remarkable speech on this occasion in which he emphasized the rapid development of aircraft with the resulting changes on world travel. The distances between countries and continents would shrink and the benefits from this would be to the benefit of all. Two years before the war, Strughold was still hoping for a positive international development:

"We can all hope fervently that this development in aviation will lead to a better understanding between nations" (27).

In that same year the British flight surgeon, Wing Commander Philip Livingston, performed an informational trip to the AMRI (Fig. 13) (28). Just before the outbreak of World War II, U.S. flight surgeon W.R. Lovelace also visited Germany to gather information on the state of Germany's aerospace medical research.

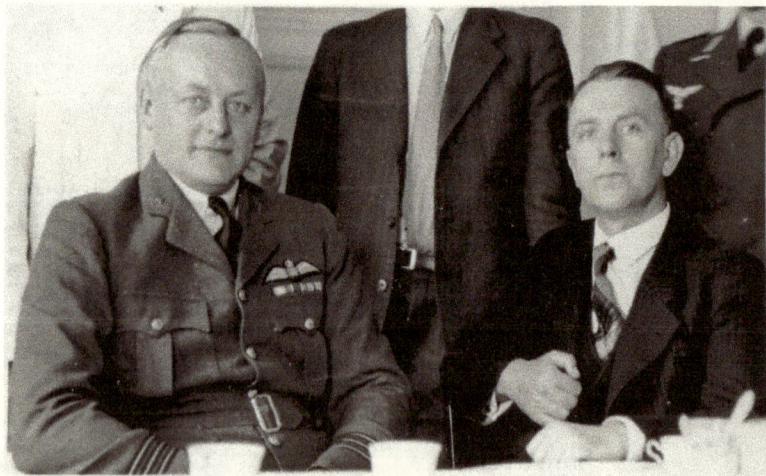

Fig. 13 Sir Livingston (left), R.A.F. in Berlin 1937. Photo private Dr. Harsch, Nbdbg.

Strughold cultivated international contacts through the employment of many foreign employees (29). In addition, he participated in several international conferences where he presented lectures. These included: The Congress of the International Academy for Medical Training in 1937 in Budapest (Hungary), the annual congress of the Aero Medical Association in New York (USA) in 1937, the International Physiological Congress in Zurich (Switzerland) in 1938, the International Sports Medicine Congress in Brussels in 1939, and the Balneology Congress in Bucharest (Romania) in 1942. Besides the regular Aviation medical lectures at the Friedrich-Wilhelms University in Berlin, Strughold presented aviation medical lectures in Budapest and Debrezcen (Hungary) in May 1941 and in Rome (Italy) in April 1942 (30). In addition, there is a letter on October 29, 1943 giving him permission to accept an invitation for a lecture tour in the winter months at the University of Sofia (Bulgaria) from the "Reich Minister for Science and Education" (31). Several international awards from that period also attest the international appreciation for Dr. Strughold. He was awarded the Order of Yugoslav Crown Class IV (Altserbian crown) in 1939 and the Commander's Cross, second Class, of the Royal Swedish award of Vasa in 1942. For his achievements in the development of aerospace medicine, Strughold was honored in 1941 with membership in the German Academy of Natural Scientists Leopoldina in Halle (Saale) (32).

Strughold's activities in research and teaching were supplemented by numerous scientific publications. He was the co-editor of several magazines since 1936, including "Aviation Medicine" (*Luftfahrtmedizin*). Strughold's first aviation physiological studies were published in the WGL periodical *Luftschiffahrt*. Luftwaffe´s first Surgeon General, Hippke, was impressed with the release of the first volume of "Aviation Medicine" (*Luftfahrtmedizin*) in 1936. The first volume was published in 1936-1937 (11 of 39 entries were from Strughold), the second volume was published in 1938-1940 (10 publications by Strughold), and the third volume was finally published in 1941-1942 (4 of 20 publications by Strughold). During the war years there were many articles not published, because they were subject to confidentiality. The most important journal publications in the field of aerospace medicine at this time are shown in Table 3 (33):

Table 3 Most important aeromedical journal publications in the 1930′s and 1940′s:

Acta Aerophysiologica (1933-34), edited by L. Brauer, Hamburg
Luftfahrtmedizin/Aviation medicine (1937-45),
    ed. by L. Brauer, H. Rein, H. Strughold
Luftfahrtmedizinische Abhandlungen/Aeromedical treatises (1936-45),
    ed. by the group of lectures in aviation medicine: edited by
    W. Knothe, A. Pickhan, G. A. Weltz
Veröffentlichungen aus dem Luftfahrtmedizinischen Forschungsinstitut
    des RLM Berlin/AMRI-Publications, Berlin (1936-1942),
    head H. Strughold
Veröffentlichungen aus dem Institut für Flugmedizin der DVL e. V./
    Publications from the DVL Institute for Aviation Medicne,
    Berlin, head S. Ruff
Mitteilungen aus dem Gebiet der Luftfahrtmedizin/Releases from the field
    of aviation medicine (1941-44), edited by. Surgeon general Luftwaffe′s M.C.
Luftfahrtmedizinische Lehrbriefe/Aeromedical teaching letters (1944-45),
    ed. by H. Strughold
Berichte und Mitteilungen der Deutschen Akademie für Luftfahrt-
    Forschung/Reports and communications of the German Academy
    for Aviation Research (1937-44), ed. by V. W. Boje and H. Loehner
Der Deutsche Militärarzt/Military Medical Doctor (1936-45),
    ed. by Waldmann, Mossauer, Hippke
Luftwissen/Air Knowledge, magazine of the Lilienthal Society

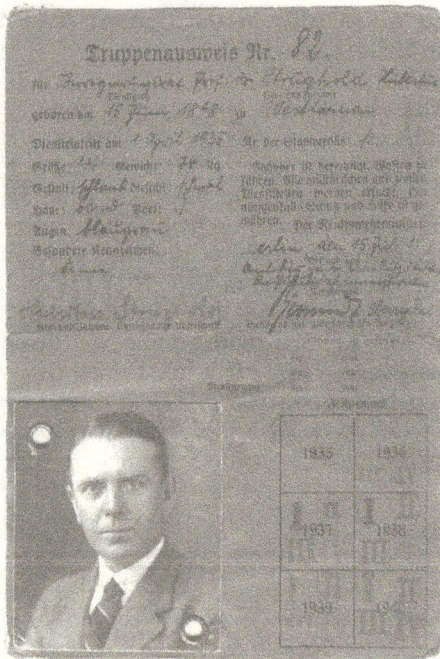

Fig. 14 Strugholds civil servant ID. Photo archive Dr. Harsch, Nbdbg.

Strughold was a member of the following societies: the Lilienthal Society (1937-45), the German Academy of Aeronautical Research (1937-1945) and the German Society for Aerospace Medicine (1943-45) (Fig. 14) (34). Strughold was the deputy chairman of the "German Society for Aviation Medicine" established in 1943. The inaugural meeting was held on April 17, 1943 in the offices of the Inspector of the Medical Department of the Air Force in Berlin-Tempelhof (Columbia Street, component S). Dr. A. Ruehl (Prague) was chairman, Dr. Anthony was the secretary, and Dr. Knothe (Jueterbog) was the treasurer. The association should serve "exclusively and directly for the promotion of public health and science". By this means it can be regarded as the forerunner of the German Society for Aviation and Space Medicine DGLRM founded in 1961 (35).

In close connection with aeromedical research was Strughold´s work in the field of sports medicine. On the occasion of the Olympic Summer Games held in Berlin in 1936, an International Sports Medicine Congress with over 1,000 participants from around the world was held (36). In the plenary hall of the Reichstag, He presented a lecture on the importance of aviation medicine (37):

"which means to enhance human performance and medical measures to prevent injury. In practice, it contributes to the improvement of the aviator's health by means of in-flight medical measures and pre-flight selection with the goal of performance enhancement and injury prevention in this new field of aviation physiology. Therefore, aviation medicine is rightly on the agenda on this occasion of the 1936 Olympics International Sports Medicine Congress, because it is the medical discipline closest to sports medicine."

In 1937, he tried to accompany the American overseas voyage of the airship "Graf Zeppelin", but was denied. The airline beat him out as a candidate, as a doctor on board was not felt to be needed (38). Another reference for sports medicine is found in the letter of the Rector of Berlin University, Hoppe. He offered to allow Lottig, Strughold and Knothe to participate at the General Assembly of International Sports Medicine Congress in Brussels (July 9-12, 1939). As representatives of Berlin University they would be present as aeromedical experts, since this congress would be making the preparations for the International Sports Medicine Congress in Helsinki, Finland in 1940 in connection with the Olympic Games. Glider flying would be performed for first time as an olympic competition. The outbreak of the second World War II, however, prevented the holding of the Olympic Games in 1940 (39).

The war driven research came under more political control, as could be shown in the following example (40):

"In the fall of 1944, my two colleagues, Dr. Heinrich Rose, a medical officer in the Air Force, and Ms. Ingeborg Schmidt examined the effects of Vitamin A on night vision. They found that with adequate fat intake, vitamin A - administered in normal doses – would improve night vision. Another investigator found that very high doses of vitamin A ingested in a special solution seemed to improve night vision in a way never seen before. These results could not be verified by my team. Some time later my superior office received a letter from an SS-institution (*SS-Sicherungs-Hauptamt*), in which my staff and my institute was charged with sabotage. Some letters were exchanged between the participants, the contents of which were unknown to me in detail. I never heard any more about it. The fact remains that my two research assistants were attacked by the SS, just because they could not confirm the findings of another researcher. A process that at the level of science is unacceptable."

With the *"Gleichschaltung"* ("co-ordination") of government, scientific, social, and economic institutions and organizations in Germany after 1933 through the Nazi-regime, a unification of control of all relevant areas was established and liberal tendencies were eliminated (41). Under these oppressive circumstances, not all German scientists were unified with the Nazi ideology. Within a limited framework, individual freedom could be maintained until the end. In the next five years (1933-38) nearly 1/3 of all German professors lost their jobs. Strughold did not join the Nazi party even though there was a clear advantage to him such as obtaining a professorship. Strughold tried to keep his international contacts despite difficult circumstances. For example: he sent publications from his Institute to the exiled Jewish Professor Max Mayer. In these times of religeous opression, Strughold continued as a professing Catholic. In the selection of his staff, Strughold attached special importance to their ethical and moral standing. He explained it this way: "During the war years I was able to pursue my work undisturbed. They did their best to push me into the Nazi party, but neither I nor anyone in my circle was a permanent staff member of the party - only the AMRI´s janitor and the keeper were Nazi-party members. One day, two representatives from the Air Ministry were there to investigate this situation. The conversation began in my office, and they indicated that they were impressed by the contribution of my institute for aviation. But to me the real reason for their visit was clear.   I knew that some of the leading men wanted me to have my workspace in the party, but I was determined that I was not one of them and would never be" (42).   He tried, whenever possible for himself and his institute, to continue to have the freedom to continue scientific work. This situation was confirmed by Dr. K. E. Schaefer. He met Strughold again in 1946 at the U.S. established Heidelberg Aero-Medical Center (43):

"From many conversations with associates of Prof. Strughold, I gained the clear impression that he was most generous in the way his team had to work independently, but the entire line of research was firmly in his hand. Prof. Strughold (...) has understood to maintain his institute and the research conducted therein in the freedom to pursue a clear line of research that corresponded to its ethical principles. So I know from him that he most strictly refused to let any harmful scientific experiments to be conducted on humans."

In political and ideological respects he did not try to gain favor for opportunistic reasons with the Nazi regime. During an illness in 1942 there were plans for replacing him at the AMRI (44). Strughold maintained largely personal and academic freedoms at the institute. Helga Gauer, a secretary at AMRI from 1938 until 1940, described the environment as follows (45):

"I learned in these two years as I worked for him, that Professor Strughold was an absolute opponent of National Socialism. Instructions of the Nazi Party and the DAF as to meetings, participation of employees in the first May-political commitments, and similar events were not followed by his staff directly by his order. Sharp criticisms by the National Socialist government of the institute's members regarding their activities, which often took place in private meetings, always found that Professor Strughold gave his staff his undivided support. In the two years that I was working at the Aviation Medical Research Institute, I never experienced it even once, that Prof. Strughold or any of its employees or assistants used the strictly ordered so-called 'German salute'. As a bachelor Strughold lived extremely withdrawn. Except at private functions of the institute's members and scientific meetings of interest, Prof. Strughold to my knowledge avoided all other official events."

Strugholds political opponent behavior is also testified by relatives and close friends (46). Professor Hugo Spatz, who held official positions at the AMRI in the field of brain research since 1937, described Strughold (Fig. 15) as follows (47):

"Prof. Strughold is a bachelor and lives reclusively. His interest is strictly limited to his scientific work area. The agreement between colleagues and subordinates in the institution was very much cordial and Prof. Strughold was universally liked. "

Strughold was represented in three formal organizations: From 1937 until the war's end he was a member of the NSA (National Socialist People's Welfare) and the Civil Service Association (RDB), but not in the National Socialist Teachers Alliance (NSD). Since 1937, he was a paying member of the National Socialist Flying Corps (NSFK), from which he resigned in 1943 (48). He neither held any office nor was integrated by any formal functions in these institutions. The membership was automatically obtained through the German Air Sports Association (DLV), which he joined in 1930, and was automatically transferred as part of the incorporation (*Gleichschaltung*) in 1937 into the NSFK (49).

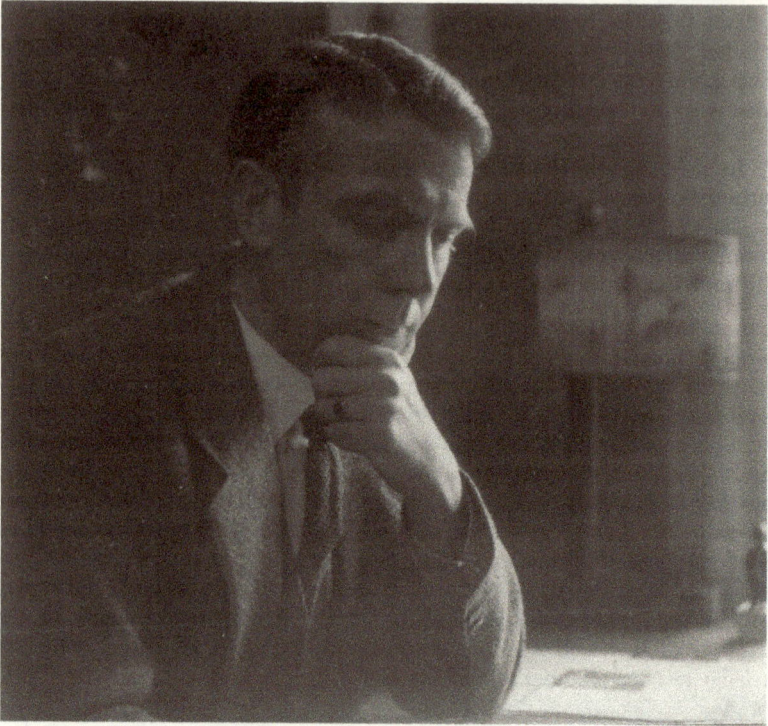

Fig. 15 Hubertus Strughold in the 30′s. Photo archive Dr. Harsch, Nbdbg.

Due to the increasing Allied bombing effects on Berlin, the relocation of parts of the AMRI was necessary. As the bombing raids were concentrated on the western part of town, Strughold moved into an eastern district. A short time later the house was destroyed by fire:

"During an air raid, I was looking like a mole in the garden. There I felt secure because only a direct hit could endanger someone."

The institute was moved to the Berlin-Tempelhof Airport in 1943. At the end of June in 1944, Strughold notified the Medical Faculty of the Friedrich-Wilhelms University in Berlin that he had shifted the bulk of the institute since the beginning of the year to the castle Welkersdorf at Greiffenberg in Silesia. A part of the Institute remained in Berlin (NW 40, Scharnhorststr. 35) and Strughold continued to personally deal with all matters necessary at regular weekly intervals by traveling to Berlin (50).With the approach of the "Eastern Front", the AMRI had to relocate again to the Physiological Institute of the Georg-August-University in Goettingen, where the physiologist Hermann Rein was still in charge. A good friend of his told him that the Russians wanted him and intended to get him to Russia. He advised Strughold that he had better get out of Berlin immediately. Heeding this warning he left in a hurry and began walking back to his old home in Westphalia, where his sister lived. Sometimes he rode with farmers whom he had never met in wagons and hid out at night in barns in haystacks (51).

The exact circumstances of the late promotion of Professor Strughold to a Colonel in the Lufwaffe is not known. He became an *Oberstarzt* in the Luftwaffe only in 1945, probably for tactical reasons (to get benefits as a POW). The reasons why he did not previously hold a military position are understandable in part - from the perspective of the lecturer Dr. K. E. Schaefer (52):

"Prof. Strughold has always refused to join the Air Force as a military officer. This was against considerable pressure from the higher authorities who were very persistent, so as to preserve his semi-official status as a civilian. As a civil servant Prof. Strughold did not have to follow the same laws and orders as a Wehrmachts officer (Fig. 16). So he was not in the chain of command and did not have to follow direct military orders given by superior officers. Prof. Strughold understood it in that way, that this was needed to preserve his institute and the research conducted therein, and the freedom to pursue a clear scientific line that corresponded to its ethical principles."

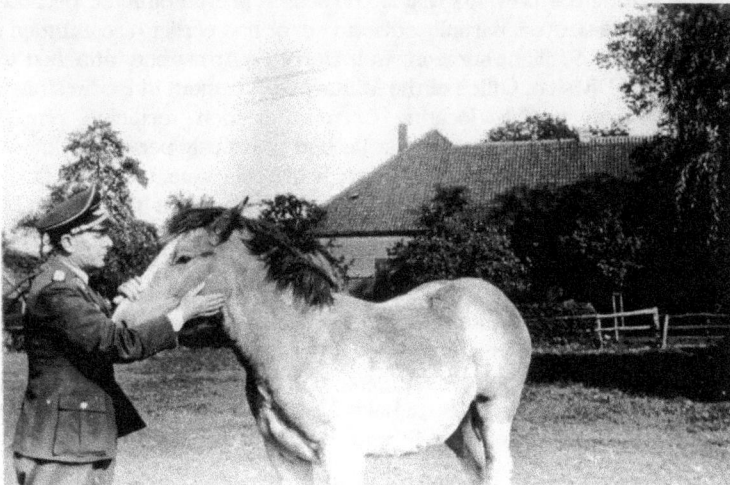

Fig. 16 Strughold in the uniform of a civil servant while at a breake taking a course given by the military. Photo archive Dr. Harsch, Nbdbg.

Chapter 5. A New Beginning: Goettingen, Heidelberg and Nuremberg (1945-1947)

As AMRI was relocated to the university town of Goettingen, Strughold moved his residence there in February 1945. He was hosted by the physiologist Hermann Rein, who was running the physiological institute as part of AMRI (1). This area, however, was soon occupied by British forces and the Institute staff, including their "guests" were taken as prisoners of war (2): Strughold was placed under house arrest on April 15, 1945 and was a prisoner of war for the next six months. In this interruption of his scientific career he could still see some positive aspects. He had time for the study of the history of medicine and felt that this was particularly instructive to him. Prof. Dr. A. E. Kornmueller, head of the KWI Brain Research Institute requested from the British military government that he be allowed to host Strughold at the physiological institute at that time. It can be assumed, that Strughold may have become a Luftwaffe Colonel in the final weeks of the war in order to obtain the "privileges" of becoming a prisoner of war (3).

With the end of the war aeromedical research came to a year-long hold. The Allied powers tried to gain German "know-how" for themself to get advantageous knowledge. An expert team from the U.S. Army Air Force was looking at German universities, laboratories and research and military institutions that had carried out research projects commissioned by the Luftwaffe during the previous years. The search proved difficult, because the facilities were destroyed, partially outsourced, or had earlier discontinued their work (4). The U.S. flight surgeon, Col. Harry G. Armstrong, attached to the Armed Forces Division, Office of the Military Government in Berlin since early June 1945, had trouble locating German aviation medicine physicians, including Strughold, a colleague that he had previously personally known. In Berlin he received information from Strughold's colleague, Ulrich C. Luft, who had already been interrogated by Soviet specialists, that the former AMRI director should be far west in Goettingen. Armstrong had met with Strughold at the New York Congress of Aviation Medicine in 1937, when the German scientist became an honorary member of the U.S. Aero Medical Association. During the war years, for obvious reasons, there was no contact between the two scientists who both edited pioneering aviation-medical textbooks in their home countries. The Soviet side was trying to gather German aviation physicians as well, especially Strughold. The Soviet flight surgeon General A. Platanow has been looking for Strughold for an academic "career" in the USSR (5).

Meanwhile, a British team of experts lead by Sir Brian Matthews, interviewed the aeromedical specialists in Goettingen. Interviews by the U.S. specialists followed. The final report from the experts evaluating aviation medical issues (the "CIOS" or Combined Intelligence Objectives Sub-committee) estimated that the German state of knowledge was low, because the research would have suffered through war-induced isolation (6). This assessment was not shared by all of the experts. The U.S. initiated the establishment of Strughold and a select group of scientists in Heidelberg to work on the newly created Aviation Medical Center (AMC) of the U.S. Army Air Force (USAAF) (7).

Armstrong noted that the collaboration with the German specialists would be valuable for the U.S. Army Air Force:

"We had the chance to bring the results of five to six years of the work of several hundred scientists with us" (8). Strughold left Goettingen in late October to relocate in Heidelberg in the sector of U.S. responsibility (9). The time in Heidelberg (1945-1947) played a key role for the future development of space medicine. Under U.S. directives, the leading German scientists and technicians from the aviation medical sector were brought together in one place. In this group a leading role was assigned to Strughold. Subsequent employment contracts for the U.S. ensured the continuity of their work and formed the basis of later space biomedical research in the Western world. For example, the acceleration physiologist Otto Gauer and astrophysicist Heinz Haber published the epochal paper "Man Under Gravity-Free Conditions" in this postwar Heidelberg era (the first published paper on the issue of space medicine). Both were inspired by a lecture by Pascal Jordan given on extraterrestrial research that had been presented in 1946 (10) (Fig. 17). This group also included Wernher von Braun. However, until their meeting in the U.S., no contacts between Strughold and Wernher von Braun occurred in Germany during the war.

Before the end of the war, Major-General Malcolm C. Grow, senior flight surgeon of the Strategic U.S. Air Forces in Europe, suggested the post-war exploitation of German technical expertise in aviation medicine by a specially department to be created in Germany. Selected German scientists and technicians could pursue their work under American leadership, and a limited amount of additional research could be continued on outstanding projects (11).

44

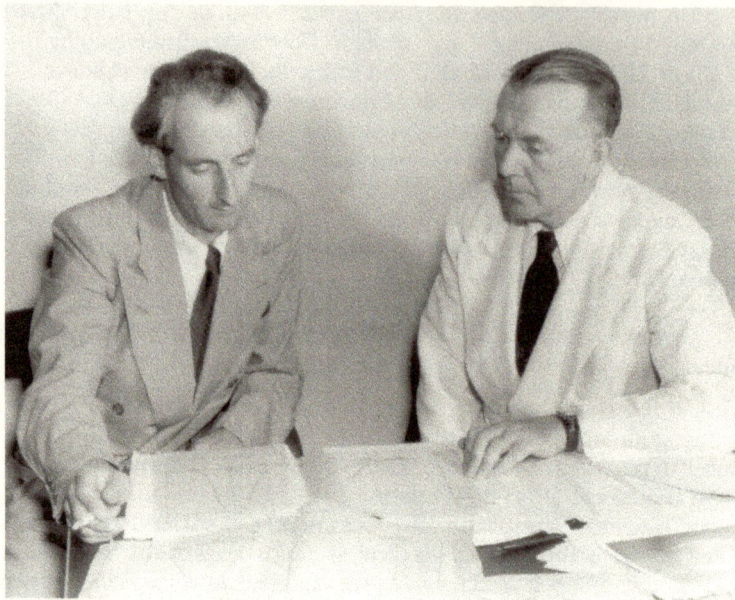

Fig. 17 Heinz Haber and H. Strughold in scientific discussion on Monography papers.
Photo archive Dr. Harsch, Nbdbg.

In the summer of 1945, the premises of the former Heidelberg Kaiser Wilhelm Institute (KWI) for Medical Research was considered an appropriate location for the establishment of the Aviation Medicine Center (U.S. AAF Aeromedical Research Center: AMC) and two aeromedical working groups to implement the project were identified (12). In early September 1945, a wing of the local office of the military government occupied KWI for this purpose (13). The first staff meeting of the AMC occurred in November 1945 and was led by the U.S. Army officers Sheeley, Benford and Burchell. At this time there were already several German aviation medical practitioners there (14). Strughold himself had joined the group on November 1, 1945 (15).

In 1946, a document with a photograph of part of the German and American academic staff of the AMC can be seen (16). At the AMC, four working groups were set up, with Strughold, Ruff, Benzinger and Henschke as leaders (17). The German scientists were tasked with the documentation of existing knowledge and the collection and analysis of unpublished aviation medical research findings and experiences. As a result of the war a lot of documents and scientific reports were lost, but here they were partially reconstructed. Until November 1, 1946 a number of research projects were conducted at the AMC. The "Intelligence Division" was busy with the translation, review and evaluation of approximately 2,000 German documents with aviation medical content. The work was then send to the "Air Surgeon," for further distribution to U.S. agencies (18). A comprehensive compilation of the German aviation medical research activities in the war years was planned as the "Survey of German Aviation Medicine, 1939-45" to be published in the fall of 1947 and then released in the U.S. (19). Edward J. Baldes and Earl H. Wood were ordered to support the "Aeromedical Monograph Project", and in June 1946 Strughold joined the team as an expert in German aero-medical publications (Fig. 18). Strughold was responsible for the review of the incoming manuscripts, the translation of the manuscripts, and was editor of the final product. Information and documents came from all four of the occupation zones. His U.S counterpart with jurisdiction of the monograph was Major W. F. Sheeley. The target group was flight surgeons and researchers in the Anglo-Saxon aeromedical community. Relocation was proposed for continuation of the work as the responsible were faced with many problems: Several well-known publishers and printers were not meeting the U.S. ideas on the scope and extent of the work due to a lack of capacity and materials within Germany. Even the translation options on the AMC staff were limited (20). Therefore, Col. Hall decided that the printing should take place in the U.S. and not in Germany. The work of the Heidelberg AMC ended on March 15, 1947 with what many considered to be a premature closure. The monograph was completed at the School of Aviation Medicine in San Antonio, Texas, where German translators were used (21). The extensive work was published in 1950 and for a long time was a standard textbook for the "residents" at the USAF SAM (22). In a letter dated April 27, 1951, Strughold commented the work to the University of Heidelberg with the following revealing words (23):

"It is my opinion, that the high level of German medical research, which in the early postwar years was unpublished, could now be distributed around the world in the right light."

A total of 56 renowned German scientists contributed to the two-volume pamphlet "German Aviation Medicine in World War II " (24). Strughold wrote the introduction concerning the contributions, development, and organization of German aviation medicine up to 1945. He also wrote the sensory physiological contribution, "The Mechanoreceptors of Skin and Muscles under Conditions Flying" and "Intermittent Light" (25).

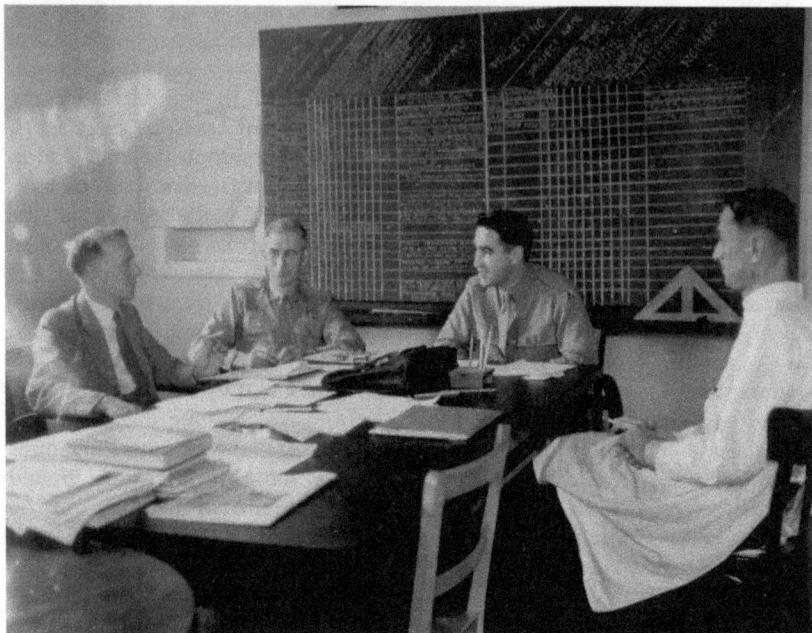

Fig. 18 US and German aeromedical specialists in discussion on the Monograph project. Strughold is on the far left, Benzinger on the far right. Photo archive Dr. Harsch, Nbdbg.

A close collaboration existed between the AMC and the scientists in Heidelberg with other scientific groups in the Western occupation zones. For example, there was contact with the working group headed by Wilhelm Ernsthausen at the AMC branch office of the former Berlin Helmholtz Institute (26). Various scientists and technicians in the three western zones were frequently visited (Fig. 19). In November 1946 alone, three multi-day missions were listed for Strughold. These were meetings concerned with the development of the anthology project, but also some preliminary discussions in order to coordinate further activities of German scientists in the U.S. (28). The AMC was the steppingstone for several German and Austrian experts to migrate to the USA (29): In a document dated January 17, 1947 Strughold can be found among others to be eligible for transportation in the United States as an expert as a part of "Operation Paperclip" (Fig. 20) (30).

47

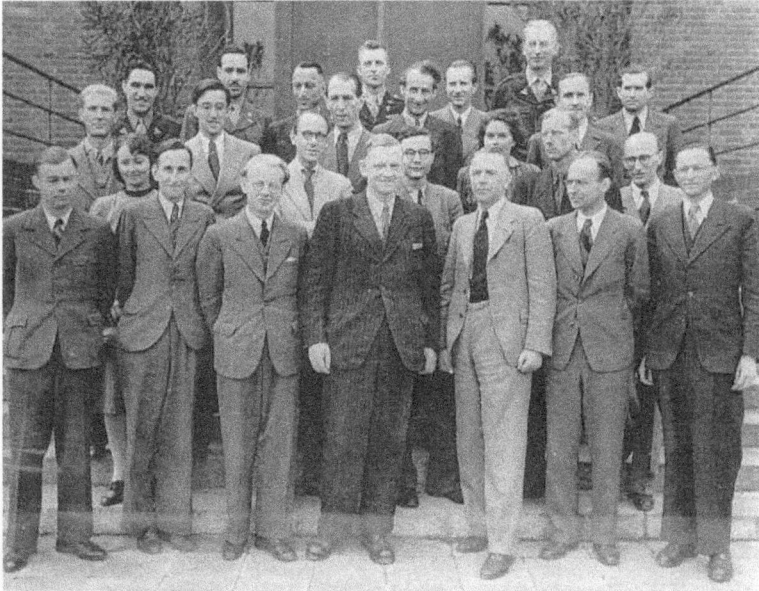

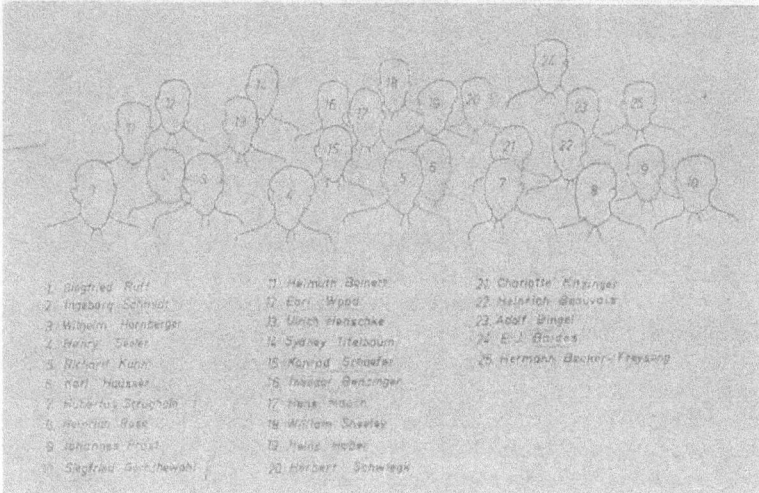

Fig. 19 Group photo of personnel at the US AAF Aero Medical Center in 1946.
Photo archive Dr. Harsch, Nbdbg.

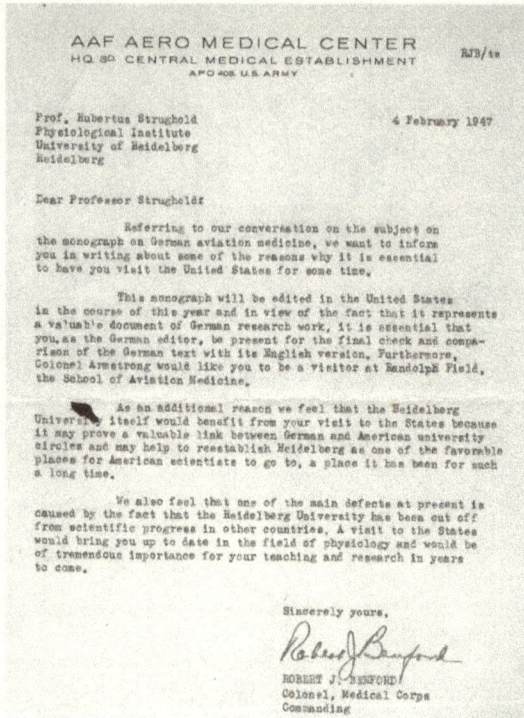

Fig. 20 Official US AAF invitation for Strughold for a continuing research visit to the US dated February 4, 1947. Photo archive Dr. Harsch, Nbdbg.

On the other hand, the United States prosecuted the excesses of Nazi medical research in one of the Nuremberg judicial proceedings ("Doctors' Trial") (31). A controversy erupted because of the events in Nuremberg and the associated blame on the German medical profession in general. The World Medical Association called for the collective guilt of the entire German medical profession concerning the crimes committed under National Socialism. This was rejected, but resulted in the German Medical Association sending an observation mission to the Nuremberg Doctors' Trial headed by Mitscherlich (32). He had published a paper "The Dictates of Misanthropy" (*Das Diktat der Menschenverachtung*). This paper had provoked criticism in many medical circles, as there were concerns that a public discussion of the unethical medical behaviour of a minority could harm the reputation of the medical profession in general (33). The Heidelberg AMC specialists Ruff, Schaefer, Becker-Freyseng, Schroeder and Benzinger were arrested. Strughold prepared depositions for the trial (34). He was never arrested or interrogated in connection with the doctor trials (35). This topic is further discussed in the concluding chapter on the ethical aspects of medical activity of Strughold.

Chapter 6. Resettlement in the United States (1947-1950)

Hubertus Strughold was appointed as the chair of physiology at the Ruperto-Carola-University in Heidelberg on September 21, 1945. He succeeded Professor J. D. Achelis, who was retiring for political reasons. Professors H. Rein (Goettingen), H. Weber (Koenigsberg) and H. Schaefer (Bad Nauheim) were all originally proposed for this appointment. Professor Rein, Director of the Physiological Institute at the University of Goettingen, refused the appointment in a letter dated April 8, 1946 and recommended that Strughold be named for the post (Fig. 21) (1):

"For immediate representation I would highly recommend for you to think of Prof. Strughold. I know that he is vividly discussed in various other places and would like to think that he could take over as acting representative for the next term without further notice. His lectures are excellent and he is indeed a man of great prestige in the world. His Westphalian deliberation, however will attract attention in Heidelberg, but is a thoroughly estimable characteristic in the team of colleagues. You absolutely must get to know him personally and then would quickly understand my sympathies. "

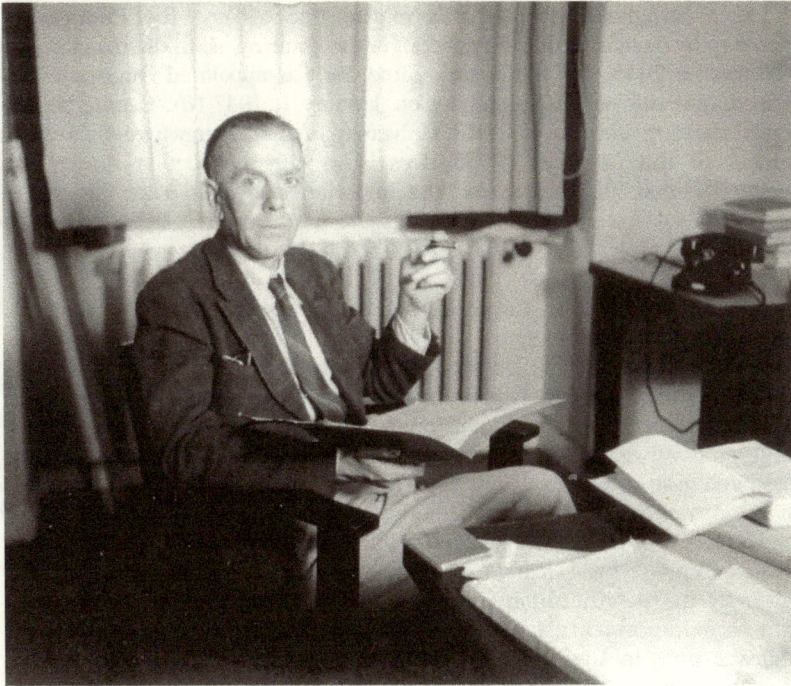

Fig. 21 Hubertus Strughold in his Heidelberg office 1946/47.
Photo archive Dr. Harsch, Nbdbg.

The Faculty of Medicine of the University of Heidelberg at first assigned Professor Weber the highest priority for the appointment, since Strughold had agreements with the U.S. Military government that could not be rescinded. However, after the U.S. considered the situation, they gave Strughold a "release" and Strughold was favored for the replacement (2):

"Prof. Dr. Strughold's work on the sense-physiological field and his other scientific research is well-known. He is regarded as a good teacher with a good personality and character. Politically, he was, as far as we know, uncompromised. His cooperation with the U.S. authorities also points in this same direction. Major William F. Sheeley has also indicated that he expected an appeal by the faculty for the appointment and that Strughold's appointment would lead to a particularly harmonious and mutually beneficial cooperation between the faculty and the U.S. Aeromedical Center."

Major William F. Sheeley, chief negotiator for the Heidelberg Aero Medical Center, assured the faculty that the U.S. authorities would not exert any pressure on the issue. It should be decided entirely by the medical faculty alone (3). The "head of the Baden school administration" asked Strughold in a letter dated July 28, 1946 if Strughold would occupy the Chair of Physiology (4). After Strughold accepted this request, he became the Professor of Physiology by resolution of the President of the country's sixth district of Baden in November 1946 (5). At the same time, he was appointed Director of the Institute and started his assignment on January 1, 1947 (6). During his six-month teaching assignment at the University of Heidelberg, Strughold was a member of the Academy of Sciences. The only publication during this transition period was the article "The importance of oxygen for life" in the university magazine in 1948, which was the first time that he discussed an astrobiological topic.

In early 1947 Col. Robert J. Benford, Director of the Aeromedical Center, desired that Strughold should spend research time in the USA. Strughold explained to the Dean of the Faculty of Medicine, Professor Kurt Schneider, that this was an opportunity to establish new contacts and would therefore be of benefit to the Physiological Institute. The work at the Institute, however, would not be affected by his limited absence (7). In devastated postwar Germany, the opportunities for any academic career were limited. Any activity abroad, particularly in the U.S., seemed advantageous. The University of Heidelberg decided to allow Strughold to take this scientific sabatical to revive pre-existing contacts with U.S. universities. At Heidelberg University the denazification process of the teaching staff in the postwar years played an important role. As part of the reopening of the Heidelberg Medical Faculty in Aug. 1945, 9 of the 16 professors were forced to retire for political reasons (past Nazi connections) (8). The Heidelberg German civil court for denazification (*Spruchkammer*) stated in a document dated October

18, 1946 that Strughold did not need to undergo the denazification process as he was regarded as completely politically uninvolved (Fig. 22) (9).

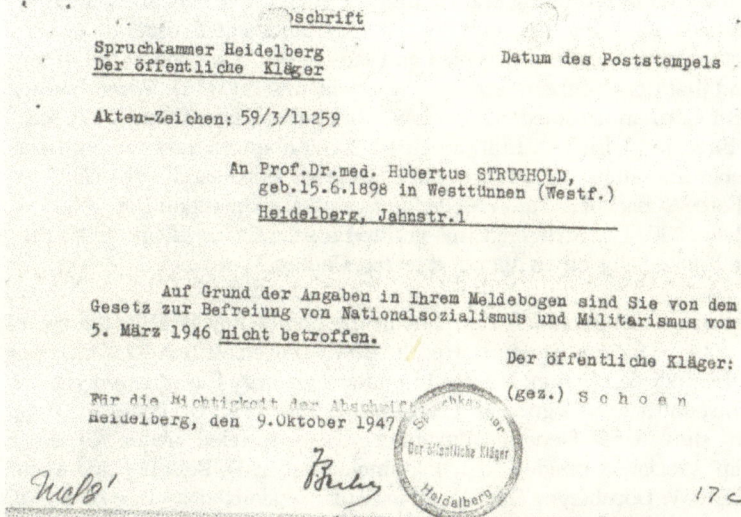

```
                          )schrift

Spruchkammer Heidelberg                    Datum des Poststempels
Der öffentliche  Kläger


Akten-Zeichen: 59/3/11259


         An Prof.Dr.med. Hubertus STRUGHOLD,
            geb.15.6.1898 in Westtünnen (Westf.)
            Heidelberg, Jahnstr.1



       Auf Grund der Angaben in Ihrem Meldebogen sind Sie von dem
Gesetz zur Befreiung von Nationalsozialismus und Militarismus vom
5. März 1946 nicht betroffen.

                                    Der öffentliche Kläger:

                                           (gez.) S c h o e n
Für die Richtigkeit der Abschrift
Heidelberg, den 9.Oktober 1947
```

Fig. 22 Hubertus Strughold in his Heidelberg office 1946/47.
(University Archives Heidelberg, Harsch 2004: A-13)

Many German scientists migrated in significant numbers to the United States after the war's end. This led to a growing gap at German universities, where already the "denazification" that was in progress led to a shortage of qualified academicians and scientists. In the article "Invitation to the USA" in the Goettingen University newspaper in 1947, the renown scientists, Hermann Otto Hahn and Hermann Rein, critizised the process of "scientist export". This "brain drain" increased the evident shortage in research and teaching areas at German universities. As the East-West confrontation evolved over time, Strughold stated that the presence of German scientists in the U.S. during this critical world situation would be of benefit for Germany and the German scientific community for several reasons (10).

The German rocket engineer Wernher von Braun was one of the first persons to receive a labor contract to come to the United States of America. However, it took more than a year before the first aviation medicine specialist followed. The USAF document, "Fifty Years of Aerospace Medicine" (1968) states that the recruitment of German physicians was not an easy task, as they were more reluctant than the other scientists (11). In 1959 Armstrong stated, that the recruitment of aeromedical specialists was a lengthy and cumbersome process. It was not until 1948 that adequate recruited scientists were in place to perform significant scientific research. The USAF School of Aerospace Medicine (SAM) at Randolph Field, Texas would acquire more than 30 "paperclip" specialists by the 1950s (12). Col. Paul Campbell was directly involved in recruiting and clearing German physicians and scientists for aerospace medicine research in the U.S. and stated that all of the scientists were "very carefully studied and screened ... I am convinced in my own mind that none of them were in any way blemished" (13). Several other prominent German aeromedical specialists, including Hans-Georg Clamann, Konrad Buettner, Ulrich C. Luft, Siegfried J. Gerathewohl, and the brothers Fritz Haber and Heinz Haber, were also assigned as research physicians to the Air Force School of Aviation Medicine as a part of Operation Paperclip. In September 1948, Dr. Strughold was granted a security certificate from the Joint Intelligence Objectives Agency director, Captain Wev.

Hubertus Strughold left Germany at the end of July 1947 at the age of 49 years (14). The sea voyage started in Bremerhaven with New York, New York as the final destination. He was hired for temporary U.S. duty on July 12, 1947. The contract was signed on February 14, 1947 (15). On board the troop transport ship "USS General Alexander" there traveled about 20 other "Paperclip" specialists besides Strughold, including Dr. D. Beischer and Major General Dr. W. Dornberger (16). Daily scientific sessions took place on-board, during which Strughold talked enthusiastically about the possibilities of manned space flight. Clamann stated that Strughold was the first person in Europe to speak about aerospace medicine (17). Kirsch and Winau (1986) stated that during his time in Heidelberg, Strughold had already inaugurated the concept of space medicine.

During the contract period Strughold was on leave from the University of Heidelberg. The U.S. expected a positive outcome from Strughold's employment. His expectations were as followed (18):

"I have ideas and plans for an academic career in the field of physiology and aviation medicine in the U.S., as this cannot be done in Germany. There are also excellent conditions for starting application-oriented research over here. Furthermore, the U.S. is the only free country that is still able to preserve the freedom and the ancient culture of Western civilization, which seems to now be threatened. My intention is to support the U.S. with my scientific skills and experience. I am familiar with the American way of life through my education in Westphalia and my past learning and research at several U.S. universities."

Strughold arrived on August 3, 1947 in New York City and in the evening caught a flight on a B-25 transport aircraft to the AAF base at Randolph Field, Texas. His first accommodation was in the U.S. military housing complex (BOQ T262) at Randolph Field. Later he lived along with other German scientists in the small community of Schertz, a few miles from Randolph Field (Fig. 23). With the relocation of the school to Brooks AFB which also was close by, he moved into the Menger Hotel in the historic town center of San Antonio, where he continued to live up until his marriage to Mary, in the 1970s (19).

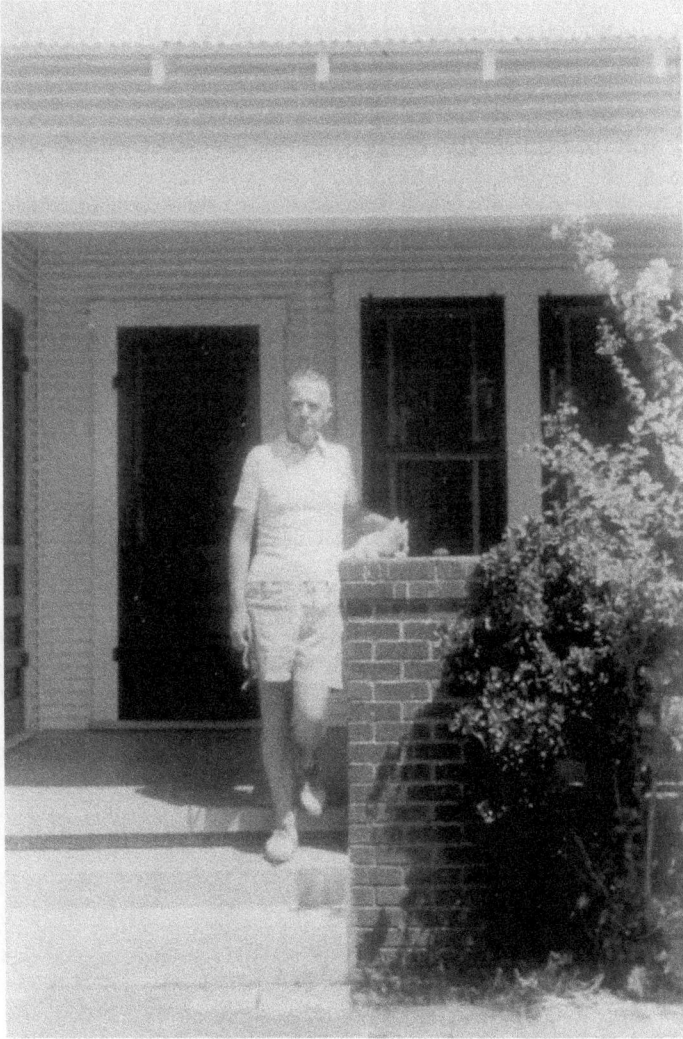

Fig. 23 Cat lover Hubertus Strughold at his home in Schertz, Texas. Photo archive Dr. Harsch, Nbdbg.

Shortly after his arrival at Randolph Field (just northeast of San Antonio, Texas) he informed the University of Heidelberg that his U.S. residency would probably be of longer duration. In the beginning of 1948 he made another request for an extension of his leave in detail (20):

"About 14 days before the question about my return to Heidelberg was to be discussed by the Head of the School of Aviation Medicine, I was asked if I could stay forever in America. I have not accepted this offer because of my duties in Heidelberg. Then the question was raised whether or not I could arrange with the University of Heidelberg to stay for at least another few months. After I thought about this for several days, I agreed, hoping that the faculty would approve of it retrospectively. I asked the School commander to inform you by airmail immediately. Here's why:

1st: Time was lost for the first months here due to the frozen post-war situation. Now things are thawing out and I think that in terms of food supplies for the Heidelberg students, a significantly better response can be expected. Therefore, I would not like to leave too early.

2nd: I can continue the ongoing scientific research here and this would not be possible in Heidelberg.

3rd: The fact that my deputy, E. K. Schaefer, has guaranteed that the Institute can be operated without difficulty.

4th: In February, March and the first half of April in Germany there are always university vacations.

5th: Here at Air University there are now 2-3 seminars weekly with presentations from all the areas of medicine by relevant disciplines that are brought by plane from the various universities throughout the country. By this means I can inform myself about the state of medical research in the U.S., without having to make any time consuming trips. Therefore, I have here the best conditions for my goal of bringing physiological education in Heidelberg up to date and combining the entire European and American knowledge in my areas of expertise. And this opportunity, which currently is not available to any other German physiologist, I want to take full advantage of."

Strughold thought that he could be of bigger use to Germany and its students through the extension of his U.S. stay. He strongly argued that as a result, the opportunity could be used to close the long years of isolation of Germany and close the resulting gaps. This conclusion had become clear to him only when he was actually in the U.S., and it was hoped that in the near future more professors would have the chance to get a comparable job. Strughold also visited the Mayo Clinic, where he received reprints, textbooks, training books and other publications for teaching at the Heidelberg University. At this point, he thought of returning to Germany in March 1948 (21). In Oct. 1948, Strughold sent a report (in the files of the Physiological

Institute) concerning the installation ceremony of General Dwight David Eisenhower as the President of Columbia University. In it he thanked the rector of Heidelberg University for the great honor that he had been given by the agency in charge of this. Strughold stressed that this invitation to a German university by the U.S. was the first of its kind after the war: Heidelberg was one of 34 foreign universities represented. At this ceremony Strughold did not wear a traditional graduation gown, but was dressed in American style clothing.

Another reason for Strughold prolonging his stay was to continue his editorial work on the handbook of German aviation medical research which began in 1946 in Heidelberg. The publication was not completed until 1950 in the USA. In these times of increasing confrontation between the U.S. and the USSR, it was also advantageous to keep Strughold away from possible soviet contact by isolating him in Texas. Strughold had received research contracts of growing importance and eventually was entrusted in 1949 with the leadership of the newly established space-related medical department at Randolph Field in Texas. Meanwhile, he was still engaged in the organization of food aid - especially for Heidelberg. At the end of 1947 he informed the rector of Heidelberg University, Prof. Dr. W. Kunkel, that Gen. H.G. Armstrong had written a large number of letters appealing for German food aid. During the 1947-48 food crisis, Strughold supported aid to the University of Heidelberg by these means (22). He had a particular concern about the situation of the students, especially those in the Soviet occupied East. They were cut off from any financial support being sent to them, so that Dr. Hoepke (the Dean of Heidelberg University) did not know how they would survive until the end of term exams (23). In a letter dated April 18, 1948 and in an earlier telegram, Strughold informed the dean that he wouldn´t come back for the lectures for the summer term. He regarded it as a necessity, to stay "in this time of trouble", as a representative of the German university in the U.S. (24):

"Things developed in the way, that my continued presence in this country is still needed. I have decided to stay, after careful consideration, although I personally feel very sorry not to lecture any more in Heidelberg. However, this is made easier for me as I am now able to support the University of Heidelberg more effectively. To support the University in food matters from here seems to me to be more important than giving lectures, as I do have a good deputy over there replacing me effectively. I have received from Heidelberg, as well as from other universities, reports on the almost disastrous food situation now occurring that threatens to wipe out all academic life."

The University expressed gratitude to Strughold for his support in the food aid. However, they judged his absence as unfavorable for the situation of the Physiological Institute and the students' education. Hoepke pointed out that he expected him back in the summer, as the institute did need his leadership (25). In the faculty meeting on May 13, 1948 this topic was discussed and Strughold was requested to return by September 1948:

"The faculty is in great difficulty, if you stay away any longer." (26). After Strughold replied on October 6, 1948 without explanation that he would not come back that year and requested an extension of his deployment until June 30, 1949, the Faculty of Medicine decided to set him an ultimatum for his return by March 31, 1949. At the same time, Prof. Dr. Hans Schaefer was officially announced as the commissioner. In addition to his visiting professorship status he was inaugurated as the deputy director of the Physiological Institute (27). In April 1949, Strughold announced his resignment from the Institute's directorship: "After much serious consideration I have agreed to stay in the U.S. for some time. This decision did cost and still costs me the most difficult willpower, especially because teaching in the Department of Physiology at the University of Heidelberg has captivated me more than any previous phase of my life. Especially with the possibility of building a physiology department with newer concepts and teaching students, it made it hard for me to go to America. Since I am here now for 1 3/4 years, the tasks that have been given to me have enlarged and last month I was given a special assignment. I, therefore, share the concern with the medical school that I was not able to return to the current summer term. I also understand that the Medical Faculty cannot be kept without a decision any longer. Nevertheless, I would ask that I can continue to be a member of the Medical Faculty. The reasons I would like to explain on my planned visit in August / September of this year (1949). "

Strughold wrote his official resignation letter on August 30, 1949. The President of the country district of Baden, Department of Education and Religion, accepted his service termination (28). The Dean of the Medical Faculty later honored Strughold overseas activities:

"He was in action in America for the interests of the University of Heidelberg on several occasions. He met several times with the personalities of American public life and was helpful in the establishment of research contracts, allocation of food-aid, etc. Although he achieved benefits for the university, the Medical Faculty was initially not favourable concerning his request for con-tinuation as a faculty member" (29).

However, the dean requested for Strughold to obtain the status of a Honorary Professor in his letter to the Department of Culture and Education dating January 19, 1950 (30):

"Strughold will stay overseas, because he is regarded abroad as the most prominent representative of German aviation medicine, and because he is appreciated in this capacity by the Americans. Through this appreciation he can be very helpful for the German cause. It must be, therefore, in the interest of the faculty and the University of Heidelberg, to keep a connection with such a man by a more or less loose association, allowing him from time to time to share his experiences with the German students."

The Army Air Force and the School of Aviation Medicine were both in a phase of reorganization in 1947. In September 1947 the U.S. Air Force (USAF) was set up as an independent branch of the armed forces (31). Many American scientists left the armed forces after the war, resulting in gaps that were filled in by German scientists (32). In 1952, the nineteen German scientists (Table 4) were allocated to the USAF SAM (33).

Table 4 "Paperclip" specialists assigned to USAF SAM in 1952:

"Paperclip" specialists	Arrival in U.S.	Area of work
Dr. Bruno Balke	-	Physiology
Abraham G. A. Bingel	-	Neurology
Dr. Konrad J. K. Buettner	1947	Bioclimatology
Dr. Paul Cibis	-	Ophthalmology/ Radiology
Dr. Hans Georg Clamann	1947	Physiology
Dr. John Siegfried Gerathewohl	1947	Ophthamology / Physiology
Dr. Herbert B. Gerstner	1950	Radio biology
Dr. Heinz Haber	1947	Astrophysics
Dr. Fritz Haber	1950	Aircraft engineer
Bernhard Hoelscher	1949	Physiology
Dr. Kurt Kramer	1948	Physiology
Richard Lindenberg	-	Neurology
Dr. Ulrich Cameron Luft	1947	Physiology
Dr. Werner K. Noell	1947	Neurophysiology
Dr. Oscar L. Ritter	1950	Radiobiology
Dr. Heinrich W. Rose	1947	Ophthalmology
Dr. Ingeborg Schmidt	1946	Ophthamlology
Dr. Hubertus Strughold	1947	Physiology
Dr. Juergen Tonna	1947	ENT

Colonel Harry G. Armstrong, commander of the School of Aviation Medicine, placed Strughold into the position as an scientific adviser (34). Strughold continued his editorial work on the handbook, "German Aviation Medicine in World War II". He was also responsible for monitoring, supervising, and integrating the activities of the German scientists at the SAM. Other areas of interest were: the selection of appropriate terminology for aerospace medical research reports, paleontological development of the Earth's atmosphere with special consideration of oxygen and carbon dioxide, and physics and physiology of space (35). In 1936 Strughold requested a harmonization and standardization of terms and methods in aviation medicine. Just 12 years later (1948) he joined H. F. Adler, A. W. Heterington and Ulrich C. Luft under the chairmanship of W. F. Sheeley in forming a "Nomenclature Committee", that was established by the SAM commander (36).

Strughold's stay in the U.S. was at first intended to be limited. The possibility of returning to Heidelberg was, however, shrinking every month as he prolonged his deployment. He was given the feeling that he was pioneering a new research field of aerospace medicine - similar to 20 years ago in Wuerzburg in the case of aviation medicine. The decision to stay in the U.S., was decisively influenced by Armstrong. On November 10, 1948, at the USAF SAM at Randolph AFB, Texas, the first Space Medicine Symposium on "Aeromedical Problems of Space Travel" took place (37). This meeting was arranged by Armstrong and dealt with the medical problems of space flight. It was the first of its kind in the world and as Strughold later stated, it was "sensational". Around 700 attendees were counted at this event, including invited scientists from various universities. Armstrong made an introduction to this historic theme, H. Haber spoke about the astronomical aspects of manned spaceflight and Strughold spoke in a visionary way about the possibility of an interplanetary flight to Mars (38). At that time he stated (39): "This new field of space medicine will play the same role in the next 30 years as did aviation medicine in 1920 and the following three decades."

In 1949 Strughold was commissioned by Armstrong to create long-term plans to improve coordination at USAF SAM. Strughold recommended the creation of a space medical department, which was based on joint discussions with H. Haber (40). The proposal was implemented through the establishment of the Department of Space Medicine on February 9, 1949 at USAF SAM. A few months later Hubertus Strughold became its first director (41). Working groups for medical science, astrophysics, engineering and bioclimatology demonstrate the extensive range of research areas at this pioneering new department. The head of the working groups were Strughold, H. Haber and K. Buettner. After only a brief period as head of the department, Strughold reported in August 1949 to the dean of the Medical Faculty of Heidelberg, Prof. K. Bauer, about a contribution to aerospace medicine in the magazine "Newsweek" (42):

"I have been doing this for some time, but it has only just begun early this year to adopt an official, tangible form. (...) The future achievement of contact with another celestial body, undoubtedly will be the greatest achievement of mankind on a technological and physiological field. The physiological pioneering work to make this possible represents a new stage in medical and physiological research. Even if we ignore the actual goal, namely extra-terrestrial flight, it still offers the study of zero gravity, the study of cell physiology from differing conditions as they exist, for example, on Mars, and a completely new perspectives on terrestrial physiology. It involves different conditions, which we overlook in the terrestrial physiology simply because there is no need for these issues, and yet it seems to me that these things are gaps in our normal physiology that need to be filled. One can also say that aerospace medicine offers a new platform for viewing physiology, which is novel and attractive for young students".

Strughold´s and his colleagues' research was initially recorded in some professional circles in a negative light and they were laughed at as a "bunch of abstract thinkers": No practical relevance for Space Medicine could be seen for the foreseeable future (43). Otis O. Benson, Jr. succeeded Armstrong as the school commander in June 1949. Benson was also open minded towards aerospace medicine and a continuity of work could still be expected (44). Strughold knew him from the Aeromedical Center at Heidelberg.

Two years after leaving Germany, Strughold visited his home for the first time in 1949. The trans-Atlantic flight in August took him from Washington D.C. to Frankfurt and two months later in the opposite direction. He experienced severe desynchronization of his own body biorhythms which prompted him to do further research on this issue. This eventually resulted in the publication of the book "Your Body Clock" in 1971 (45). An important goal for Strughold's trip to Europe was to recruit German scientists to work in the U.S. (46). Having Heidelberg specialists Cibis and Tonndorf already on the SAM team, Strugold was able to convince the experimental surgeon, Bernhard Hoelscher, who worked in the field of stress research, to leave the Heidelberg Institute of Physiology and to take a job in San Antonio, Texas (47).

On March 3, 1950 leading scientists and technicians met at the Chicago Executive Club for a noon luncheon, including members of the Department of Space Medicine at USAF SAM. The meeting was chaired by Andrew C. Ivy. Harry G. Armstrong, Wernher von Braun, Hubertus Strughold, Heinz Haber, Paul Campbell and Konrad Buettner presented their research and further developmental possibilities. Dr. John P. Marbarger was asked to organize a following meeting entitled "Biomedical Aspects of Manned Space Flight" at the University of Illinois. The crowded lecture hall was overflowing with over 300 people. An introductory film clip, "A Study of Rocket Flight," was shown followed by introductory remarks by the Vice President of the University, A. C. Ivy. Strughold presented, "Physiological Considerations on the Possibility of Life in Extraterrestrial Conditions". The conclusion was a summary presentation by the USAF Surgeon General Harry G. Armstrong. Strughold was enthusiastic about the apparent success of the event and encouraged Marbarger to publish the lectures. This conference led to discussions to form a permanent space medicine organization. Only a short time later, the same scientists (17 in all) met at the 21st Annual Meeting of the Aviation Medical Association (AMA) on May 31, 1950 at the Palmer House in Chicago, Illinois. At this informal meeting the Space Medicine Branch of the AMA was formed. It was chaired by A. C. Ivy. The following German scientists were among the founding members: K. Buettner, F. Haber, H. Haber, U. K. Henschke, H. J. Schaefer and H. Strughold. Strughold's presentation dealt with the international state of space medical research (48). On May 13, 1951 the Space Medical Branch (now the Space Medicine Association) of the Aero Medical Association (now the Aerospace Medical Association) was founded and since then annual meetings have been held. Strughold later served as Secretary-Treasurer, Vice-President and, in 1959, as the President of that organization. The Hubertus Strughold Award was instituted beginning in 1963 by the Space Medicine Branch of the Aerospace Medical Association (49). It is presented each year for dedication and outstanding contributions in advancing the frontiers of Space Medicine and for sustained contributions to further the goals of the Space Medicine Branch (now the Space Medicine Association).

Chapter 7. School of Aviation Medicine (1950-1960)

In the early 1950s the Space Medicine Division of the USAF School of Aviation Medicine (SAM) published over 130 documents, highlighting the fundamental importance of this institution in the emerging field of space medicine. Many of these pioneering publications were authored by Strughold, such as "From Aviation Medicine to Space Medicine" (1952), "Where Does Space Begin - Functional Concept of the Boundaries between Atmosphere and Space" (1951) and "Atmospheric Space Equivalence" (1954). With the founding of the Space Medicine Division at the USAF SAM a new frontier was entered and there was a need for basic definitions and international standardization. An important role in this new field of medicine was played by the journal of the Aero Medical Association, the "Journal of Aviation Medicine" (1). Another relevant publication on space medicine at this time which contained many works from Dr. Strughold and other researchers at the Space Medicine Division was "Space Medicine - The Human Factor in Flights Beyond the Earth" by J. P. Marbarger (1951) (2). In 1951 Von Braun stated that the time was right for aerospace medical research, as there were no technical problems which needed to be solved to make manned space flight reality, but only the limitations of the human organism (3). Strughold seriously directed his focus to determine the possibilities of space medicine, realizing that a journey to the Moon or Mars were not prime targets for the U.S. Air Force. But he also realized that it would be a big mistake to overlook the fact that there existed only small steps from stratospheric to interplanetary flights, which he termed space equivalent flights (4).

The public also followed the development of space flight with increased interest. Beginning in March 1952, "Collier´s" magazine published eight editions publicizing the future of manned space travel. Three of the editions contained space medical contributions by H. Haber and Strughold (5). In August 1955 "The National Geographic Magazine" published an article entitled "Aviation Medicine on the Threshold of Space" which also featured Dr. Strughold (6). The public interest was intensely focused on space travel by a popular TV series produced by Walt Disney and released in March 1955. This television documentary, "Man in Space", ran for eight episodes and featured space stations, men performing what is now termed EVA from a spacecraft, and the landing on a runway of a space shuttle with chilling accuracy. Willy Ley, Wernher von Braun and Heinz Haber were obtained as scientific consultants. Heinz Haber was responsible for the medical aspects and possible problems of manned space flight. Ernst Stuhlinger also later joined this expert group. ABC-TV broadcasted the first show in March 1955 entitled "Man in Space". In December 1955 this was followed by "Man and the Moon". A third show was entiteled "Mars and Beyond" and was broadcast after the Sputnik-shock in December 1957 (7). Disney became focused on space travel through the 1952 articles in Collier´s magazine. He was fascinated by the belief of the scientists, who convinced him of the possibility of manned space travel. Strughold later said that Disney was the one who brought the idea of space travel close to the American people. Strughold also worked several times on the television series. He appeared with Col. Henry M. Sweeney on the 6th series of a 13-part TV documentary series called "Doctors in Space" produced by the Public Broadcasting System (Fig. 24). Strughold also participated in the 1961 documentation, "The Moon", which appeared on National Educational Television (8).

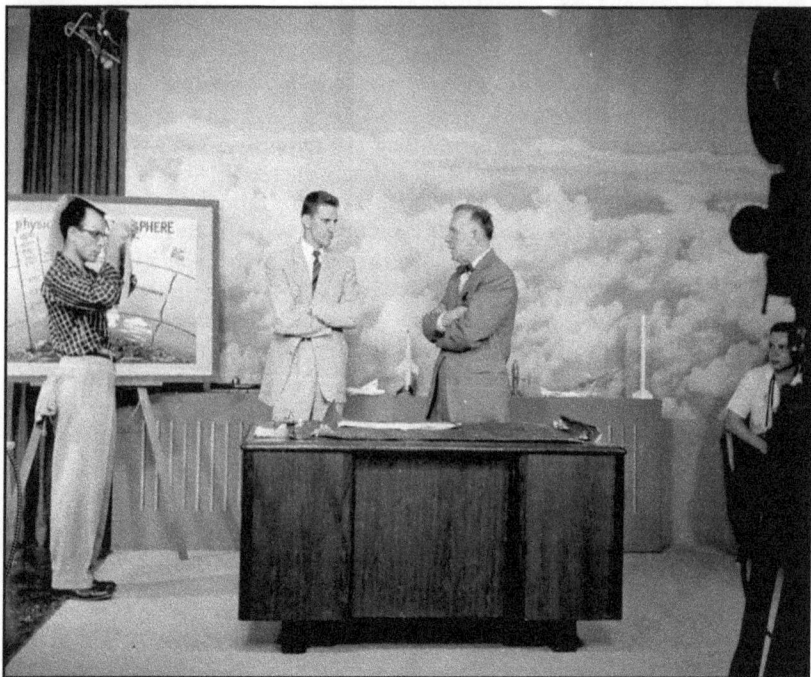

Fig. 24 Strughold at the "Doctor´s in Space" TV show. Photo archive Dr. Harsch, Nbdbg.

Hubertus Strughold was appointed as a Professor of Aerospace Medicine at the "Air University" of the USAF SAM in 1951. In 1958 he was the first one (and so far the only one) appointed as a Professor of Space Medicine (Fig. 25). This fact, as well as his other accomplishments, have led people to give him the title of the "Father of Space Medicine" (9). When Strughold presented his lecture "The Man on the Threshold of Space" in the 1950´s before the Sputnik launch, his audience seemed amused after the first few minutes: "They thought that this was a continuation of the cocktail party held the night before" (10). Strughold had already experienced similar reactions with an audience during his Wuerzburg physiology lecture before the Lindbergh flight in 1927, when people also did not take his vision of routine transatlantic flights as being serious (11).

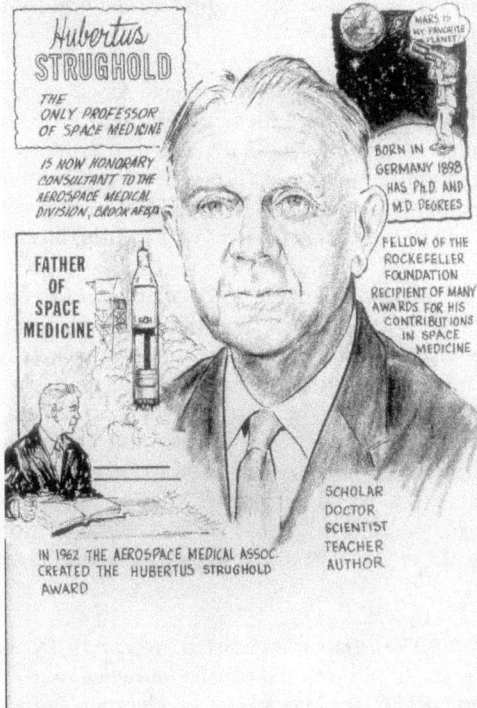

Fig. 25 Sketch of Hubertus Strughold, The Father of Space Medicine.
Photo archive Dr. Harsch, Nbdbg.

In November 1951 a symposium on "Medicine and Physics of the Upper Atmosphere" was held in San Antonio, Texas (12). Strughold was unimpressed by the unspectacular title of this historic event. He suggested a renaming of the event to "The Physical Environment of Airmen at Very High Altitudes" to interest more scientists about the actual progressive character of the symposium (13). The convention was held November 6 - 9, 1951 at the "Air University" at the School of Aviation Medicine (SAM) at Randolph AFB, Texas. Numerous scientists from various disciplines attended with a total of 400 participants. Dr. Wernher von Braun was present, however, he was not among the speakers. Stuhlinger and Ordway (1992) explained that this was because of rivalries between the branches of the US armed forces (Dr. Von Braun was assigned to the Army). The following book "Physics and Medicine of the Upper Atmosphere" (1952) was classified as a "milestone" by Strughold. The Catholic researcher even called it a "bible of scientific space medicine". Dr. Ivy wrote the foreword and contributions were made by W. von Braun, H. Haber, H. Strughold, P. A. Campbell and K. Buettner. Strughold contributed the article "Basic Environmental Problems at the Highest Regions of the Atmosphere as seen by the Biologist" (14).

At the annual meeting of the Aero Medical Association in Washington, D.C. on March 19, 1952, the Space Medicine Branch (SMB) annual meeting was also held. Paul A. Campbell was the chairman, the vice-chairman was Dr. John P. Marbarger, and the secretary of the society was Strughold. He was also the bibliographer and first treasurer of the SMB. Strughold gave on this occasion a speech on the statuts of space-related medical literature (15).

At the time of the installation of the Department of Aerospace Medicine at the USAF SAM, other installations were also getting started to be involved with manned space flight. Preliminary animal experiments in suborbital space flights were performed by the Aeromedical Field Laboratory (AML) at Wright-Patterson AFB in Dayton, Ohio. The German Paperclip Project scientists Otto Gauer, Ulrich Henschke, Henning von Giercke and Erich Gienapp were all assigned to this US Air Force research center. Other important aerospace medical centers were the Naval School of Aviation Medicine at Pensacola, Florida, where Hermann J. Schaefer and Dietrich Beischer worked, as well as at the Naval Medical Center, Bethesda, Maryland, where Theodor Benzinger was employed.

In the early 1950s, laboratory-based research by ballooning and biomedical experiments in aircraft and missile launches were conducted (16). Dr. J. P. Henry, head of the Biophysics Unit Acceleration Branch of the USAF, was involved in the first primate flights beginning on June 18, 1948 in White Sands, New Mexico (17). The main problem in biomedical research was considered to be zero gravity and especially the physiological effects during prolonged duration weightlessness, which actually raised additional questions (18). For brief suborbital flights there were the recent results from aircraft and missile launches. For longer-term orbital or inter-planetary flights the data were so far non-existent. A document of the first animal studies can be found in the archives of USAF SAM, Brooks AFB, Texas. This 10-page working paper dated June 21, 1949 was in German language and titled "Animal Experiments in Rockets" It dealt with the technical requirements of the biomedical missile launches. The Germans researchers H. Strughold, K. Buettner, H. Haber, H. G. Clamann and J. W. Prast were mentioned as staff personnel. The following is an excerpt from the paper (19):

"The force of gravity can be visualized as a ubiquitous environmental factor. It can be analyzed experimentally only with unusual methods, and then established only for a relatively short time. The modern development of aviation and the expected progress in the near future of rocket technology, however, require a detailed study of the physiological effects of a gravity-free condition (g = 0). The preceding considerations teach that missile flights are currently the only way to realize the gravity-free condition for longer periods experimentally. This suggests the idea to conduct animal experiments on the physiological effects of a gravity-free state with rockets. A number of scientists from the SAM, which is interested in conducting such experiments were discussing this with scientists and engineers of the group of Wernher von Braun in El Paso. "

To clarify the effect of weightlessness on the human organism, these short-term in-flight studies were complemented by prolonged underwater immersion tests. No evidence of significant cardio-respiratory adaptation phenomena that would preclude space flight were found with any of these research methods. Also, the effects of weightlessness on sensorimotor functions and the vestibular system were of interest and always a favorite subject of Strughold (20). Gerathewohl, Stallings and Strughold reported at the 27th Annual Meeting of the Aviation Medical Association on April 16, 1956 in Chicago, Illinois concerning the "Sensorimotor Performance During Weightlessness. Eye-Hand Coordination." Parabolic flights in a T-33A jet aircraft of up to 30 seconds duration were performed on seven volunteers to obtain this data. After only six exposures to parabolic flight, adaptation processes could be detected (21). In the research area of the acceleration and deceleration effects on the human organism, John P. Stapp at Holloman AFB, New Mexico conducted research using rapid acceleration/deceleration rocket sleds close to the limits of human performance. Altitude physiological experiments were also performed (22). The sleep-wake rhythm of the space traveler was also of main research interest as well as radiation effects. These issues required additional data from biological experiments using orbital space probes.

Wernher von Braun published his book "The Mars Project" in 1953. Interestingly, Strughold published his book "The Green and Red Planet," in the same year. In this book, the possibility of life on Mars was discussed by him from a physiological perspective (23). He also began in that same year with a "private" Mars experiment using the best known simulated Martian conditions for biological experiments. He bought a thermometer with an appropriately low temperature range, and collected lava stones covered with lichens and mosses from Grant, Arizona in a jar. Overnight, the material was put in an ice-filled vessel and during the daytime at room temperature. After 14 days, the lichens were still alive, but Strughold acknowledged that only one part of the environmental conditions on Mars had been simulated. He discussed these results with the research director of the SAM, Dr. H. M. Sweeney, whereupon Strughold was asked to organize a lab to continue investigations. The results were published in 1958 with two co-authors from the Microbiology Department, R. B. Mitchell and I. A. Koistra. In the following years, Strughold continued to be interested in the question of the possibility of life on Mars.

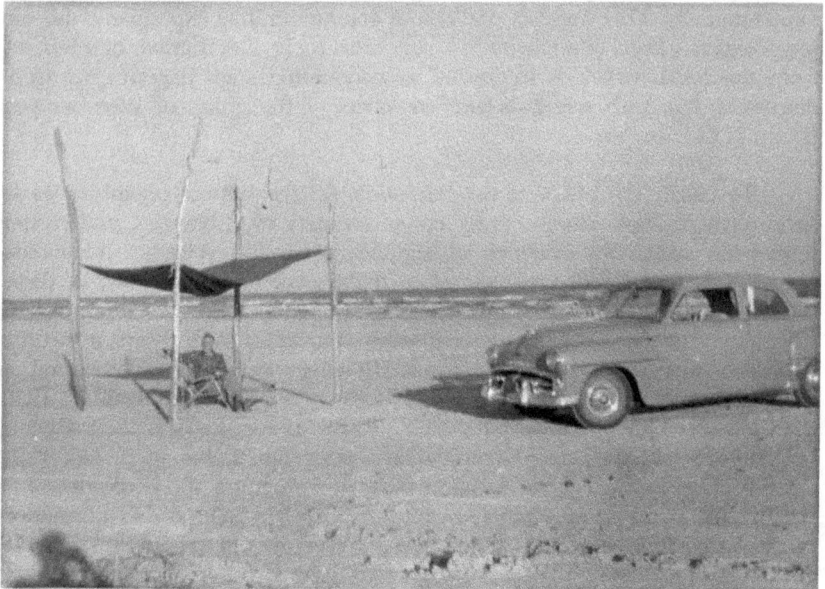

Fig. 26 Strughold at Port Aransas, Texas 1953. Photo archive D. Harsch, Nbdbg.

Strughold kept his international contacts despite the huge demands placed upon him by his research (Fig. 26). He closely watched political developments, especially in Germany. In a letter to the Heidelberg dean, Dr. Hoepke, he expressed his concerns (24):

"We hear and read in the press that everything is fine in western Germany on the whole. Hopefully the splitting of Germany will end soon, before the eastern part is completely Sovietised and Russified."

On July 20, 1956 Strughold became a U.S. citizen. This was followed by a presentation of honorary citizenship by the State of Texas (25). At this point, due to the status of the German scientists, an additional requirement was needed. The German specialists working at the USAF SAM initially had no official status. A regular entry in the United States took place only when they crossed the border with their families into neighboring Mexico and then returned immediately (this occurred in 1949). Five years later they could apply for U.S. citizenship (Fig. 27).

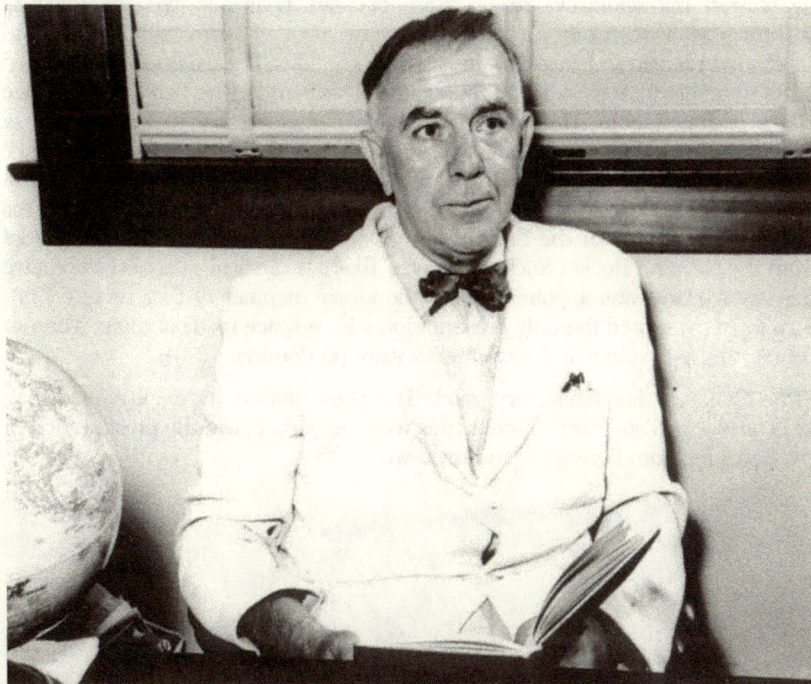

Fig. 27 Strughold at his office. Photo archive Dr. Harsch, Nbdbg.

Out of the more than 30 German scientists and technicians who came to the USAF SAM immediately after WWII only 13 remained by 1953. After a few more years, there were finally only seven that remained: H. Strughold, H. G. Clamann, B. Balke, H. W. Rose, S. J. Gerathewohl, H. B. Gerstner, and O. L. Ritter. Some of the German specialists left the lower-paid civil service job in order to take higher income jobs in the private sector or other institutions of the United States. Only a few went back to Germany (26). The loss of the scientists who had initially contributed to the build up of the USAF SAM was painful (27). An equivalent replacement in the United States was hard to find. In general, they already held higher income jobs and didn´t give up their present positions of responsibility and research projects for a lower income job with the USAF. Because of this, the USAF in 1953 planned a visit for Strughold and Clamann to travel to Europe to "interview" German specialists and to recruit them to work in the US. Clamann was also joined by Col. H. M.

Sweeney on this trip in November 1953. They were able to convince four specialists to come to the US for a job. A trip to Europe for Strughold is documented in 1954 (28). He arrived on August 1, 1954 in Wuerzburg, where he started his scientific career three decades before at the Physiological Institute as a research assistant. Here he met up with old friends and continued his trip to Innsbruck in Austria (Fig. 28). The "Main-Post" reported in its issue dated August 12, 1954 about his visit under the heading of "Space Flight within Reach". He stated that space flights are not just a product of imagination as they are already at work on the details to accomplish this. Strughold attended the fifth annual meeting of the International Astronautical Federation (IAF). On August 8, 1954 in Innsbruck he was honored for his outstanding service in the field of space exploration with the Oberth Medal from the German Rocket Society (he was the first medical specialist to receive this award) and was appointed as an honorary member of that society (29). Strughold presented the only presentation with a space medical topic. Themes concerning astronomy and astrophysics were predominant (30):

"The Congress has been very good. The presentations were of a very high level, and scientists from ten countries were present. I gave the presentation of Dr. Schaefer from Pensacola and my own."

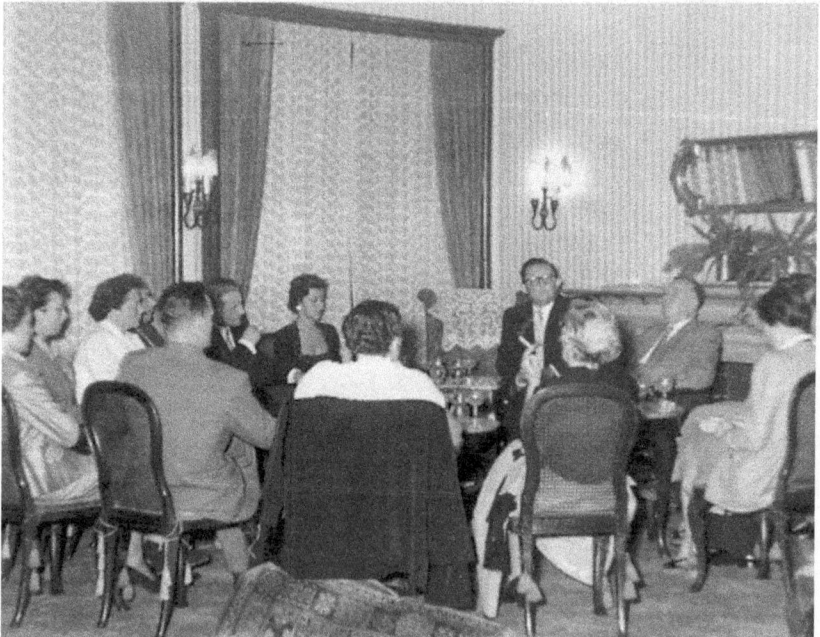

Fig. 28 Strughold with friends in Germany in 1954. Photo archive Dr. Harsch, Nbdbg.

Strughold concluded his trip by a visit to relatives in Westphalia. He maintained contact with colleagues and friends all over the world. His family he supported at all times and especially in times of economic hardship (31).

In 1956 Strughold had already spoken extensively about manned space flight (32). The course of development of manned space flight, he outlined after the Sputnik launch (1957) would take the following four steps (33): 1. Space equivalents (suborbital) flights; 2. Satellite flights; 3. Moon ventures and 4. Interplanetary enterprises. In 1958 he presented the status of space-related medical research in the article, ´Man in Space: Aerospace Medical Research as a Pioneer´:

"The problems of space flight in the last nine years were the subject of theoretical and experimental investigations in this new area of medicine that is a logical extension of aviation medicine. Space medicine is involved in all of the medical research aspects covered during the flight beyond the atmosphere, the so-called astronautics. It is a sector of 'Bioastronautics', that is researching the possibilities of life in the universe, how they will even meet people from our planet in the future perhaps. The task of space medicine is to secure the livelihood of people in space and help them in the exploration of space and other celestial bodies, and how to retain their performance capability and not suffer impairment in their well-being."

His scientific achievements were widely recognized, but in the late 1950´s there were also critical voices concerning his career in Germany. In 1958 he was claimed by a magazine in the U.S. of having abused detainees for his research. This assumption was rejected as untenable by a study by the Justice Department (34). Nevertheless Strughold was exposed recurrently to similar charges thereafter.

Hubertus Strughold sponsored an astrobiological meeting at the Lowell Observatory in Flagstaff, Arizona. It was chaired by Albert Wilson and held on June 15, 1957 during the "International Geophysical Year". Wilson introduced Strughold with these words:

"For doctors, pilots and rocket specialists, Dr. Strughold needs no intro-duction, but today he is a visiting astronomer"(35).

In the summer of 1957 Strughold traveled once again to Europe. With him on board the "SS United States," was the famous American film director, Walt Disney, who stated to Strughold:

"Throughout my life, I have been a witness to numerous changes and discoveries, so that if somebody would say to me that I would be a witness to a manned space flight to the moon over the next five to ten years, I would believe this."(36).

Two weeks later, the USSR launched its first satellite, "Sputnik". Strughold began his visit to Europe in the Sauerland region in Hespecke at the home of the folklore writer Anna Kaiser (1885-1962). Strughold's sister, Mathilda, worked at this place as a housekeeper and secretary (37). Strughold called this place his "Tusculum" (quiet country estate) (Fig. 29). During this visit he also met his brother, Joseph, who lived in the vicinity. Thereafter, he visited General Armstrong in Wiesbaden, followed by visits to friends in Wuerzburg and Heidelberg. In early October he traveled to Spain, where he attended the 8th International Congress of the International Astronautical Federation on October 6 - 12, 1957 in Barcelona (38):

"It was the most dramatic meeting that I had ever attended. Celebrations on the one side, anger on the other, they stood in solidified blocks. I chaired a working group, which discussed the medical problems of space flight. David G. Simons spoke about his experience in the stratospheric 'Man High' balloon flights, which had taken him that same year to over 100,000 ft. altitude. At this meeting there were more than 500 delegates from 25 nations present and altitude and space research was discussed."

Strughold then attended an astronautical congress in Rome, where he gave an astrobiological lecture, "The Life Zone or Ecosphere in our Solar Planetary System." That was followed by a meeting in Germany where Strughold met with David G. Simons at a press conference in Wiesbaden. Besides the formally invited six reporters, there were many media representatives from around the world due to the large public interest that had developed concerning space flight. A Soviet reporter asked if all of the medical problems had been resolved for manned space flight. Strughold terse reply was:

"Not one!" (39).

However, in a later interview in 1957, he stated that the tremendous space medical challenges are not impregnable. In the German newspaper "Essener Tageblatt" he was cited (40):

"Based on our research results, I would say that this problem is solved in medical terms. The difference between ascent to high altitude in a balloon and a rocket is only acceleration."

71

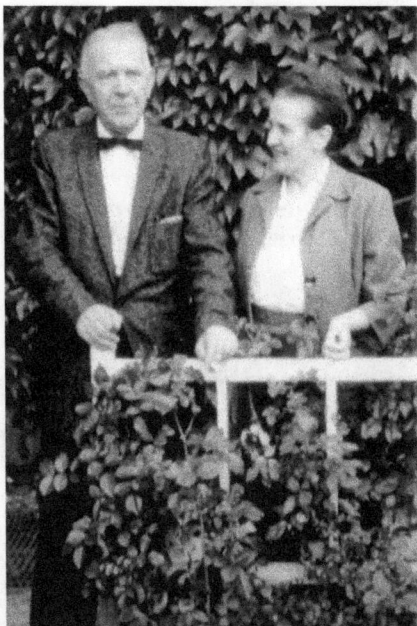

Fig. 29 Strughold and his sister Mathilda in Germany. Photo archive Dr. Harsch, Nbdbg.

Strughold returned to America via Frankfurt and Paris not by plane but onboard the" HMS Queen Elizabeth" (41). He noticed the effects of desynchronization on the passengers biorhythms, and outlined his findings in a field report in November 1957 in San Antonio, Texas (42).

Another milestone in the basic biomedical research carried out at SAM was the study of prolonged isolation. The project began in 1952 with the idea from Strughold that a kind of "space capsule" should be tested in the laboratory (he termed it the "sealed cabin simulator"). The plans were based on the work of K. Buettner from a paper, "Bioclimatology of the Manned Rocket." F. Haber completed the construction plans in December 1952. In the summer of 1954 the cabin was delivered completed to SAM. H. G. Clamann equipped and tested it at the Department of Physiology and Biochemistry together with his assistant, R. W. Bancroft. The investigation began in 1956 with a one-day test run with airman D. F. Smith. Two doctors monitored pulse, respiration, temperature, humidity and CO_2 (43). Then a pilot, Donald G. Farrell, performed a prolonged isolation test on February 10-16, 1958. The United States appeared to be disadvantaged and falling behind in the space race after the launch of Sputnik. These series of space simulation experiments was a huge media success. For seven days the successful progress of the simulated "trip to the Moon" were widely circulated in the press reports (44). Upon termination of the experiment in the "Space Cabin Simulator", Farrell was welcomed "back to Earth" by the Republican Majority Leader (and later President) Lyndon B. Johnson on February 16, 1958 who expressed the gratitude of the nation (Fig. 30 a and b) (45). It was not clear from the beginning whether the first attempts at space flight should be carried out using a man. It was widely felt that the reliability of the entire system should be checked out first on animals (dogs), which Strughold ironically judged in his characteristic way:

"I doubt that Lyndon Johnson would have wanted to shake a dog's hand" on return from moon (46)."

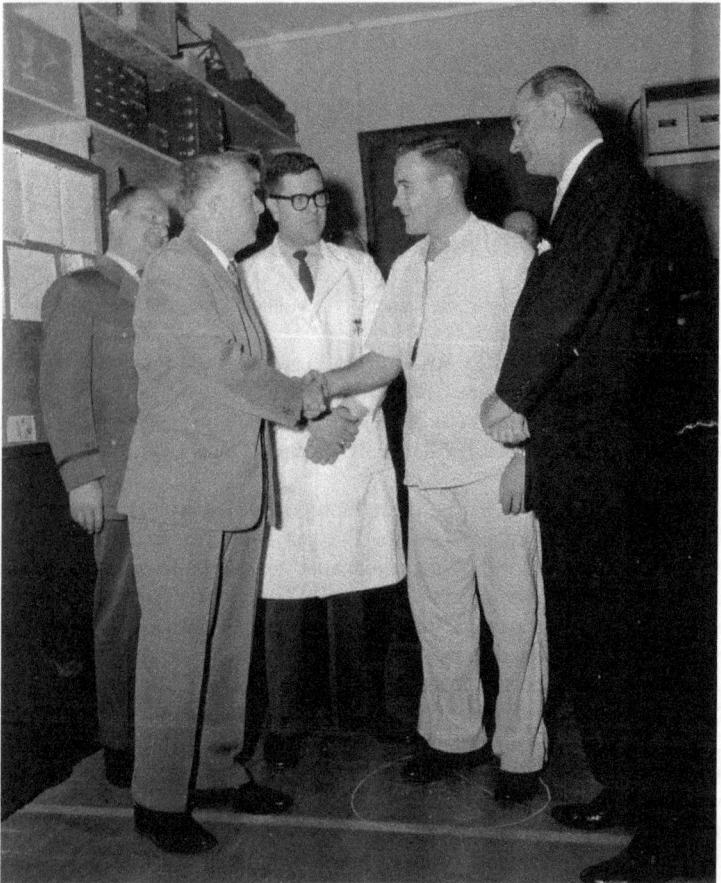

Fig. 30 a Lyndon B. Johnson welcomes Airman Donald Farrell back "home".
Photo archive Dr. Harsch, Nbdbg.

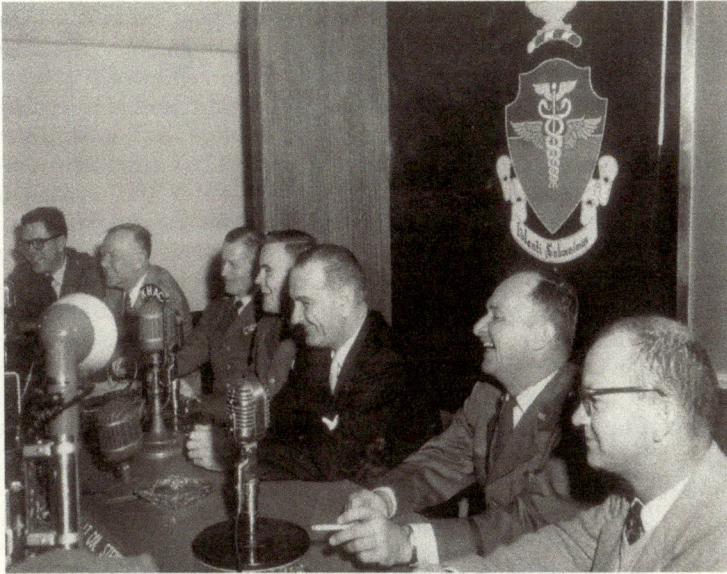

Fig. 30 b Press Coneference at SAM, Brooks AFB in 1958
        Photo archive Dr. Harsch, Nbdbg.

The subsequent press conference was very successful for the SAM staff. Lyndon B. Johnson, who as a vehement and influential proponent of the idea of space flight expressed this explicitly:

"If we fail to master the space race first, then we will be in all respects only a second-best country" (47).

Strughold, Benson and Farrell were invited for lunch by L. B. Johnson to the U.S. Senate on February 23, 1958 by Johnson to the U.S. Senate. Here Strughold outlined in front of more than 100 people the state of space-related medical research (48). The closed system of the Space Cabin Simulator provided a miniature prototype of a future space craft cabin (Fig. 31). The capability for maintaining the temperature and humidity was available along with a device for the recovery of drinking water from body fluids. With this closed ecological system it was possible to investigate metabolic and respiratory parameters. Attempts were made to examine the aspects of biorhythms, day/night cycles for space missions and the effects on organisms in a cycle range from 18 to 28 hours were examined. Great importance was placed on studying the psychology of the long duration isolation. The chamber pressure could be varied and investigated with changes in the atmospheric composition. Strughold and H. Haber named the experimental arrangement an "Astronautilus", a prototype of a "living room in an artificial satellite" (49).

On May 5, 1958 Strughold made a presentation before the "House Select Committee on Astronautics and Space Exploration" in Washington, D. C. He suggested that aerospace medicine should be represented in research and education at all universities. In addition the scientists should be enabled to visit domestic and foreign institutions. These ideas had a biographical background and represented his expirience from the 1920´s and 1930´s in the field of aviation medicine. Strughold further suggested the creation of a translation and distribution center for foreign literature. He also called for the introduction of the metric system in the United States. He felt that the rapid advancement of the USSR in the field of rocketry had become possible only because the German rocket construction plans were metric and could be used immediately without any time consuming and expensive conversional work. He also urged a limitation of the administrative burden on researchers which he considered as indispensable. Strughold also noted that in the scientific fields in the United States there were too many committees involved, so that it often happened that totally incompetent people were urged to give their consent (50).

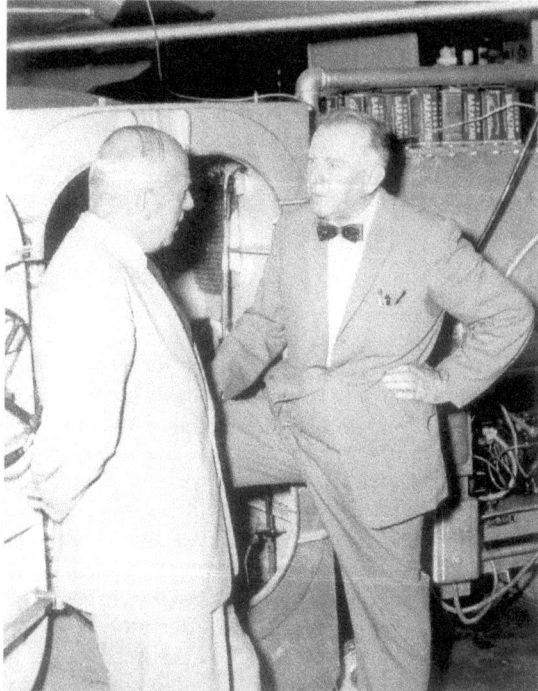

Fig. 31 Strughold and Dornberger at the Space Cabin Simulator at School of Aerospace Medicine. Photo archive Dr. Harsch, Nbdbg.

In 1958 Strughold attended the second symposium on Bioastronautics. He was the chairman of the meeting which lasted from November 10-12, 1958. Some 800 participants met in San Antonio, Texas (51). Van Allen presented the discovery of the radiation belt of the Earth, which eventually was named after him. Krafft Ehricke discussed the possibility of a manned Moon landing, to be used as training for future interplanetary travel and Strughold talked about astrobiology. Wernher von Braun was one of the speakers as well. Lyndon B. Johnson noted (52):

"Now we have reached a new front - the 'vertical front' as you choose to call it - the space frontier for the layman. The scientists assembled here are the pioneers of this new front. They lead their nation, and humanity, to approach this new front, which is so vast that it can never be settled completely and does not seem static or fixed. The 'Space Frontier' is above all a relentless front."

The year 1958 brought Strughold several awards. Among others, he was honored for his pioneering research with the "USAF Distinguished Civilian Service Medal in Gold" at the Jet Age Conference in Washington, D.C., the highest honor the Air Force presents to a civilian (53). In an article in the "New York Times" on March 20, 1958 it was abundantly stated (54):

"While the struggle continues for research funds, working men like Professor Strughold quietly work for the future of humanity. (...) Was not King Ferdinand and Queen Isabel of Spain warned against giving Columbus so much money? "

In the ending decade at the USAF SAM a further challenge was emerging, helping select the first astronauts from the ranks of U.S. test pilots for the U.S. space program. At the end of January 1959, the selection of the prospective Mercury Program astronauts was announced. However, the first medical examinations were carried out under the direction of the Lovelace Clinic in Albuquerque, New Mexico, as NASA wanted a civilian entity to be involved to maintain a non-military aspect to the now civilian space program. Dr. Charles A. Berry, who had been at SAM since 1956, was promoted in 1958 as the head of the Department of Aviation Medicine. During this time he was involved in the selection of the first seven astronauts. He later transferred to NASA as the head of medical operations" (55).

The 10th anniversary of the creation of the Department of Space Medicine at USAF SAM was celebrated on February 9, 1959. This occasion was used to review the past achievements of space medicine over the last decade which was now on the threshold of manned space flight as well as to discuss the outlook for future progress. The meeting attracted 400 participants. Gen. Armstrong was present in the audience, as well as the German founding members, Strughold, H. Haber and Buettner. President Eisenhower sent the following congratulatory telegram to the school commander:

"The scientific leadership of this department continues the tradition of outstanding medical research. The benefit of this research will accelerate the time for the onset of humans in space" (56).

The speakers at this scientific meeting philosophized about the development of future opportunities in the next decade, which would lead to the first humans to land on the moon (57). In the first year of the founding of the Department of Space Medicine, the estimated time for the development of space medicine research and for the beginnings of manned space travel was too conservative and was quickly overtaken by the rapid developments of the U.S. and Soviet space programs. According to Strughold in 1959, the dreams of the past were already now a reality (58). Strughold's department had very modest financial means in its beginning in 1949, but now, a decade later, was able to operate under far more favorable conditions (59).

Chapter 8. School of Aviation Medicine (1961 - 1968)

In April 1958, the Surgeon General of the USAF created an "Ad Hoc Committee" on space medical research. Strughold and others met on April 16, 1958 to develop a 10-year plan for research projects (1). In 1959 the newly created USAF "Aerospace Medical Center" (AMC) of the "Air Training Command" (ATC) moved to the south of San Antonio and relocated at Brooks AFB. Strughold was installed as the chair of the "Advanced Studies Group" of the AMC in 1960. In 1961 the school was renamed, the "School of Aerospace Medicine" (2). The research work at the AMC included the following areas: issues concerning the capabilities of perception in flight, medical flight safety, preventive and clinical aviation medicine, aviation medical aspects of radiation, aerospace physiology, biomedical aspects of microwave radiation, and astrobiology. Since 1960, SAM conducted an annual instruction course, "Lectures in Aerospace Medicine". This week-long event was held to provide medical officers of the United States and its allied forces, as well as civilian scientists from universities and industry, with the latest information concerning scientific progress in the field of aerospace medicine (Fig. 32) (3).

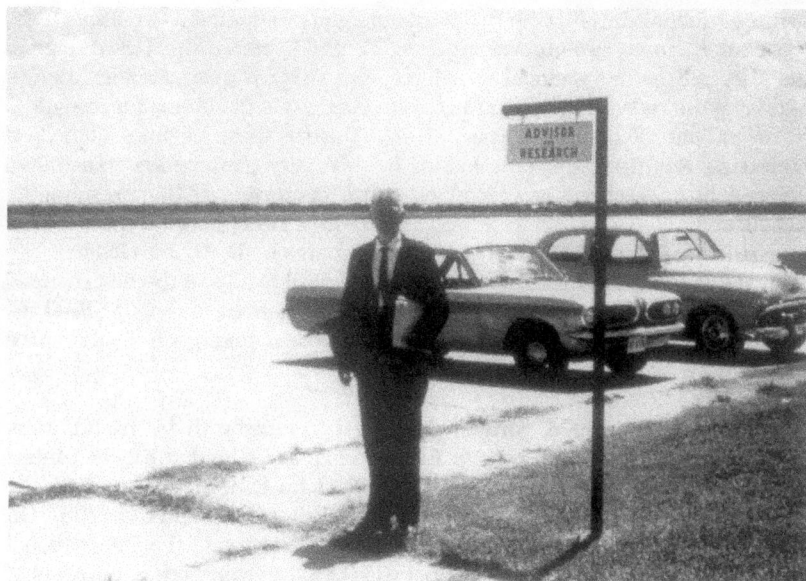

Fig. 32 Strughold's parking place (Medical Advisor; his car in the back).
Photo archive Dr. Harsch, Nbdbg.

On November 1, 1961 the USAF Aerospace Medical Division (AMD) of the Air Force Systems Command (AFSC) was established with an expansion of its roles and responsibilities. The first commander was Theodore C. Bedwell (8). The AMD had a threefold mission: teaching and clinical work in the aeromedical field, coordinating aerospace medical research and development in the U.S., and finally, to support the national space program being rapidly developed by NASA (9). Strughold was installed in February 1962 as the chief scientist (Advisor for Research) and was appointed Chairman of the Advanced Studies Group of the AMD at Brooks AFB, Texas. Even after his retirement, he remained as a consultant to this institution and continued to be in close association with it (10).

His responsibilities included: advising the school commander, representing the school and commander at relevant conferences, evaluating and suggesting research projects in the field of space medicine and astrobiology, and reviewing selected works (11).

During a committee discussion at the Nevada State Medical Association in early 1961, Strughold predicted that the Soviet Union would soon attempt a manned spaceflight (12). The first orbital flight was accomplished by the Soviet cosmonaut Yuri Gagarin in April 1961. The U.S. astronaut, Alan B. Shepard, followed this with a 15-minute suborbital flight in May 1961. President Kennedy announced on May 25, 1961, before the U.S. Congress that the goal of the national space program was a Lunar landing, thereby launching the race to the moon (13). John Glenn was the first US astronaut to fly an orbital flight in February 1962. During these flights, biomedical monitoring was used and downloaded by telemetry. Parameters transmitted included body temperature, blood pressure, heart rate (ECG), respiration, speech characteristics, brain waves (EEG) and heart sounds. At the 12th International Astronautical Congress in Washington, D. C. on October 1-7, 1961, the focus of the meeting were the biomedical results of the first manned space flights. Two members of the Academy of Sciences of the USSR, O. G. Gazenko and V. G. Yazdovsky, presented the recent findings from the space flight of German Titov (14).

In September 1963, Strughold traveled together with his friend, Mary Webb Dalehite, from New York to Europe (11). He attended the 14th International Astronautical Congress in Paris (12). John Paul Stapp, met with the couple at the Hotel Astor in Paris for breakfast on September 25. On September 26, Strughold attended the scientific meeting of the International Academy of Astronautics. There he met with H. Oberth and other members of the society. The theme of this congress was to look back on the space travel activities of the past two years and to discuss future developmental opportunities (13). Strughold then traveled by train to Rome, where he attended the 6th International Congress of Aviation and Space Medicine from

October 1-5, 1963 (14). Strughold was received with other scientists by Pope Paul VI. for a papal audience (15). Strughold had been invited by the chairman of the "German Society for Aviation and Space Medicine" (DGLRM), Heinz von Diringshofen, to attend their first meeting in Germany. Von Diringshofen stated, that the newly founded society already had 100 members, but out of them were 55 high school teachers (16). At this first meeting of the DGLRM from October 8-9, 1963 at the Physiological Institute in Munich, Strughold was awarded an honorary membership for his "far superior merit in the field of aviation and space medicine". Bedwell congratulated Strughold for this honour, stating "Your pioneering leadership has affected the scientific work on both sides of the Atlantic" (17). The conference was attended by more than 200 participants, among them H. J. von Beckh, Col. J. P. Stapp, P. A. Campbell and S. J. Gerathewohl (18). Strughold then visited the German Air Force Institute of Aviation Medicine (FlMedInstLw) in Fuerstenfeldbruck (Fig. 33), that was headed by Col. E. A. Lauschner (19).

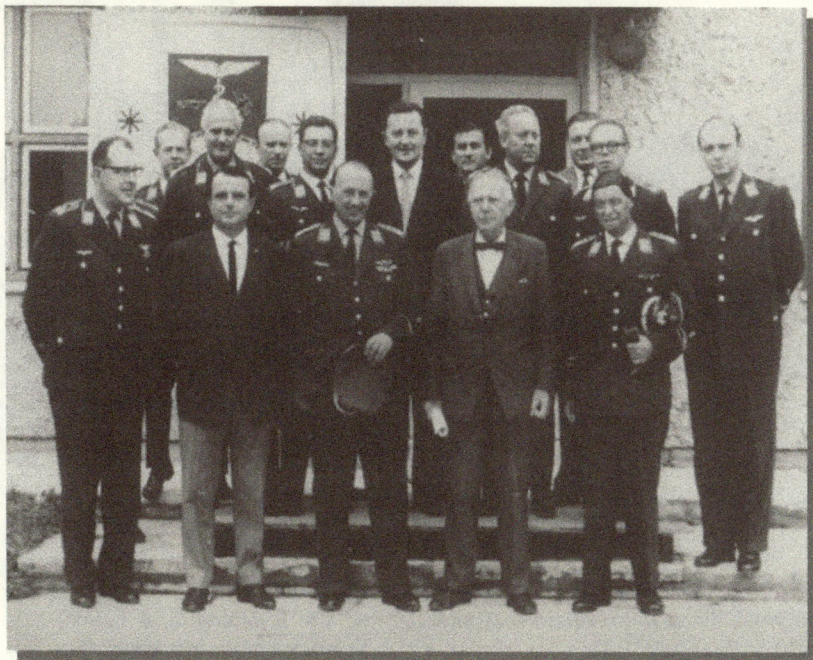

Fig. 33 Strughold in front of the clinical building of the German Air Force Institute for Aviation Medicine in Fuerstenfeldbruck (close to Munich) in 1963: Ebeling, von Beckh, Kohler, Strughold, Lauschner (first line). Photo Archive Dr. Harsch, Nbdbg.

The U.S. President, John F. Kennedy, visited Brooks AFB on November 21, 1963 for an inauguration ceremony of a new complex of buildings of the AMD. Kennedy made one of his last official speeches here (the next day he was assassinated in Dallas, Texas). In this speech, Kennedy paid tribute to the contribution of the scientists for the development of aerospace medicine (Fig. 34 and Doc. 7) (20). He was briefed on the status of the Apollo project and devoted his attention to the ongoing trial of the Space Cabin Simulator, where four subjects had simulated a long duration "space flight" (21).

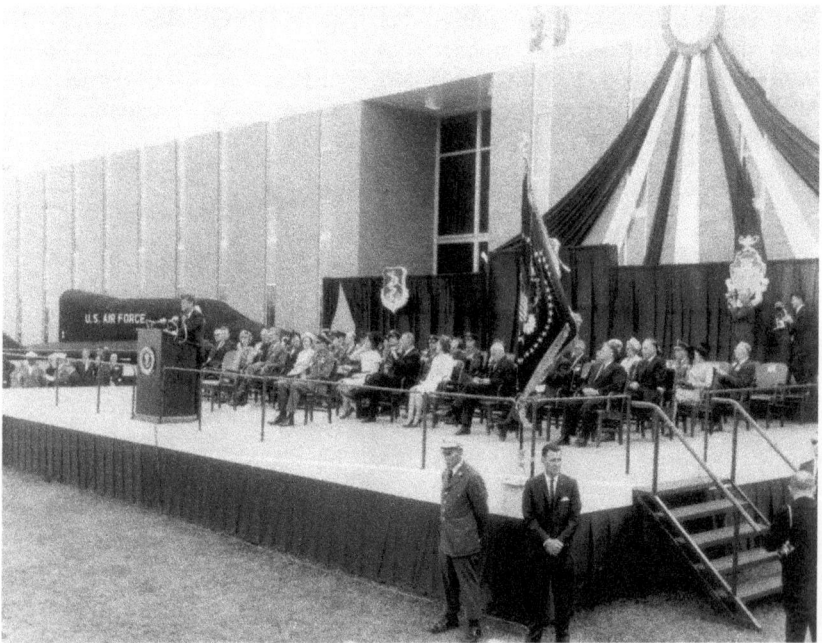

Fig. 34 Inauguration ceremony with President Kennedy in 1963 at Brooks AFB; Strughold at the back right. Photo archive Dr. Harsch, Nbdbg.

The following year, the third bioastronautics Symposium (3rd International Symposium on Bioastronautics and the Exploration of Space) was held at the USAF SAM (22). Wernher von Braun wrote to Strughold (Fig. 35) (23): "Although I could not participate at the symposium, I was extremely pleased to receive the congress-book and to survey the surprisingly large variety of presentations. They reflect a tremendous growth rate and lead to satisfaction, if you compare it with our humble beginning in 1951."

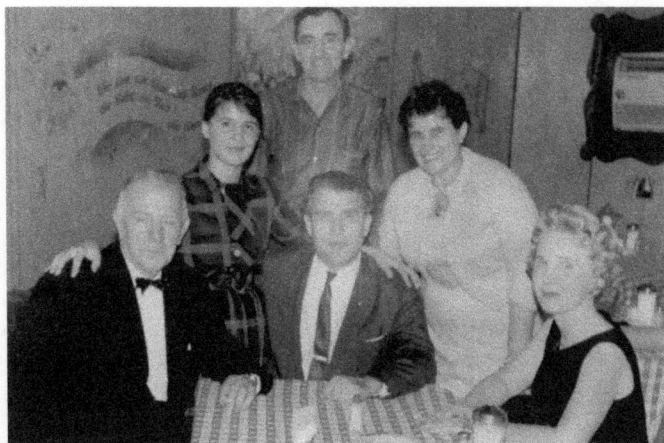

Fig. 35 Hubertus Strughold with Wernher von Braun in 1961, Mary Webb Dalehite on the right. Photo archive Dr. Harsch, Nbdbg.

At the end of August in 1965, Strughold was present as an observer for the "Gemini T-5 flight" at the NASA Manned Spacecraft Center in Houston, Texas. Here he met with Dr. Charles A. Berry and was briefed on the astronauts' medical status (24) (Fig. 36). Strughold was convinced that after this flight time of eight-days, that people could be expected to survive a two-week space flight and still stay physiologically intact. Dr. Berry wrote the following letter of thanks to Strughold 1966 (25):

"Dear Strugi: I have so many things for which to thank you for that I do not know where to begin. First, and most of all, I would like to express my gratitude for your pioneering efforts to provide a basis for the things that we could achieve with our current program. This success was only possible through the visionary work by scientists, as you are, which began many years ago, when it was not foreseeable where the path would lead. Your personal support and advice to me were always a constant source of guidance and will power."

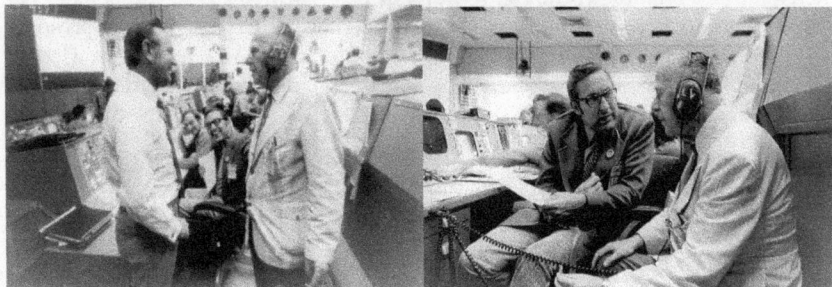

Fig. 36 a and **b** Strughold at NASA's Mission Control. Photo archive Dr. Harsch, Nbdbg.

From the results of the "Bio-Instrumentation" monitoring and telemetry, Strughold expected a benefit for Earth medicine:

"And it's not too utopian, that it will soon be possible, that a physician can send an ECG over a satellite link to a specialist for diagnostic evaluation and discussion," said Strughold in 1961. Because space research was so expensive, any question of immediate profit was prevented from the outset. Strughold reflected that not all research approaches would directly be useful for Earth medicine. Space medicine was similar to aviation medicine, however, in that it could lead to results in the future in other more practical medical areas (26).

The Nobel prize winner, Max Born, however, was more critical. He stated that space travel was a big triumph of the mind, but it was a tragic failure of good sense (27).

In the last year of USAF service, Strughold still took part in numerous conferences. At the World's Fair in June 24-27, 1968 (HemisFair) in San Antonio, Texas, the "Father of Space Medicine", Dr. Strughold, welcomed the "Father of the German Economic Miracle", Dr. Ludwig Erhard. Strughold participated as co-chair at the "Fourth International Symposium on Bioastronautics and the Exploration of Space" on June 24-27, 1968 at Brooks AFB, Texas. The event was titled "Beneath the Sea, Across the Ocean, Around the World, Now to the Moon, And next to the Planets." It also was the 50th anniversary of the USAF SAM and the 20-year anniversary of the Department of Space Medicine. Strughold lectured on aspects of the planet Mars in a presentation, "Planetary Environmental Medicine". His final discussion about the future of space exploration was recorded by ABC-TV (28). In September at the same location, the "Third Symposium on Modern Concepts in Civil Aviation Medicine" of the Civil Aviation Medical Association (CAMA) also took place (29).

On September 30, 1968, Strughold retired at the age of 70 years and after more than 20 years of service for the USAF. He remained a consultant (Honorary Consultant) working for the AMD with his own office in the headquarters building (30). His retirement ceremony was held on October 5, 1968, where many presentatives from academia and industry were present (31). Strughold's successor as chief scientist of the AMD was Hans Georg Clamann. Twenty-five years earlier he was Strughold's deputy at the AMRI in Berlin (32).

Chapter 9. Retirement (1969-1986)

In 1961, Strughold was visited by the son of his childhood friend from Germany. Guenter Oberdorf was from Westphalian Rhynern and remembered his meeting with his "Godfather" in San Antonio, Texas (1):

"It was a nice time. Professor Strughold showed me the Institute and the Space Cabin Simulator. On the large parking lok in front of the AMC Strughold amused himself by steering his 'Chevi' with both feet. His briefcase was placed on the gas pedal serving as a cruise control. On the public street however, he drove his automatic car in an over-cautious manner. He was known throughout the city for his slow driving. A traffic cop yelled to him in jest: 'Get out of this intersection, Prof!´ At the hotel Menger we then had good food to eat. Strughold then allowed himself an extra helping of his favorite pudding. His home I did not see, however – he said, there was nothing to see, just stacks of books and cats."

More personal impressions conveyed the newspaper "Welt"-journalist, Baerwolf, in his 1995 book, ´The Martian Factory´ (2):

"I met Strughold in the early sixties for an interview at the Menger Hotel at the old Spanish town of San Antonio where he lived permanently. A parrot squawked constantly in the venerable hall 'Strugi, Strugi' whenever the old man with the white mustache passed. While drinking a "Dortmunder" beer in the subtropical garden of the Menger hotel, and it had to be a Dortmunder beer, because he came from Westphalia, he talked to me about the planet Mars, which fascinated him so. And he was deeply convinced, that the flight of people to the planet Mars would be the greatest achievement and biotechnological development of mankind."

The US-officer Schriever met Strughold in 1958 when both worked together on a production of a television documentary about space and remembered:

"Strughold smokes a pipe and speaks slowly, but he is very receptive. … He was an eternal optimist. He never saw the impossible."

Strughold's office was simply decorated, but had an eye-catcher: an old Indian headdress. Other accessories pointed to his fondness for Egyptian, Greek and Roman Art. He presented Roman coins with joy to his friends. He worked often while having good food, preferably in a Viennese coffeehouse, where the atmosphere inspired him (3).

His hobbies included "numismatics", collecting coins, as well as "semantics", the return of the words on its origin. In this way Strughold was able to read, understand, and speak many languages (but not fluently). In a letter to the family of the Austrian acceleration physiologist, von Beckh, who lived in Alamogordo, New Mexico, Strughold shared his joy over the sponsorship of their first child:

"I assume that you have given her a name that fits excellently into the Space Age" (4).

Another story illustrates Strughold's ties to the living world: During an interview, he was asked if he wanted to accompany the journalist for some fishing. Strughold replied ironically: "No thanks", as he preferred to study them, "Fish are my friends!" His home in Schertz, significantly, housed countless cats. Glasgow (1970) describes an incident when Strughold dined with friends at the Dinner Club. One of the guests watched as he took ice from a drink and slid it seemingly at random under the sofa. As the process repeated a short time later, however, the stunned visitor asked him for the reason for his behaviour. Strughold said in all seriousness, that he was watching a mouse, which obviously lived underneath the sofa. Although it could live off the crumbs of fallen down food, it would not be able to find water in this environment. In this situation he was now providing the necessities for survival of the mouse.

Strughold continued working scientifically after retirement. He kept his office at the USAF SAM and later he moved into a study in the library (5).

Strughold attended the manned Lunar landing on July 20, 1969 as a guest at the NASA control center. These first steps of man on another celestial body was the fulfillment of a lifetime dream of the scientist (6). Former U.S. President Lyndon B. Johnson, who witnessed the Apollo 11 launch at Cape Canaveral, Florida, was notified by Strughold after the successful completion of the mission with the following letter of congratulations (7):

"My dear President. On the occasion of the hugely successful conclusion of the Apollo 11 flight, I would take the liberty to congratulate you. Without your support before and during your White-House-era this outstanding achievement in human history would not have been possible. I remember your presence in the final stages of the eight-day experiment of the space cabin simulator with airman Farrell at Randolph, which gave us a tremendous boost at a time when aerospace-medicine was commonly regarded as illusory. I had the honor of being in the 'Mission Control' center in Houston during the flight to the moon and watch daily the recorded heart beats and breathing activity of the astronauts. This represented the summit of my professional life. Again congratulations and thank you for your early support of our space-related medical research. Dr. med. et phil. Hubertus Strughold"

L.B. Johnson replied on August 30th 1968:

"Dear Dr. Strughold: Yours are the skilled hands of the physician, the keen brain of the scientist, the loyality of a trusted public servant and the warm heart of a friend. Your thoughtfoulness – remembering my birthday – adds to my growing admiration. You have my best wishes. Sincerely, L.B.J."

Strughold congratulated also the first man on the moon in another letter (8):

"My dear astronaut Neil Armstrong: A space-famous prophet once said: 'The Earth is the cradle of the mind, but you cannot stay in the cradle forever.´ Today, the human mind is on the moon: Thanks for your first steps on its surface. I bring my congratulations in deep admiration."

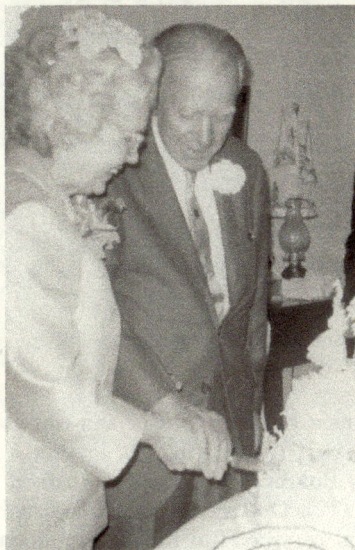

Fig. 37 Strughold and Mary Webb Dalehite.
Photo archive Dr. Harsch, Nbdbg.

On March 6, 1971, Hubertus Strughold married his longtime girlfriend, Mary Webb Dalehite (Fig. 37). The two had first met at the birthday celebration of their common good friend, Tamara Boubel, on June 26, 1959. Ms. Dalehite was in charge of public relations at Kelly AFB, Texas as a "civilian information officer" (9). Strughold lived in the 1960s at the Menger Hotel. The couple moved thereafter to 202 East Mayfield in San Antonio, Texas (9).

Even in retirement Strughold continued to write reports, attend meetings and to give countless interviews. In 1971 he published his 82 page book, "Your Body Clock," which he dedicated to his wife Mary. In 1975 the article, "Biological and Physiological Rhythms", by Strughold and H. B. Hale appeared in the "Foundations of Space Biology and Medicine", in which U.S. and Soviet scientists expounded upon the state of their field of knowledge (10).

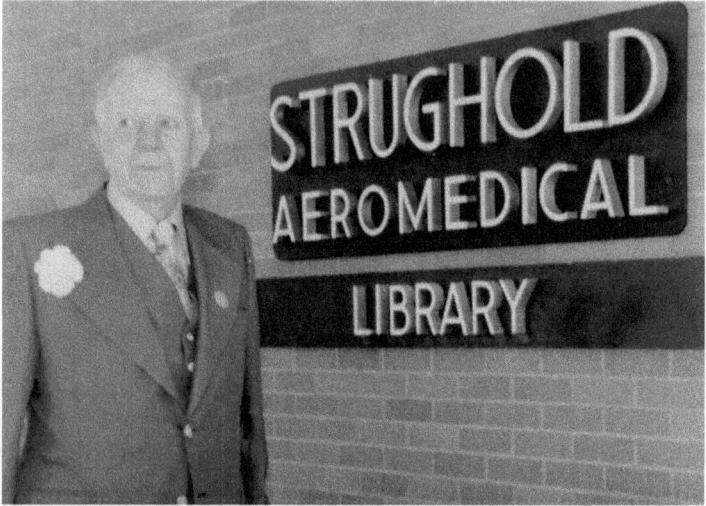

Fig. 38 Strughold at the USAF Aeromedical Library at Brooks AFB.
Photo archive Dr. Harsch, Nbdbg.

Hubertus Strughold was a visionary thinker and was able to experience many of his predictions coming true during his lifetime (11). The USAF "Aeromedical Library" at the Brooks AFB, Texas was named in his honor on January 19, 1977 (Fig. 39) (12). On October 6, 1978 Strughold's name was inducted in the third annual ceremony in the "International Space Hall of Fame" at Alamogordo, New Mexico. He was the 43rd person so honored. He said that it was the greatest honor of his life (13). He stated in his acceptance speech (14):

"Now the International Space Hall of Fame in Alamogordo is my galactic home on earth."

Continued close ties to Germany characterized the U.S. citizen, Strughold, during his retirement. At the annual scientific meeting of the German Society for Aviation and Space Medicine (DGLRM) on November 6, 1974 in Fuerstenfeldbruck, the creation of a "Hubertus Strughold Prize" was proposed by the society's president, surgeon general Prof. Dr. Heinz S. Fuchs (Fig. 39) (15).

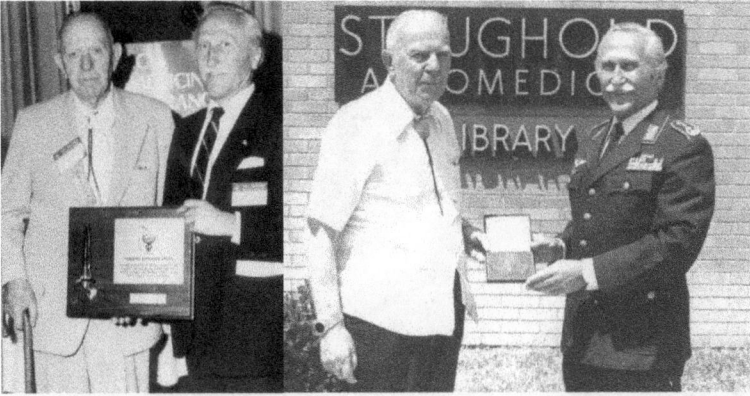

Fig. 39 a and b Strughold and the President of the Space Medicine Branch of the Aerospace
Medical Association, General H. S. Fuchs, with the Strughold Award in 1978.
On the right: General Fuchs presenting Strughold the DGLRM-medal honoring
the "Father of Space Medicine" in the mid 70′s. Photo archive Dr. Harsch, Nbdbg.

The mayor of the Westphalian city of Hamm and a parliament-member
of the *Bundestag*, Dr. Rinsche, sent Strughold a letter dated May 26, 1971
with warm greetings on the occasion of the annexation of Strughold's village of
birth, Westtuennen, into the community of Hamm:

"In your old home town, we are proud of the high regard with which you have
obtained in America. I would like to congratulate you and express my appreciation."(16).

For his 85th Birthday in 1983 Strughold was awarded the Grand Cross
of Merit of the Federal Republic of Germany. The Consul General, Joachim R.
Vogel, presented the award by saying that Strughold received this not only for
his scientific achievements, but also for his contribution to increasing German-
American understanding and friendship. He is the living example of what
could bring about an individual with ties to two countries (Fig. 40) (17). The
newspapers "San Antonio Light" and "San Antonio Express" reported on the
event. Strughold's health was already significantly impaired, but it did not
prevent him from giving the following statement (18): "I hate to dwell in the
past. But I do love thinking about the future and what the Space Shuttle will
eventually be able to do. And there is my favorite planet, of which I am still
dreaming about, Mars!"

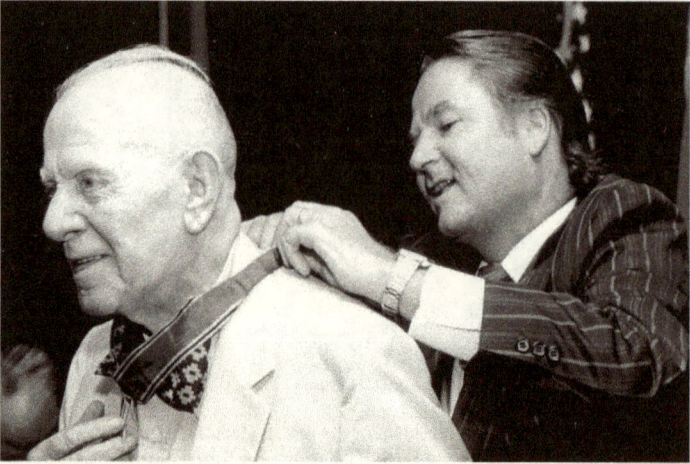

Fig. 40 Strughold receiving the Grand Cross of Merit of the Federal Republic of Germany in 1983. Photo archive Dr. Harsch, Nbdbg.

The Senate of Texas proclaimed it to be "Dr. Hubertus Strughold Day" on his 87th Birthday on June 15, 1985 (19).

Strughold, who had long lived as a bachelor, found in Mary a loving wife, who cared for him in times of severe disease (after two strokes). On September 25, 1986 Hubertus Strughold died at the age of 88 in his adopted home of Texas. He was buried at the cemetery "St. Herbertus Loring Funeral Home" near the Brooks AFB, Texas. The "Father of Space Medicine" found his final resting place in a modest atmosphere – according to his way of life (Fig. 41) (20).

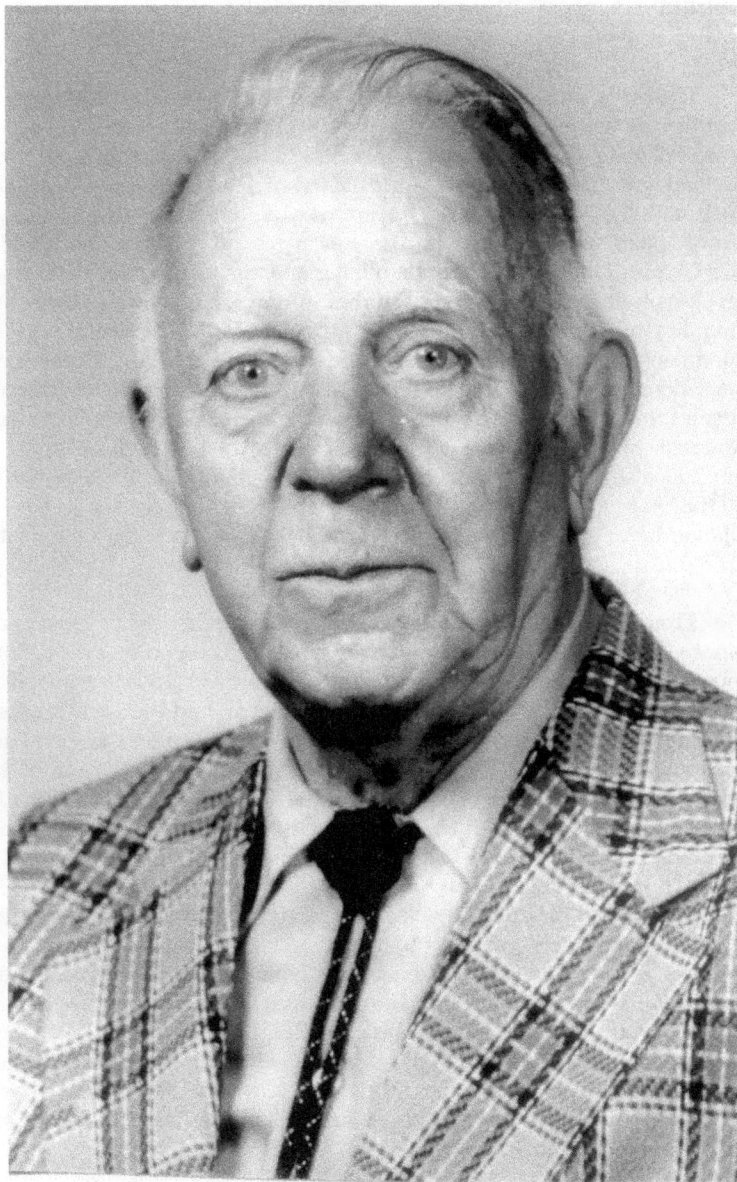

Fig. 41: Portrait of Hubertus Strughold. Photo archive Dr. Harsch, Nbdbg.

Chapter 10.   Strughold´s Scientific Work

Hubertus Strughold life's work included an unusually wide range for a scientific physiologist of the 20th century (1). Strughold's name is inseparably connected with German aviation medicine and early space-related medical developments in the Western world (2). John Pickering, an U.S. radiation expert, noted that the U.S. space program would have had a less advantageous starting point with respect to the Soviet Union without Strughold (3). After Charles Lindbergh's transatlantic flight, Strughold aspired to work in the aerophysiological field. Laboratory studies were complemented by experiments using hot air balloons, aircraft and small airships. The results of these experiments found their way into the scientific journals of aeronautical associations. Publications in aeromedical writings dominated his journalistic activities until the end of World War II. In the second half of the 20th century numerous publications in English followed. In total, Strughold wrote more than 200 scientific papers, including 20 in the "Journal of Aviation Medicine" and the "Journal of Aerospace Medicine" (4). During the post-war period in the "Citation Index", over 400 references to Strughold´s publications can be found (6).

From his pen also came popular-science books like "The Green and Red Planet - A Physiological Study of the Possibility of Life on Mars" (1953) and "Your Body Clock - Its Significance for the Jet Traveler" (1971) . Strughold was co-editor of the book "Outline of Aviation Medicine" and the "Atlas of Aviation Medicine." He was also the editor of the two-volume "Compendium of Aerospace Medicine" (1977 and 1979). Together with O. O. Benson he edited the "Physics and Medicine of the Atmosphere and Space" (1960). With C. H. Roadman, and R. B. Mitchell he published "Bioastronautics and the Exploration of Space" in 1964 and 1968. Numerous studies of Strughold were translated into French, Italian, Japanese, Russian, Spanish and Chinese (7). Strughold worked in various medical and scientific organizations on both sides of the Atlantic and was an honorary member and advisor of several professional associations (8). He also was honored by numerous institutions during his lifetime, with an extraordinary number of awards. By the end of World War II, these included not only German awards for his scientific achievements, but also those from Yugoslavia, Hungary and Sweden. After his emigration to the U.S., he was given further awards, led by the "Hermann Oberth Medal" of the German Rocket Society and the "Great Federal Cross of Merit" from the Republic of Germany (9).

In 1977 he was inducted in the "International Space Hall of Fame" in Alamogordo, New Mexico. The library at the USAF SAM, Brooks AFB, Texas was designated the "Strughold Aeromedical Library". Strughold maintained contacts with U.S. and foreign universities throughout his life. At the USAF

SAM he was named Professor of Space Medicine in 1958 - the first and still the only professor to be so named. He attended countless meetings in the military and civilian sector and was always a valued speaker (10). Many civil organizations, representatives from aerospace industries, representatives of airlines, and other technical enterprises consulted him. On television and radio the "space doctor" was also found to be present. A lively correspondence with people and institutions around the world included scientists, military officers, astronauts and presidents (11).

Strughold discovered during his medical studies, an interest in physiology, where he received his doctorate and later qualified as a professor. Promoter of this devotion to his scientific career was his teacher, Max von Frey in Wuerzburg. The focus of Strughold's scientific papers in the early 1920´s was concerned with sensory physiology. In his dissertation (medical theses to receive the doctorate) on the effects of the agents Diphenylarsinchlorid and Aethylarsin dichloride on human skin (two chemical weapons used in World War I) he tested the influence of these compounds on pain, pressure sense, and temperture sense (12). Further investigations were related to other neurophysiological considerations. At the suggestion of the Freiburg physiologist, P. Hoffman, Strughold examined the absolute and relative refractory periods of reflexes. In addition, attention was focused on the dependence of the refractory phase of facilitation and its relationship with clonus (13). In the years 1923-1929 Strughold published some 25 basic papers on these subjects. Until the end of World War II, another 15 papers followed on neurophysiology, partly on the effects and influence of hypoxia. The transition to the aeromedical focus of his research was made by his paper, "Flight Physiological Studies: The sense of touch (pressure-sense of the skin) at low oxygen pressure"(1929). Here his previous sensomotoric findings were applied to the extreme situations encountered in aviation. The altitude dependence on the threshold of sensation was detected using the effects of hypoxia (14). He noted during hypoxia that the sense of orientation and movement in the room changes without the loss of skin sense. Strughold demonstrated this in a self-experiment in 1928, when he blocked his pressure perception in his buttocks by injection of a local anesthetic (15).

The Berlin physiologist, Nathan Zuntz (1847-1920), who was quoted in some early papers by Strughold, pointed out that experienced pilots could fly with more situational awareness as they felt every fluctuation of their airplane with their buttocks (16). In the 1950s, Strughold discussed the neuro-sensory and physiological effects of weightlessness. Experiences were gained using parabolic flights, immersion tests in water, and later with prolonged immobilization in a slight head-down position. This all served as the basis for future investigations in the context of prolonged stays in space (17). In 1957 his neurophysiological work, "Mechanoreceptors and Gravireceptors" was published in the Journal of the Astronautical Society of the United States. An essay was published in the handbook "German Aviation Medicine World War II" (1950) on the same theme. The last article on this topic by Strughold was released with the title "Mechanoreceptors, Gravireceptors, Accelero-receptors" and was published in the second volume of the "Compendium of Space Medicine" (Strughold, 1979). Here a functional link between the mechano-receptors and the vestibular apparatus was postulated by him. He wrote in April 1948 to the Goettingen physiologist Hermann Rein (18): "You may be also interested to know that our common skin neurophysiological research papers from 1923-1930 are in very high regard in this country" (19).

As head of the AMRI in Germany, Strughold published in the journal "Medical World" in November 1935 about the tasks of aviation medicine in the German Luftwaffe. By 1945, he had published more than 40 aeromedical papers. He was also the co-editor of two manuals and an atlas. An outline of the altitude effect (hypoxia) was made by him on the basis of experimental procedures using tendon reflexes: Tolerance times while exposed to hypoxia (reserve time) were also tested at altitude while performing strength tests, which were used to understand the mechanisms of altitude adaptation. In his 1938 paper about neurophysiological exams, Strughold focused on standardization of the physiological nomenclature, which is essentially still valid today (20). Strughold inaugurated the concept of "*Zeitreserve*" (Time of Useful Consciousness), in 1937 which he defined as the time from the end of additional oxygen breathing until the onset of neurophysiological disorders (21). Strughold defined the natural living zone and the supplemental oxygen zone (4,000 - 11,000 m) as well as the zone higher in altitude requiring additional atmospheric pressure (22). The breathing of pure oxygen in altitude flights was demonstrated to be harmless, as his assistant researchers Clamann and Becker-Freyseng examined in risky self-experiments. The lack of oxygen and the reserve time was realised as having a key influence in rapid and explosive decompression flights in altitude chambers from about 3,000 up to 15,000 meters within a few seconds (23). For high altitude missions the need for emergency oxygen equipment and the need for an immidiate descent (emergency dive) if decompression occurred was postulated. In the article, "The Medical Problems in the Substratosphere" Strughold made requirements for pressure suits and pressurized cabins for high altitude flights in the stratosphere (24). A measure of the altitude/hypoxia effect on the central nervous system was demonstrated by the writing sample produced by the exposed subject. Further studies took advantage of the electroencephalogram. Strughold published in 1942, "The derivation of brain action currents, a method to study altitude sickness" (1942). The thermal, mechanical and chemical effects of the high altitude environment became more important in World War II. Together with Gauer, Opitz, and Palme he analysed parachute jumps and reserve times at high altitudes (1942). They recommended not to open the chute until reaching oxygen sufficient lower altitudes (25).

Through his residency in the U.S. during 1928-29, Strughold acquired the ability to look and to think through scientific and political boundaries. He had a big influence on the development of aerospace medicine (26). After World War II, the most basic and important aviation medical matters were largely resolved. New rocket technology, however, required an intensification of biomedical research in regard of the possibilities of a manned space flight. The appearance of the first artificial earth satellite in 1957 spurred further research activity (27). Strughold regarded weightlessness as the preeminent phenomenon of space travel (28). This problem was first discussed by astrophysicist Heinz Haber and acceleration physiologist Otto Gauer at a seminar at the Heidelberg Aero Medical Center in 1946 (29). Together with Fritz Haber, Heinz Haber, and Konrad Buettner, Strughold published the paper "Where Does Space Begin - Functional Concept of the Boundaries Between Atmosphere and Space" in 1951. In this article it was first described, that the edge of space is non-stationary: Above a height of 20 km a pressurized cabin could not be operated with sufficient ambient air, so that there the use of a completely pressurized space cabin was necessary. In 1952 the article "From Aviation Medicine to Space Medicine" followed. Strughold stated on this occasion that aviation medicine was the parent discipline of space medicine (30). Other important papers of Strughold were: "Living Room in Space" (1954) and "The Medical Problems of Space Flight" (1955).

During his naturalization process in the United States, which occurred in 1956, he published over 40 books and articles. He also introduced the terms, "Astrobiology" and "Bioastronautics" in the scientific world. He also suggested the development of "Spatiography" (31). In 1947 he gave a lecture at Heidelberg University on the importance of oxygen for life, which was well received. It was the world's first lecture on astrobiology (32):

"We see that the main problem of Astrobiology is also only an oxygen problem. And here - in relation to the oxygen and the given biological development opportunities – there is Earth again in the center. Insofar, Ptolemy was right. I think my dear audience that you share with me the view that the oxygen in its function as a living fabric attracts our attention - I want to say: deserves our sympathy, because it is the element that's in the truest sense of the word is of all importance, although it is invisible and we can´t detect it with our senses. And the concern with it is one of the most appealing, for it leads us back to the enigmas of life in the cells of humans, animals and plants, it takes us to the heights of the Himalayas and to the depths of the oceans, to the structure of the atom and to the expanses of space."

Strughold began studying the ecology of other planets for the U.S. Air Force beginning in 1947 (33). In 1951, his work appeared on "Physiological Considerations on the Possibility of Life under Extraterrestrial Conditions", followed by "The Possibilities of an Inhabitable Extraterrestrial Environment Reachable from the Earth" (34): This preliminary work culminated in the

1953 book, "The Green and the Red Planet "(35). The first symposium on "Problems Common to Physics and Biology" at the "Astronomical Society of the Pacific" and the "International Mars Committee" was held on June 15, 1957 in Flagstaff, Arizona. The main focus was on Mars research, including the "Mars-experiments" by Strughold, who exposed lichens to large temperature fluctuations in a refrigerator (36). Astronomical research at that time gave evidence of a seasonal change of color of the Martian surface, which could result from seasonal changes in vegetation. Picking up on this hypothesis, Strughold investigated the possibility of plant life under Martian conditions. In later works by him he pointed out that Mars may have life. Although it was though to be arid, water could be present in the Martian polar caps. He also pointed out that there may be also an ice sheet (sub-surface frozen hydro-sphere) under the dust layer, with water in liquid form below (aquatic bio-sphere) (37).

Another area of interest of Strughold was the biorhythm (chrono-biology). He was probably the first to realize the medical effects of flights that occurred over several time zones (38). Strughold experienced psycho-physiological effects during a time zone flight in 1949 when he first flew from the U.S. to Europe and two months later when flying back in the opposite direction. He observed differences in the desynchronization of his "internal clock" (39). His first work on this, "Physiological Day-Night Cycle in Global Flight" appeared in 1950 in the "Journal of Aviation Medicine." He stated that the biological sleep-wake rhythm was synchronized as a kind of conditioned reflex with cosmic events (circadian rhythm). The biorhythm occurred in the context of flight operations with "time-scheduled" tasks such as the Berlin Airlift of 1948 causing serious impacts. In the German "Journal of Medical Education", Strughold's contribution "Metabolism clock goes wrong" appeared (1963). After time zone flights involving jet aircraft, travellers experienced an increase in pain sensitivity, predisposition to hallucinations, and emotional incontinence. The "New York Times" reported in 1961 about the dangers of jet-tourism (40). The London "Weekend Review" spoke of "jet lag" as the "Strughold Syndrome". The speech for the inauguration of the "Strughold Aeromedical Library" on January 19, 1977 was closed by Strughold with the words (41): "God bless you and your body clock."

During his education, Strughold completed nine years of Latin and five years of Greek. He held both languages, especially in the nuclear and cosmic age, to be of the utmost importance, as the evolving science have a great need for proper names and those languages were very likely to result in a universal understanding (42): "New words are very important in this field. It should be understood internationally and the press should adapt to it and transmit it to the public. I remember the time not long ago when I had to explain the word 'orbit'. Nowadays, with the exposure from the press, radio, and television, the public has naturally embraced the word into its vocabulary. Appropriate words can accelerate progress, inappropriate words can unnecessarily hinder progress. Really good words can act as catalysts."

The so-called "Astroglossary" was stuffed with Strughold's neologisms (word inventions) (43). Already for 30 years he had dealt with questions of nomenclature. In his work, "On the question of unification of terms and methods in aerospace medicine", Strughold developed guidelines for this purpose (44). After his arrival in the United States in the 1940´s, Strughold was a member of the nomenclature committee at SAM, Randolph AFB, Texas. His focus was not only on the standardization of scientific language, but also of the scientific units. The temperature measurement in the U.S. in degrees "Fahrenheit" he regarded as outdated. The USAF Aerospace Medical Division was a pioneer on the road to standardization. A directive of the USAF from 1964 prescribed the use of the metric system in research, teaching and publications. In 1973, the Aerospace Medical Association and their magazine "Aerospace Medicine" adapted to the metric system. Strughold stated, that what is good on the Moon, of course, should also apply to the Earth (45).

Chapter 11. The Controversy of Hubertus Strughold during World War II

Dr. Hubertus Strughold was an early pioneer of aerospace medicine. He was educated in Germany and was the Director of the Aeromedical Research Institute of the German Air Ministry in Berlin during World War II. After the war, he was brought to the U.S. as a part of "Operation Paperclip" and was instrumental in the early development of space medicine. He was a founder of the Space Medicine Branch (now Space Medicine Association) of the Aerospace Medical Association. His contributions were so fundamental that he is called "The Father of Space Medicine" and the Hubertus Strughold Award is given yearly by the Space Medicine Association for individual achievement in space medicine. Following his death, criticism of his possible involvement in World War II atrocities has emerged and most of his honors have been removed.

World War II Atrocities and Investigations

At the Nuremberg Trials, three sets of medical experiments that were cruelly and in-humanely performed on prisoners by German physicians in the aviation medical field were brought to prosecution. These reprehensible experiments were conducted at the Dachau concentration camp. They involved prisoners who were subjected to hypoxia in altitude chambers, subjects immersed in ice water for long periods, and subjects forced to drink seawater. Many of the subjects of the hypoxia and ice water experiments did not survive (1).

Hypoxia Experiments (see expanded document in Appendix 1)

The hypoxia altitude chamber experiments were initially approved by Dr. Weltz, the Director of the Institute for Aviation Medicine in Munich, and conducted by his assistant, Dr. Rascher (who had conceived of the idea and had obtained permission from *Reichsfuehrer SS* Himmler). The civil Department for Aviation Medicine in the German Experimental Institute for Aviation (DVL) in Berlin-Adlershof with Dr. Ruff and Dr. Romberg collaborated. A mobile altitude chamber was provided by the Experimental Institute for Aviation (DVL) directed by Ruff and was transported to Dachau in great secrecy. In the Nuremburg Trials, Ruff testified as to the high level of secrecy involved, but that Dr. Hippke

(Luftwaffe surgeon general) was aware and had given approval of the Dachau experiments (2). Rascher and Romberg conducted the experiments, while Weltz and Ruff were their respective superiors in charge, although Weltz turned Rascher over to Ruff's supervision (3). Dr. Lutz (a high altitude researcher at the Munich institute) testified at the Nuremburg Trials that he was asked to do research at Dachau and refused and described several secret meetings at the DVL between Weltz, Ruff and Romberg which no one else was allowed to participate in (4). Dr. Strughold was at one time approached by the SS in 1942 and also asked to participate in experiments using concentration camp prisoners, but he refused (5).

Weltz and Ruff initially kept the experiments secret, but later conducted a private screening of a film to selected individuals at the Air Ministry including Dr. Benzinger (6), who worked at the Rechlin Test Center, 130 km northwest of Berlin. His superiors were with the Air Material Command, and he was not a part of Dr. Strughold's staff in Berlin (7). Ruff reported on the experiments by Romberg and Rascher at the 9th Scientific Meeting of the German Academy of Aviation Research on November 6, 1942. Strughold was not mentioned as an attendee; however he was a member of this scientific organization. At this meeting the aeromedical community was briefed about the rescue possibilities by parachute at high altitudes. In the official text it was not mentioned that some of these tests were performed at Dachau or that deaths occurred (8).

Dr. Rascher, a reserve captain in the Air Force with the equivalent rank of a *Sturmbannfuehrer* in the *Sturmstaffel* (also better known as the SS, a fanatically racist political and military organization), performed both official experiments under the responsibility of the Luftwaffe and his own private experiments with the intention of obtaining a Ph.D. degree for his research. These private experiments were responsible for all of the deaths of the subjects in the hypoxia experiments and were only reported to Himmler (9). When Romberg assisted Rascher in a series of additional experiments to find out how long test subjects could withstand extremely high altitude, several deaths occurred. Romberg immediately reported these unplanned tests to Ruff who intervened with the Luftwaffe to get the mobile altitude chamber removed from Dachau. Rascher tried to get the chamber returned through SS channels, but was unsuccessful (10). He and his wife were both executed under Himmler's order just before the end of war (11).

Drs. Ruff, Romberg, and Weltz were arrested and prosecuted at Nuremberg. All three were acquitted due to the lack of any direct evidence of participation with Dr. Rascher's private experiments (12). Dr. Benzinger was arrested and interrogated, but not prosecuted (13).

Hypothermia Experiments (see expanded document in Appendix 2)

The freezing experiments were conducted by Dr. Holzloehner (who committed suicide at the end of the war), who was a physiologist from the University of Kiel, assisted by Dr. Finke (Luftwaffes *Oberarzt* at the Westerland Hospital), and again by Dr. Rascher. They had permission from the Luftwaffe Field Marshal Erhard Milch (who was prosecuted in Nuremberg and imprisoned until 1954) and *Reichfuehrer-SS* Heinrich Himmler (who committed suicide at the end of the war). The head of the Luftwaffe´s Medical Corps was Luftwaffe Surgeon General Dr. Hippke and he was also possibly involved (who was not prosecuted at Nuremberg as his location was not known at the beginning of the Trials).

As already shown in the hypoxia experiments, there was an "official series of experiments" performed because of the Luftwaffe´s interest, but also a second series of experiments performed separately by Dr. Rascher. Beginning in August 1942, Holzloehner conducted experiments in collaboration with Dr. Finke and Dr. Rascher utilizing human test subjects. These were the Dachau experiments where several deaths occurred. A report for the Luftwaffe's medical corps was therefore not officially published. Implementation of the results from the entire series of hypothermia experiments was deemed necessary by the Luftwaffe to handle the problem of hypothermia in the sea-downed aircrews and to develop a method of re-warming with the further development of appropriate protective clothing (14).

The results of these experiments were not distributed to the Luftwaffe, but were partially presented at a conference, the "Medical Problems of Sea Distress and Winter Emergencies" on October 26,1942 in Nuremberg and then again two months later in Berlin (the Second Conference of Special Medical Consultants from 30th Nov. to 3rd Dec. 1942 at the Military Medical Academy). There is no list of the participants of the second conference in Berlin. There is no evidence that Strughold was present at the Berlin meeting. However, over 90 German scientists and physicians attended the first conference, the Nuremberg Winter-

Symposium, including Dr. Strughold. According to one of the participants: "The afternoon session of the first day seemed to end, as the leader of the discussion announced outside the program that the following presentation was top secret and anyone who would speak about it outside the meeting or to anyone other than the conference participants, had to reckon with his execution" (15).

Dr. Holzloehner lectured on the "Prevention and Treatment of Hypothermia in Water" at the Nuremberg conference. In addition several presentations by other researchers were conducted on the bio-climatological, physiological and pathological basics of thermal regulation and hypothermia as well as other topics of practical importance. Strughold participated at this meeting and gave the following comment after a series of three presentations by Jarisch, Weltz and Holzloehner. Commentaries were then given by Rascher, Benzinger, Denecke, Lehmann, Wezler, Groose-Brockhoff, Deuticke, Schwiegk, Knothe, von Werz and finally by Strughold:

"With regard to this experimental scientific research, but also for the orientation of the sea distress service, it is of interest to know what temperatures are to be counted on in the cases concerned during the various seasons. Dealing with this subject, valuable material with descriptions and sea-charts are already available. The following are the most important literature findings. At the same time, details about the content of the salt in the water are to be found there."

The comments were not, therefore, directed specifically to Dr. Holzloehner's presentation, but were concerning the whole series of lectures. The reaction of the audience to the Holzloehner presentation remains controversial. Some written sources state, that not all of the participants realized the unethical character of the investigation and believed only the results of distress units were presented (16). For many of the conference participants it was not obvious that the Holzloehner presentation was based on human experiments. In the presentation he did not specify that prisoners were used and he was not explicit that deaths occurred during the experiments (17). It became evident that these were not only the results of animal experiments or observations from the German Armed Forces distress service, when the nature of the trials was clarified after the official end of the lecture series and outside of the official program by Dr. Rascher (18).

After the presentation at the Nuremberg conference by Holzloehner and the remarks that followed by Rascher, Drs. Strughold, H. Rein and F. Buechner protested against the conduction of the human experiments with the highest ranking Luftwaffe officer at this conference, Dr. Anthony (19). None of these protests were officially documented as they were oral objections only, but several individuals published accounts in the post-war period that the protests occurred and that there were also other individuals at the conference who disagreed with these unethical experiments (20). The famous physiologist, Dr. Otto Gauer, also attended this meeting and later in life told his student, Dr. Kirsch, that all of the top researchers present disapproved of Rascher's experiments and behavior.

A critical debate flared up following the statement of Mitscherlich in 1946 (21), that none of the 95 conference participants, most of whom were notable representatives of science, protested against the human experiments. Rein and Buechner discussed on several occasions that this was absolutely not true. Rein stated: "The author of the book (Mitscherlich) was not present at the meeting. He would not have forgotten the bitterness and indignation of the scientists who were attending this meeting. The initiator of those experiments, an SS doctor (Rascher), was immediately recognizable to all as a pure sadist. His 'scientific' staff member (Holzloehner), who was also a speaker of that session, was scientifically outlawed from this day forward. Three of those present declared that such experiments are completely meaningless and unscientific and should therefore be omitted. That this was presented in a ´top secret´ meeting seems not to be clear to the author Mitscherlich. It is important that in the conference documents there is a letter from Himmler where he stated: 'People who refuse even today to perform these human experiments, would rather let brave German soldiers die from the effects of hypothermia, I see this as high treason and I will not be afraid to call the names of these gentlemen at the appropriate locations.´ The fact that the official record of this memorable session contains nothing about it, only proves how they worked and that no one dared, in such attempts, to inaugurate the real representatives of the science " (22). One of the conference speakers, Buechner, accused Holzloehner of the "ethical impossibility" of his human experiments. Buechner stated in his 1965 book, "Plans and Coincidence. Memoirs of a German University Teacher" (23) that "In the foyer Hermann Rein, Hubertus Strughold, and myself (Buechner) and also other doctors one after another objected to the senior medical officer of the Luftwaffe emphatic objection to Luftwaffe doctors participating in such experiments in cooperation with SS officers."

Sea Water Drinking Experiments (see expanded document in Appendix 3)

The sea water experiments were approved by Dr. Becker-Freyseng (a former assistant of Dr. Strughold's several years before the experiments took place) and conducted by Dr. Beiglboeck (from the Department of Aviation Medicine in the Surgeon General's Office of the Air Force). Both were not from Dr. Strughold's Institute at the time of the experiments. Dr. Schaefer (from the Medical Experimental and Instructional Division in Jueterbog) was under Dr. Strughold earlier in the war, but was detached by order of the Surgeon General of the Air Force (Dr. Schroeder, who had replaced Dr. Hippke) to work on the sea water experiments because of his expertise in making sea water drinkable using silver. He attended a planning meeting on the experiments in May 1944 at the German Air Ministry. At the Nuremberg Trials, Dr. Schaefer testified that he opposed the experiments, but was threatened that his behavior would be considered an act of sabotage (24).

The 40 designated test-subjects were brought specifically for this experiment from the Buchenwald concentration camp. They were transferred to Dachau with the prospect of an improvement in their conditions. The tests were designed to last for 12 days, but were canceled in many instances when health problems occurred in test subjects after less than a week. There were no deaths among in the prolonged exposure to salt water experiments, but serious complications and injuries did occur (25). Because of the torturous, unethical character of the experiments, Dr. Schroeder was convicted and sentenced to life imprisonment at the Nuremberg Trials, Dr. Becker-Freyseng was convicted and sentenced to 20 years, and Dr. Beiglboeck was convicted and sentenced to 15 years. Dr. Schaefer was acquitted.

Information for the Nuremberg medical trials came from multiple sources, including Himmler's private files that were found intact at the end of the war. Personal files from the different institutes (which were all heavily bombed) were missing and are claimed by Bower (26) to have been destroyed as the war came to an end, possibly as part of a cover-up. Twenty three physicians and high ranking officials were prosecuted for war crimes at the Nuremberg Trials. Of these, seven were executed, five were given life sentences, and four were convicted with lesser sentences. In all, eight physicians were arrested for war crimes related to aviation medical experiments (27). Of these, one was unprosecuted, four were acquitted, and three were convicted (28). Although Dr. Strughold has been said (29) to be on an Army Intelligence list of suspects in 1945 before the end of the war (Central Registry of War Criminals and Security Suspects), he was never arrested or prosecuted. The purpose of the list was to identify people who were wanted for interrogation and not necessarily for arrest, He did testify by affidavit in the trials concerning character references with the other defendants. During his testimony he stated that he disapproved of the secret studies conducted by Dr. Rascher (30).

Dr. Leo Alexander (Maj., U.S. Army) investigated the medical experiments on concentration camp inmates as a Nuremberg Medical Trial Expert (31). After a two year investigation, he produced a 220 page report for the Nuremberg Trials, "The Treatment of Shock from Prolonged Exposure to Cold, Especially in Water". The Alexander Report (32) is very detailed in exactly who was involved in Dachau and the abundant evidence that was collected from Himmler's cave depository of SS materials captured in Hallein, Germany. Dr. Strughold reported to Dr. Alexander (33) that he knew about the human experiments from the Nuremberg Winter-Symposium and stated that although he thought that prisoners had been used, he disapproved of such experiments in non-volunteers on principle. "I have always forbidden even the thought of such experiments in my Institute, firstly on moral grounds and secondly on grounds of medical ethics." Strughold and the other aviation medicine doctors told the Americans that the Dachau experiments were not only unimportant, but also of dubious scientific value (34). Dr. Strughold related to Dr. Alexander that he did not know about the hypoxia altitude experiments until they were announced on the radio at the end of the war in connection with Dr. Rascher (35).

The Hypoxia Experiments on Children at AMRI- Berlin (see expanded document in Appendix 4)

Another non-criminal but unethical medical experiment has also been associated with Dr. Strughold. In 1993, Koch (36) reported that six children ages 11-13 from the psychiatry clinic in Brandenburg-Goerden were tested in an altitude chamber using oxygen-reduced gas mixtures (mild hypoxia). We can assume that there was no informed consent. These tests were carried out at the Strughold directed Aeromedical Research Institute (AMRI) in Berlin on September 17, 1943. The altitude was up to 6,000 m. The trial managers were in the chamber with the youths and they could add oxygen if required at any time. There were no seizures observed and no injuries reported.

The biologist, Dr. Hans Nachtsheim, performed research during the war on epilepsy in cooperation with Dr. Ruhenstroth-Bauer from the KWI (Kaiser Wilhelm Institute) for Biochemistry. The director of this institute was Dr. Adolf Butenand, a Nobel Prize winner from 1939. About 150 hypoxia experiments were performed on rabbits beginning in the spring of 1943. This research was sponsored by the German Reich Research Council. Use of the AMRI altitude chamber inducing epileptic seizures in animals (rabbits) had started in June 1943. Dr. Karl Brockhausen made 6 epileptic children available for the experiments at an altitude chamber of the AMRI on one day, September 17, 1943. The children were 11 to 13 years old and were exposed to an altitude up to 4,000 to 6,000 m. The experiments "failed", as no seizure occurred.

The introduction of a 1944 article by Ruhenstroth-Bauer and Nachtsheim on animal experiments stated (37): "For the experimentally working clinicians treating patients the methodological possibilities are always limited, as they should take the patients well-being into consideration. Only in exceptional cases, a researcher could dare in one patient a trial in the interests of future patients, whereof he cannot predict anything certain."

Dr. Gerhard Ruhenstroth-Bauer stated in 2000 (38). "Together with Professor Hans Nachtsheim, I carried out experiments with epileptic adolescents. I would like to stress that in every case Dr. Nachtsheim, a Luftwaffe doctor, and I went up into the vacuum chamber with the children. For each participant with nausea, immediately a supply of oxygen could be applied or the exam could be canceled. This did not occur in any case: on the contrary, the children talked almost cheerfully among themselves and also with Dr. Nachtsheim. Since no seizure occurred, we finished these experiments and had the impression that the problem concerning "oxygen deficiency in epileptic adolescents" was finished. Now, after more than 60 years, this assumption turned out to be wrong. In my correspondence with Mr. Klee (39) I was made aware of the fact that the institution in Goerden represented an "euthanasia" institution. Understandably, this revelation shook me hard." However, others have pointed out that the psychiatric wards were quite well known during the war as questionable treating facilities (40). Though it is mentioned that no test subject was hurt, Beddies (41) reports that in one test subject a facial cyanosis of the mucous membranes is mentioned as well as a mild dizziness.

The medical historian, von Schwerin (42), concludes: "The experiments with the children from Goerden are not comparable with those of criminal medical experiments that are known mainly from the concentration camps where the death of the subjects participated was anticipated. These experimemts are rather an example of biomedical experimental practice on a daily basis. But the limits of this practice were being exceeded in National Socialism and the boundries stretched".

As the author Schmuhl (43) stated in 2003: "As the available sources testify unanimously, the experiment did not produce any tangible result - it did not succeed in inducing an epileptic fit in the children through low pressure. Consequently it did not cause them any suffering - but Ruhenstroth-Bauer and Nachtsheim could not have foreseen this. According to Nachtheim's account, the children were subjected to a low-pressure situation that corresponded to an altitude of 6.000 m (not to mention the mental strain of being locked into the vacuum chamber). According to the knowledge available to altitude medicine at the lime, at this altitude tile onset of threatening conditions had to be expected even for adults - all the more so for children. Moreover, there was no possibility of resorting to any previous experience with epileptic humans in low pressure situations. Furthermore, Ruhenstroth-Bauer and Nachtsheim knew from the animal experiments that young epileptic rabbits reacted to low pressure with violent, often fatal convulsions -and they expected (and hoped !) that the children would react like the rabbits. In other words: the scientists knowingly accepted the risk that the children could be placed in fatal danger. Ruhenstroth-Bauer's reassuring statement that he himself, Nachtsheim, and an additional physician of the Luftwaffe had been in the vacuum chamber with the children and had been able to abort the experiment at any time - as could the children themselves - thus fails to get at the root of the matter. Nonetheless: the low-pressure experiments by Nachtsheim and Ruhenstroth Bauer ignored the Reich Health Council's regulations on human experiments from the year 1931 as a matter of course. For the most part, these regulations, as adduced elsewhere, had already been ignored by research back in the 1930s. Yet this experiment marked a further boundary crossing as the experimenters unscrupulously subjected the children to an incalculable health risk, even accepting a potentially fatal outcome of the test - and all of this *needlessly*, for the utilization of the vacuum chamber was by no means imperative."

Dr. Strughold was the head of the institute providing the infrastructure (the AMRI altitude chamber) on September 17, 1943. He was not part of the experiments and did not use its results to our knowledge. The children were not harmed or seriously endangered according to the literature. However, these kinds of experiments were against the medical ethical understanding in Germany as published in 1931. There is no evidence that Strughold knew of, approved of or allowed the children experiments to take place at the AMRI, but it has been assumed. For this reason the scientific prize named after Dr. Strughold by the German Society for Aviation and Space Medicine (DGLRM) was terminated, a decision made in Germany by the DGLRM in 2004.

Criticism of Dr. Strughold

Dr. Strughold's World War II record did not become a public issue until 1958, when a magazine article charged that he used prisoners in his German research. This charge was disproved by a Justice Department investigation. This 1958 investigation was discontinued when the Air Force stated that Strughold already had been "appropriately investigated" (44). The allegations resurfaced in 1974, when the Immigration and Naturalization Service (INS) investigated him for allegations of Nazi war crimes and considered possible deportation (45). Dr. Strughold publicly stated at the time that "I was completely cleared when I came over here. I was cleared before I came here, before I was hired." The investigation was terminated several months later due to lack of evidence, although the New York Times claimed (46) that there was possible CIA intervention. The INS Director Leonard Chapman reported that inquiries to the military and other federal agencies had disclosed "no derogatory information" and therefore the INS considered the case closed (47). In a San Antonio newspaper article in 1974, Dr. Strughold stated that an investigation into whether he was a Nazi war criminal was "idiotic". It was "nonsense and false to even think that I had ever been a Nazi. It is so fantastic; I always have allied myself with the enemies of Hitler in those days in Germany. I sometimes had to hide myself because my life was in danger from the Nazis" (Doc. 9). The Department of Justice – Office of Special Investigations reopened the investigation again in 1983, but this was terminated upon Dr. Strughold's death in 1986.

Several popular books have been published that have commented on the Strughold controversy. In "The Paperclip Conspiracy, The Hunt for Nazi Scientists" (1987) (48), the reporter-journalist author, Tom Bower, proposed that the U.S. military, in seeking to gain the scientific high ground from the Soviets at the end of World War II, recruited and protected from the Nuremberg Trials, a large group of committed Nazi scientists and brought them to the United States. "Strughold's secret arrival in America in 1947 had been a carefully planned operation masterminded by Col. Harry Armstrong (49)." Again, Dr. Strughold is not accused of direct involvement at Dachau, but of knowing about the experiments and trying to cover-up for his colleagues (especially Ruff, Romberg, and Holzloehner) (50). This is based on the claim that he edited out references (51) to human experiments in the 1947 book, German Aviation Medicine in World War II (52), Bower stated, "Strughold struck out the incriminating disclosures with a blue pencil." However, others have pointed out that the very scientific purpose of such bibliographies is to clearly identify valid science and to distinguish it from the invalid. Therefore, given Dr. Strughold's strong distaste and disdain for these experiments that were not only horrendous, but unscientific, it is logical that he was keeping these experiments from being portrayed as valid science. Bower also reported that Dr. Benzinger and Dr. Lauschner (Hippke's assistant) felt that Dr. Strughold was complicit in the Dachau experiments because he frequently communicated with both Dr. Hippke (his superior) and Dr. Ruff (53). Some non-historians claim that there was an enormous amount of hard evidence linking Strughold to Dachau and that he was protected by the US government and never 'brought to justice. The statement is made by Bower, "The OSI has had an open investigation file on him (Dr. Strughold) since the early 1980's, but despite the abundant evidence of his knowledge of and complicity in the Dachau experiments, Strughold continues to live in retirement (54)."

The historian, Maura Mackowski, in "Testing the Limits" (55) stated, "Strughold did not specify that some of the authors (in German Aviation Medicine in World War II) had been tried at Nuremburg... and that some of the research results (in their presentations) were obtained from inmate test subjects." Indeed, Drs. Becker-Freyseng, Benzinger, Schroeder, Schaefer and Ruff were five of the authors (there was a total of fifty-six aviation specialists who contributed to the two volume book) and were later involved in the Nuremberg trials. The book was based upon the data collected by the Germans and edited by Strughold in 1945-1947 while at the USAAF Heidelberg Aeromedical Center. Therefore, authors appear

107

which were later involved in the Nuremberg trials. However, a careful review of the contents of the book does not show any data that was derived from inmate experiments. There is no evidence of the publication of any Dachau data in this book. Becker-Freyseng, Benzinger, Schroeder and Ruff wrote about subjects that were unrelated to any of the Dachau studies. Schaefer wrote about thirst using data not obtained from Dachau. Possible references to Dachau could have been edited out, such as the Schaefer paper on thirst with no incorporation of the unethical experiments. In fact, the deletion of any data or presentation based upon inmate experiments was used by Bower to criticize Strughold (see above). An article concerning brain pathology was written by Spatz, "Brain Injuries in Aviation", from the Kaiser Wilhelm Institute. There is suspicion that Spatz was involved in unethical brain research involving concentration camp inmates (56), but it would be unrelated to this article.

In "The Nazi Hunters" (1988) (57), the importance of the Dachau hypoxia experiments is vastly over inflated, saying that the results of the experiments allowed the Germans to be able to fight the Allied Air Forces at higher altitudes. The use of supplemental oxygen at high altitudes had been discovered using legitimate studies at The AMRI before 1941. Roth in "Deadly Heights" (58) claims that Luftwaffe concern over high altitude parachute use drove the Dachau hypoxia studies, but again this had already been determined by legitimate studies (see Appendix 1).

Dr. Eckart, a historian from the University of Heidelberg, has been a long-time critic of Dr. Strughold. He puts forth several claims (59): The neuroscientist, Hallervorden, worked at the Kaiser Wilhelm Institute (KWI) for Brain Research in Berlin-Buch together with the neuro-pathologist, Hugo Spatz. It is claimed that they also conducted brain autopsies on murdered concentration camp inmates. Spatz was also connected to Strugholds AMRI institute (external Department for Brain Research). Eckart also believes that the low pressure experiments of Rascher should be interpreted as a part of a physiological research network, which was extended over many physiological research institutions throughout the Reich territory. This included the Institute of Physiology at the University of Goettingen under the direction of Hermann Rein. That institute was coordinated by Strughold through the AMRI. Eckart also believes that through his contacts with Hippke, Benzinger, Schaefer and Ruff, that Strughold was aware of the Dachau atrocities. There is no claim by Eckart that Strughold directed, participated, or organized the Dachau atrocities, but that through his contacts would have been aware of them.

In the "Secret Agenda: The United States Government, Nazi Scientists and Project Paperclip, 1944-1990" (1991) (60), the journalist, Linda Hunt, stated, "Strughold was not arrested, interrogated, or even called as a witness at the trial, despite the derogatory information against him. It was a glaring example of how far the military went to protect him. His war time superior, close associates and a subordinate all were tried at Nuremberg" (61). "General Harry Armstrong was protecting Hubertus Strughold from being exposed to the public" (62). "The Department of the Air Force then expanded the Paperclip cover up when it proudly published translations of the German's war time research in two volumes as German Aviation Medicine in World War II. In these books the Air Force not only ignored the lessons of Nuremberg but embraced what the Nazis had done" (63).

Hunt also stated, "One scientist (Strughold) had disturbing links to Dachau experiments" (64). The "links" that Hunt presented are summarized below:

1) Although Maj. Alexander stated that Strughold told him that he knew of the freezing experiments from the 1942 Nuremberg meeting, he was suspicious that Strughold was covering up the involvement of Ruff and Holzloehner (65).

2) Benzinger (in an interview with the author) claimed that his arrest at the time of the Nuremberg Trials was "set up" by Strughold to take the heat off of Strughold's own questionable war time activities (66).

3) Becker-Freyseng's Nuremberg testimony concerning Strughold's ability to stop any experiment that he did not agree with (67).

4) Hippke and Schroeder were Strughold's superiors and he frequently advised them on research matters (67).

5) Becker-Freyseng worked afternoons at Strughold's institute (68).

6) Schaefer had previously worked at Strughold's institute on problems of how to make seawater relatively safe to drink (68).

7) Several meetings were held to plan the experiments (to make sea water safe to drink), including one at Strughold's institute (Strughold was not stationed in Berlin at the time and did not attend). The group eventually decided to use concentration camp prisoners (69).

In "Secret Agenda" (67), Hunt states that Dr. Becker-Freyseng testified at Nuremberg that Dr. Strughold knew of the Dachau experiments and could have stopped them at any time:

Meyer: "If Dr. Strughold did not agree with a specific experiment, could he interrupt it?"
Becker-Freyseng: "I would assume yes."
Meyer: "Did he have the power at his disposal?"
Becker-Freyseng: "Of course, he was the director of the institute. He could do what he wanted there."
Meyer: "If we had not agreed with the work of the doctors, could he have sent for them and said: ´You must stop that or go to another institute."
Becker-Freyseng: "Yes. That is, he would have had to report to his superiors, because it was a military institution."
Meyer: "As director of the institute he could distribute and stop work?"
Becker-Freyseng: "Yes."

The Nuremberg Trial documents do show that Becker-Freyseng was interviewed at Nuremberg regarding concentration camp experiments (70). But Becker-Freyseng had given the comments above regarding experiments conducted at Dr. Strughold's Berlin Institute, and not regarding the experiments at Dachau. Many reports and documents (including Linda Hunt's book) have wrongly claimed that Becker-Freyseng was referring to the Dachau experiments and, therefore, was implicating Dr. Strughold's involvement with those experiments (67). Review of the Nuremberg documents show that Becker-Freyseng never testified that Strughold could directly influence the events happening at Dachau (71).

Marsha Freeman, the aerospace historian who authored "The History of German Space Pioneers" (who incidentally is Jewish) is very critical of the "Secret Agenda", in which unproven incriminations of Strughold are presented and actual facts, which do not fit into Hunt's political view of the world, are omitted. Freeman rated the "Secret Agenda" as the most insidious and mendacious book about "Operation Paperclip" ever published. (72).

Maura Mackowski, in "Testing the Limits" (73) also was very critical of the sloppy criticism of Strughold by other authors. "Errors in such books (popular histories) have unfortunately been repeated by magazines, newspapers, on the Internet, and in other books by authors who have failed to do any primary-source research ... evidence has been taken out of context, misinterpreted and mistranslated".

Mark L. Kornbluh, an assistant professor of history at Washington University in St. Louis, Missouri reviewed "Secret Agenda" in the "Bulletin of the Atomic Scientists" in September 1992 (74). He stated, "American scientific recruiting teams ignored the inhumane basis of much of their work and treated Nazi scientists as both colleagues and friends. The records of the Nazi activities of these scientists were altered, hidden, expunged, or classified. U.S. officials not only ignored the fact that many of these men were Nazis; they actively concealed that information in order to shield the Nazi scientists from prosecution. They then relocated them to new homes in America, with the understanding that the recruits would then share their technology with the U.S. government. The American space program became a veritable haven of ex-Nazis. Dr. Strughold pioneered aviation medicine through gruesome experiments conducted on prisoners in Dachau".

The consequences of such efforts promoting this mass of misinformation are as unfortunate as they are compelling. Brooks AFB Aeromedical Library was named after him in honor of his accomplishments in aerospace medicine in 1977. In 1995, the U.S. Air Force removed Strughold's name after the Jewish Anti-Defamation League (ADL) protested. "Paying tribute to Dr. Strughold was an obscene mockery of the pain and death suffered by his victims," commented ADL National Chairman Richard Strassler. The basis of the claim was his presence at the October 1942 meeting in Nuremberg where the freezing experiments were presented. The letter from the Air Force Chief of Staff to the ADL stated, "We are not in a position to draw any specific conclusions beyond this (his presence at the meeting) regarding the possibility of his complicity in or responsibility for the torture of concentration camp inmates in the guise of medical research. Although available information lends some support to those, including your organization, who maintain that Dr. Strughold was aware of and in some way aided such experiments, his death and the cessation of any formal investigation or proceedings concerning him make it unlikely that this question will ever be resolved conclusively. Nevertheless, and as you suggest, the evidence of Dr. Strughold's wartime activities is sufficient to cause concern about retaining his name in an honored place on the library."

In 1993, his portrait was also removed from a mural of medical heroes in a display of the "The World History of Medicine" at Ohio State University at the request of the World Jewish Congress. The German Society of Aviation and Space Medicine (DGLRM) had an award named after Dr. Strughold but canceled it due to the controversy concerning the use of the AMRI for experiments with hypoxia in epileptic children (75). Dr. Strughold was inducted into the New Mexico Museum of Space History Hall of Fame in 1978. The museum removed him from the hall of fame in May 2006 after protests from the ADL. Mark Santiago, the director of the museum, stated that no new information had been discovered, but that Dr. Strughold's removal was based upon information previously available (personal correspondence).

In their extensive press releases at the time of his removal, the museum and the ADL stated: "Strughold gave up his right to be on any hall of fame in the 1940s, when he directed a program that experimented on, tortured and killed Jews and gypsies at the Dachau concentration camp in Germany as the Nazi director of medical research for aviation, said Susan Seligman, regional director of the New Mexico Anti-Defamation League. These experiments at Dachau ... were the beginnings of early space medical research. Strughold, who was referred to as the "father of space medicine," directed a group that participated in experiments where prisoners were frozen to near death and re-warmed to see how quickly they would recover, according to the league's documents. The ADL presented documents to the Commissioners provided by the Office of Special Investigations in the Department of Justice that placed Strughold, the Reich's Director of Medical Research for Aviation as a participant and commentator during a 1942 conference on cold water experiments conducted at Dachau Concentration Camp."

At the time of his removal from the museum, the Institute of Ethics at the University of New Mexico released the following statement: "Surely recognition in a "Hall of Fame" should be reserved for those who represent widely held values of tolerances and respect for human dignity, and surely Hubertus Strughold, whatever his scientific contributions, should not be given a place of honor when his conduct failed to uphold those basic human values."

A careful review of Internet links using standard search techniques for "Strughold" (Appendix 5) reveals many obvious distortions. Some of these are minor and others outrageous. The most prevalent (all apparently from the same original source and simply repeated or magnified) state with confidence that Dr. Strughold was a Nazi, in charge of the Dachau experiments, was protected at the Nuremberg Trials, and involved in mind control experiments with psychoactive drugs at both Dachau and later in the U.S. under the C.I.A. In other web links, he is described as the examining physician when the aliens landed in Roswell, N.M. in 1947. Most state that he worked at NASA (he was a civilian contractor for the U.S. Air Force from 1948 -1963 and was never a NASA employee or contractor).

According to Bower, a 1945 intelligence report on Strughold stated: "His successful career under Hitler would seem to indicate that he must be in full accord with Nazism (76)." However, Strughold's colleagues in Germany and those with whom he had worked briefly in the United States on fellowships described him as politically indifferent or anti-Nazi. Dr. Strughold was never a member of the Nazi party as documented by Docket 5, Military Government of Germany, September 4, 1945. This was not a trivial matter, as membership in the Nazi party would have been advantageous to professional promotion and refusal of membership when in a relatively high position was actually dangerous. The directors of the other aviation medicine research institutes in Germany were all members of the Nazi party – Ruff, Weltz, and Benzinger (77). He was a member from 1937-1945 of the National Socialist Flying Corps and the National Socialist Welfare Organization. He was also a member of a certain entity called the RDB (*Reichsbund der Deutschen Beamten*) which was the Nazi trade union for civil servants. The membership in all three organizations was of absolutely no political influence, as there were no other alternatives in those years.

There is evidence that he would not allow any members of his staff to join the Nazi party and would refuse to return the *Heil Hitler* salute. Drs. Luft and Clamann (on Strughold's staff at the AMRI) stated that Strughold had instructed them not to join any political organizations. In the 1933 election (the last free election in Germany) he voted for the Central Democrat candidate. There have been no examples of racism or anti-Semitism in his writings, publications, or in his conversations with colleagues before or after the war. His personal and moral aspects, political dimensions, and humanistic beliefs were intensely scrutinized by the Allies in the period 1945-1947 before inviting him to work for the Army Air Force in the U.S. (78). He denied involvement with Nazi experiments and told reporters in this country that his life had been in danger from the Nazis. In an interview in 1974, Strughold claimed that after Count Claus von Stauffenberg attempted to assassinate Adolf Hitler in July 1944, Strughold had to go into hiding for two weeks as he was afraid that he was on a Nazi party enemy list and would be arrested (79).

After the war, the University of Heidelburg removed most of its faculty because they were Nazi party members. Dr. Strughold was appointed as Professor and Director because he was a known and consistent opponent of the Hitler regime. In September 1948, Dr. Strughold was granted a security certificate from the Joint Intelligence Objectives Agency director, Captain Wev. This certified that he was not a member of the Nazi party and was not involved in any war crimes.

In Dr. Strughold's affidavit testimony at the Nuremburg Trials (80), which was given as character background to several of the defendants, he described his political beliefs and the consequences. He described himself as being a "declared opponent of the Nazi movement" and would not work with any researcher if they were enthusiastically pro-Nazi. Because of this, he was threatened with imprisonment and was denied the opportunity for Professorship appointments at the universities. He stayed in contact with Jewish professors who had fled the country and made "frequent skeptical-ironical statements about Hitler and his policies" to other researchers whom he trusted. He stated that he would never have worked at any level with a researcher if he felt that they advocated experiments with involuntary subjects. He also testified that other researchers with supposed anti-Nazi views or activities were denied professional advancement (for their lack of interest in political issues), accused of sabotage (for demonstrating experimental results that did not confirm previous results that had been claimed by other Nazi party sources), or were even executed.

Dr. Strughold's comments in the 1942 Nuremberg Conference minutes were interpreted by the OSI in 1983 as encouraging (or at least endorsing) repetition of the freezing experiments – this time at the correct temperatures. Review of the minutes indicate that it was not explicitly meant as a reply to Holzloeehner's presentation, but was referring to a series of presentations, including the Rascher experiments, but most of them containing data using animal experiments (81). Dr. Benzinger was deposed by the Department of Justice – Office of Special Investigations (OSI) in their investigation of Dr. Strughold in 1983. When asked what his interpretation was of the above comments, Dr. Benzinger did not think that it was meant in any way as an endorsement of the Dachau experiments. Dr. Benzinger also stated that Dr. Strughold was not involved in any of the Dachau experiments, saying, "I never had any reason to believe that" (Department of Justice, Benzinger Deposition of 11/22/83).

In 2006, in response to a Freedom of Information request, the U.S. Department of Justice released their files concerning the investigation of Dr. Strughold to the authors. Over 300 pages of documents were released and support the conclusion that there was no evidence of Dr. Strughold being involved in any war atrocities, being a member of the Nazi party, or being involved in any way to the Dachau experiments. A summary of the review of these documents is below. Research has also revealed that the organization of aeromedical research institutions in Germany during World War II consisted of a complex network controlled by the Luftwaffe (Fig. 9, page 27). Dr. Strughold's institution, the Berlin Aeromedical Research Institute (AMRI), was a peripheral institution without control of or involvement with the institutions that were involved in the Dachau atrocities. He was not the director of all aeromedical research in Germany as has been claimed by many of his accusers.

Summary of Freedom of Information Act Documents from the U.S. Department of Justice

1. A letter to Senator Javits in 1956 (this was after the first investigation) stating that no derogatory information had been found on Dr. Strughold.

2. A letter to Congressman Gonzalez in 1974 stating that after an extensive investigation, no derogatory information had been found and that the INS investigation would therefore be closed.

Letter by Commissioner L. F. Chapman (July 18, 1974) to U.S. Representative Henry Gonzalez, quoting the Senior Prosecutor, War Crimes Prosecution, Central Office, Ludwigsburg, "Results of our inquiry show that Professor Strughold was at no time a concentration camp doctor, but only Director of the Medical Research Institute of Air Travel, a branch of the Airways Ministry of the Reich. This Central Office had made a thorough study of the experiments carried out by the medical research teams operating in the concentration camps, at which time it was found no grounds for suspecting Professor Strughold of any criminal act."

3. A letter discussing an interview with Dr. Leo Alexander in 1978 that strongly stated that Dr. Strughold was not involved in any war crimes and offering to testify in his behalf if needed. This is very important as

Dr. Alexander was the lead prosecutor for the Nuremberg Medical War Crimes Trials in 1947. He spent over two years investigating and prosecuting the doctors involved in any war crimes including all of the Dachau medical experiments.

Memorandum (p.108) from the Department of Justice by Vincent L. Timbone, December 16, 1978: "Strughold, Hubertus, A6 746 941," that contains an interview of Dr. Leo Alexander by Mr. Timbone, October 5, 1978. The memo states that "... Dr. Alexander produced his post-war diary of all interviews he conducted." The memo quotes Dr. Alexander as having "made contemporaneously" his notes with the interviews, and interviewed Dr. Strughold on June 16, 1945. It is stated in the memo: Dr. Strughold first learned of the Dachau "human experiments listed as 'war crimes' at the meeting in Nuremberg..." The memo also provides: "Dr. Alexander stated that he remembered Dr. Strughold 'vividly' and Dr. Strughold was never involved in 'war crimes'. Dr. Alexander emphasized that he would, in fact, testify favorably in behalf of Dr. Strughold."

4. There was also reference to an investigation by Central Agency for the Prosecution of Nazi Crimes in Ludwigsburg, Germany in 1974 that resulted in no derogatory evidence against Dr. Strughold.

5. A report from the FBI that they could not find any derogatory information on Dr. Strughold (1949).

Memo dated January 24, 1949, by Peyton Ford, Assistant to the Attorney General, containing a dossier on Dr. Strughold, received from the Joint Intelligence Objectives Agency of the Joint Chiefs of Staff, included attachments of a letter from the Secretary of the Air Force to the Attorney General (November 17, 1948) and four Federal Bureau of Investigation reports concerning Dr. Strughold (p crm-151). Enclosure No. 495918 states "The enclosed Federal Bureau of Investigation reports reflect that no derogatory information was discovered during the course of the investigation by the Bureau."

6. A report that shows the structure of the various aviation research entities in Germany. The importance is that it was a network system and that Dr. Strughold and his institute was a peripheral player and he did not have any authority over the many other institutes.

Professor Strughold was shown to be the Director of the Aero Medical Institute within the "Air Ministry", Berlin, with Dr. Ruff as Director of a totally separate Institute, the Institute for Aviation Medicine of the German Experimental Establishment for Aviation within the "Controlled Specialist Institutes."

7. Several documents (in German) that were mainly put together on behalf of the investigation in Germany in the 1970´s by the *"Ludwigsburger Zentralstelle zur Verfolgung von Naziverbrechen "* (Central Agency for the prosecution of Nazi crimes in Ludwigsburg, Germany), concluding that no evidence of involvement was found and that the case was closed. However, several pages were of interest:

Files from the GeStaPo-archives (secret service) from Wuerzburg (*Geheime Staatspolizei* GESTAPO) of Nazi-Germany from 1935 and 1934, where he was Professor of Physiology and gave lectures on Aviation Medicine, before he became a civil servant at the Aeromedical Research Institute of the Luftwaffe in Berlin (1935).

The files are from the State-Archives in Munich (*Staatsarchiv München, Gestapo-Akte* Strughold_hubert, Nr. 15720), and were released on 30.05.1980 to the *Staatsanwaltschaft Wuerzburg.*

There is a request by the Bavarian Political Police of 18th March 1935 on reputation, family and financial situation of Strughold as a consequence of his communication with a central agency (assume that it was the HQ of Luftwaffe – *Reichsluftfahrtministerium*).

There is a statement from the Wuerzburg Police Department on 11th April 1935 on his social and financial status and his association with the University teachers association (*Gruppe Deutschnationaler Hochschullehrer*).

There is a telegram from the Wuerzburg Police to the Bavarian Political Police from 7th September 1936 that documents that no negative information on Strughold's political, criminal or other public behaviour is known. Though he was known as member in the Association of National German Lecturers, he was regarded as old-German and monarchistic oriented. He was not a member of the NSDAP (Nazi Party).

8. The transcript from the 1942 "Cold Conference". This is very important as this is the document that everyone claims implicates Dr. Strughold (see the details in the manuscript attached, "Strughold Controversy"). Reading it, there is no indication that Dr. Holzloehner's presentation involved prisoners at all. There follows multiple commentaries from various participants regarding the whole series of lectures previously given (not just Holzloehner's), including one from Dr. Strughold. It is clear that Strughold was referring to the entire group of lectures just given. His comments are very general in any case. We do know that by the end of the conference that it was realized that non volunteers were used as Dr. Strughold and two other participants protested to Dr. Hippke (the Air Force Surgeon General) concerning their use.

"Translation of Document No. NO-401, Office of Chief Counsel For War Crime, REPORT on a conference on 26 and 27 October 1942 in Nurnberg (sic) on Medical Problems Arising from Distress at Sea and Winter Hardships, sponsored by Inspector of Medical Service of the Luftwaffe, Chairman of the Conference: *Stabsartz* Professor Dr. A. J. Anthony." The report lists 95 attendees. The FOI contains an 11 October 1946 memo by the Office of U.S. Chief Counsel, U.S. Army, by H. Sachs, stating: "The meeting was called on instigation of Prof. Dr. Hippko (note: Hippke), the chief of the Medical Service of the Luftwaffe." Dr. Strughold's presentation as contained in the FOI 5 December 1946 memo by Patricia A. Radcliffe, No. 401 (excerpt from official Nuremberg (sic) staff translation), summarized the literature on temperatures contained in sea charts and various seasons important to the sea distress service, covering publications in 1915, 1902, 1921, 1927 and 1928. There is no evidence he sanctioned or participated in the "horrific" Dachau atrocities.

In 2006 a request was made to the Space Medicine Association Executive Committee to remove Dr. Strughold's name from the Strughold award which is given out annually by that organization since 1963 for "dedication and outstanding contributions in advancing the frontiers of Space Medicine". After two years of intense research, that committee met on May 15, 2008 and reviewed the investigation of Dr. Strughold, including the recently released Dept. of Justice files above. It was concluded that there was no incriminating evidence found and that there would be no attempt to remove his name from the Strughold Award. The Wall Street Journal published an article detailing the debate on November 30, 2012.

Col. Harry Armstrong (later USAF Surgeon General), Brig. Gen. Malcolm Grow, Dr. Paul Campbell, and Col. Otis Benson were directly involved with recruiting and clearing German physicians and scientists for aerospace medicine research in the U.S. They also continued to facilitate Strughold's career in the U.S. and were responsible along with other well-known leaders in the Space Medicine Branch in establishing the Strughold Award in 1963. The details of his war activities were well known to these aerospace medicine leaders who, nevertheless, held him in high esteem.

Strughold classified himself as a non-political scientist, an image that was also supported by eye witnesses. He opposed the totalitarian regimes in Nazi Germany as well as in Stalin's USSR. Strughold's publications and correspondences are free from political, ideological or racial content and paint the picture of a stable, purely scientifically active personality. Lifelong he followed a convinced Christian attitude based on a humanistic education. His political background was German nationalist with tendencies to support monarchism, in later life with cosmopolitan tendencies. He was neither perpetrator nor victim of persecution, but participated in terms of scientific support to the military effort in the totalitarian Germany of World War II. His political passivity should not be considered as system-conformity, but he chose this way into military aviation medicine as a non-Nazi-party individual trying to continue his scientific career.

It is important that future debate of Dr. Strughold's World War II activities be carried on with documented and well referenced facts and not with blatantly false information or politically inspired revisionist history. Everyone is entitled to their own opinion, but they are not entitled to their own facts. The Internet and several books criticizing Dr. Stughold have multiple distortions, misrepresentations, and assumed guilt by even casual association. It is highly unlikely that new information will become available in the future concerning Dr. Strughold as the true facts are either already known or will never be known. It is recognized that this issue will continue to be debated and will always be controversial. The Holocaust and the Nazi regime were horrific and any ties to that part of German history, whether real or remote, will always follow Dr. Strughold.

Appendix

Appendix 1. Hypoxia Experiments.

"At the beginning of WW2 German Luftwaffe ordered to stop all aeromedical research concerning altitudes of 7,300 m and higher, although various aviation medical research experiments had already penetrated to altitudes of up to 15,000 m. Pilots were forbidden to fly in altitudes greater than 7,300 m. A year later, after the 'Battle of Britain', the same Air Force facilities requested information on the medical impact of flights over 10,000 m. Fortunately, the research work at the time had not been terminated, so partial recommen-dations could be given immediately."

H. Strughold (1)

Altitude research was performed at several research facilities in Germany in the early part of World War II contemporaneously. Strughold's assistant, Dr. H.G. Clamann reported in 1939 concerning rapid decompression experiments up to an altitude of 15,000 m. Results were comparable to that of the Rechlin research group, who had reached the same altitude even two years earlier (2).

One year prior to the SS Dachau altitude experiments a paper was published by Gauer, Opitz, Palme and Strughold at the Berlin Aeromedical Research Institute (AMRI) on the topic of "parachute jump and reserve time at high altitudes" (*Fallschirmabsprung und Zeitreserve in grossen Hoehen*). The conclusion was that on exiting a plane at high altitude, the parachute should not be opened immediately: The airmen should maintain in freefall until it they reach safer altitudes (3).

The research group of the DVL in Berlin (Romberg, head: Ruff) reported at the same time concerning their altitude chamber research up to 12,000 m altitude. It was also confirmed that the immediate pull of the trigger mechanism after the jump would cause severe altitude sickness and possibly even death. Romberg recommended therefore to open the parachute only after a free fall to a safe altitude (4).

At the Rechlin Research Institute (head: Theodor Benzinger) decompression tests were performed at an even greater altitude than in Berlin. Some 400 rapid and explosive decompressions up to 19,000 m were carried out with a pressure difference of up to 60,000 m / sec. (Fig. 42) (5).

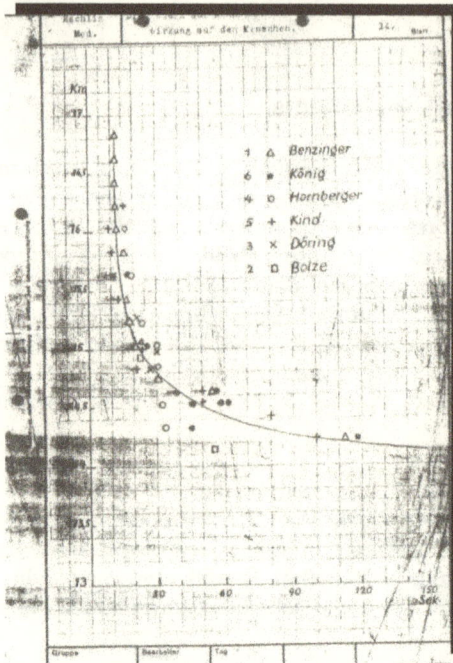

Fig. 42 Altitude exposure in seconds on humans up to 17,000 m.
Private archive T. Benzinger. Harsch, 2007 (unpublished matererial).

Besides a rapid decompression due to technical or infrastructural failure of the airframe the safe use of an ejection seat at high speed and altitude also had to be considered. The last situation resulted in the historian, Dr. Karl Roth, concluding that the Dachau human experiments were needed to solve this "rescue problem" (6). However, the Rechlin pressure "space" suite was not operational in Germany during the war years and Heinkel Corporation ejection-seats were primarily introduced in a limited number of high performance, but not high altitude planes (7).

As mentioned above (3), additional altitude experiments seemed not to be necessary from the Luftwaffe´s perspective. However the DVL Berlin did get involved by passive permission of the Luftwaffe. Why and who made this possible, still remains unclear. The record of the Dachau hypoxia experiments was as followed: SS-Untersturmfuehrer Dr. Sigmund Rascher (1909-1945), an M.D. and Nazi-member, attended an aeromedical course headed by Heinz Kottenhoff as a Luftwaffe reservist at Luftgau VII (Munich) in May 1941. He suggested utilizing inmates of Dachau concentration camps for further aeromedical experiments (8). Although the pressing questions concerning altitude rescue seemed to have already been resolved, in 1942 hypoxia experiments were performed on inmates at the Dachau concentration camp with the knowledge of the Luftwaffe´s Medical Corps Office. Himmler (SS) approved the experiments at Rascher´s request and Hippke (Luftwaffe) agreed to cooperate in case there was an operational need for them (9).

Dr. Weltz, Director of the Institute for Aviation Medicine in Munich, visited Dr. Ruff, the director of the civil DVL Institute of Aviation Medicine in Berlin in early 1942 to find out the status of the ongoing research on altitude rescue issues. There was a lack of volunteer test-subjects, therefore, they agreed to perform additional tests on "volunteering prisoners" utilizing a Berlin stationed mobile altitude chamber (10).

After the chamber was transferred south to Bavaria, the hypoxia experiments were conducted using it by Dr. Rascher (Luftwaffe´s reserve switching to the SS) and Dr. Hans Wolfgang Romberg of the civil Department for Aviation Medicine in the German Experimental Institute for Aviation (DVL) in Berlin-Adlershof. Dr. Weltz and Dr. Ruff were their respective superiors in charge (11).

At the Nuremberg medical trials it was testified that two different series of experiments at Dachau concentration camp were to be distinguished: first the official one under Ruff's supervision (Working Group Romberg/Rascher). This was – to follow the Nuremburg defense's presentation - grew out of the Luftwaffe´s practical needs to rescue aircrews that were unprotected and exposed to high altitudes. Another series of experiments, where deaths occured, were under Rascher's responsibility (12).

When Ruff heard about the casualties, he forced the termination of the experiments (13): "When I heard that Rascher carried out additional experiments under his own responsibility and with his own objectives, at which three deaths had already occurred, I requested the Luftwaffe´s Surgeon General to re-deployment of the mobile altitude chamber, as it was subordinated to the Luftwaffe Medical Corps. This was done immediately after I reported it."

Rascher tried to get the Luftwaffe mobile altitude chamber back for further experiments. The SS intervened at Milch´s Luftwaffe office but was unsuccessful (14). Hippke criticized the scientific value of the Dachau altitude tests shortly after by stating, that cold effects were not taken into account in these experiments and should therefore be continued at AMRI, a cautious distancing from Dachau (15). Also the research groups from Munich and Rechlin dissociated from the Dachau experiments (16).

The Dachau experiments were first kept secret, but later a private screening of a film to selected individuals at the Air Ministry (including Dr. Benzinger) was conducted (17). Dr. Benzinger worked at the Rechlin Test Center, 130 km northwest of Berlin. His superiors were with the Air Material Command, and he was not a part of Dr. Strughold's staff in Berlin (18).

In an historical commentary, Dr. Karl Roth (19) describes a document stating that the Dachau hypoxia experiments were discussed by Ruff and Romberg at the Scientific Meeting of the Members of the German Academy for Aviation Research (*Deutsche Akademie der Luftfahr-tforschung*). Strughold was an Academy member and it is possible that he was present, but there is no evidence of this (20). Due to his co-authorship with Dr. Ruff on the two editions of the Outlines of Aviation Medicine (*Grundriss der Luftfahrtmedizin*) in 1939 and 1944 it is also likely that he was informed about Ruff's participation in the Dachau experiments. In the 1944 textbook additional information on parachute rescue jumps was discussed, but no Dachau experience mentioned (21). Strughold cooperated in some research projects with Ruff before the war. In 1938 he recommended the adoption of Ruff's Habilitation thesis to become a university professor. Ruff however, never became a professor in Berlin. Strughold and Rein believed that this was due to his political abstinence (22). There was some rivalry between the two institutes (AMRI and Berlin DVL) and Ruff possibly expected some advantages from his Dachau research program. The biologist Hansjochem Autrum stated that Strughold refused to use concentration camp inmates for his experiments (23): "We were interrogated by the US specialists about our publications during the war Heidelberg in June or July of 1945 (Dr. Denzer and me, involved in our experiments). On this occasion Strughold told us this background. ... In (1942) a meeting was held in the main office of the SS, at which Strughold had to attend. Here he was asked whether he wanted to make these experiments in vacuum chambers on concentration camp inmates. Strughold rejected this: Animal experiments are much more meaningful, as psychological factors do not influence them. We did not hear of this macabre and horrific background before."

Rascher and his wife were both executed under Himmler's order just before the end of war (24). Drs. Ruff, Romberg, and Weltz were arrested and prosecuted at Nuremburg. All three were acquitted due to the lack of any direct evidence of participation with Dr. Rascher's private experiments (25). Dr. Benzinger was arrested and interrogated, but not prosecuted (26).

Strughold cited von Helmholtz in a 1942 article "that only the values derived on the ground of exact scientific knowledge allows the control of the forces of nature" (27).

Appendix 2. Hypothermia Experiments.

The freezing experiments were conducted by Dr. Holzloehner (who committed suicide at the end of the war), who was a physiologist from the University of Kiel, assisted by Dr. Finke (Luftwaffes Oberarzt at the Westreland Hospital), and again by Dr. Rascher. They had permission from the Air Force Field Marshal Erhard Milch (who was prosecuted in Nuremberg and imprisoned until 1954) and Reichsfuehrer-SS Heinrich Himmler (who committed suicide at the end of the war). The head of the Luftwaffe´s Medical Corps was Surgeon General Dr. Hippke (who was not prosecuted at Nuremburg as his location was not known at the beginning of the Trials). The results of these experiments were not distributed to the Air Force, but were partially presented at a conference, the "Medical Problems of Sea Distress and Winter Emergencies" on October 26,1942 in Nuremburg and then again two months later in Berlin (the Second Conference of Special Medical Consultants from 30th Nov. to 3rd Dec. 1942 at the Military Medical Academy). There is no list of the participants of the second conference in Berlin. It is unknown whether Strughold was present or not.

Over 90 German scientists and physicians attended the first conference, the Nuremburg Winter-Symposium, including Dr. Strughold (1). According to one of the participants: "The afternoon session of the first day seemed to end, as the leader of the discussion announced outside the program that the following presentation was top secret (*geheime Kommandosache*) and who would speak about it outside the meeting and to others than to the conference participants, had to reckon with his execution" (2).

As already shown in the altitude experiments, there was an "official series of experiments" performed because of the Luftwaffe´s interest, but also a second series of experiments performed separately by Dr. Rascher. Implementation of the results from the entire series of hypothermia experiments was deemed necessary by the Luftwaffe to handle the problem of hypothermia in the sea-downed aircrews and to develop a method of re-warming with the further development of appropriate protective clothing (3).

While Dr. Georg A. Weltz conducted animal studies on the issue of cooling and heating in water in February 1942, the Kiel physiology professor, Dr. E. Holzloehner, received a Luftwaffe research contract to examine the "effects of cooling on warm-blooded animals." Dr. Rascher again suggested the use of inmates from the Dachau concentration camp for this trial (4). The finding that Weltz´s animal experiments provided more extensive and reliable results than the Dachau human trials indicates the lack of need for these human experiments (5).

Beginning in August 1942 Holzloehner conducted experiments in collaboration with Dr. Finke and Dr. Rascher utilizing human test subjects. These were the Dachau experiments where several deaths occurred. An official report for the Luftwaffe's medical corps was therefore not officially published (6).

The results of the working group were presented at military medical conferences in 1942 on two occasions. Dr. Holzloehner first lectured on the "Prevention and Treatment of Hypothermia in Water" at the Nuremberg conference on "Medical Problems of Sea Distress and Winter Emergencies" (7) and shortly thereafter in Berlin (8). In addition several presentations by other researchers were conducted on the bioclimatological, physiological and pathological basics of thermal regulation and hypothermia as well as other topics of practical importance (9).

Strughold participated at this meeting and gave the following comment. These comments were made after a series of three presentations by Jarisch, Weltz and Holzloehner.Commentaries were then given by Rascher, Benzinger, Denecke, Lehmann, Wezler, Groose-Brockhoff, Deuticke, Schwiegk, Knothe, von Werz and finally by Strughold (10):

"With regard to this experimental scientific research, but also for the orientation of the sea distress service, it is of interest to know what temperatures are to be counted on in the cases concerned during the various seasons. Dealing with this subject, valuable material with descriptions and sea-charts are already available. The following are the most important literature findings. At the same time, details about the content of the salt in the water are to be found there."

The comments were not, therefore, directed specifically to Dr. Holzloehner's presentation, but were concerning the whole series of lectures.

After the presentation at the Nuremburg conference by Holzloehner and the following remarks given by Rascher, Drs. Strughold, H. Rein and F. Buechner protested against the conduction of the human experiments with the highest ranking Luftwaffe officer at this conference, Dr. Anthony (11). None of these protests were officially documented as they were oral objections only, but several individuals published accounts in the post-war period that the protests occurred and that there were also other individuals at the conference who disagreed with these unethical experiments (12). The famous physiologist, Dr. Otto Gauer, also attended this meeting and later in life told his student, Dr. Kirsch, that all of the top researchers present disapproved of Raschers experiments and behaviour (personal communication with Dr. Harsch).

The reaction of the audience to the Holzloehner presentation remains controversial. Some written sources state, that not all of the participants realized the unethical character of the investigation and believed only the results of distress units were presented (13). For many of the conference participants it was not obvious that the Holzloehner presentation was based on human experiments. It became evident that these were not only results of animal experiments or observations from the German Armed Forces distress service, when the nature of the trials was clarified after the official end of the lecture series - outside of the official program - by SS-doctor Rascher (14).

A critical debate flared up following the statement of Mitscherlich in 1946, that none of the 95 conference participants, most of whom were notable representatives of science, protested against the human experiments. Rein and Buechner discussed on several occasions that this was absolutely not true (15). Rein stated: "The author of the book (Mitscherlich) was not present at the meeting. He would not have forgotten the bitterness and indignation of the scientists who were attending this meeting. The initiator of those experiments, an SS doctor, was immediately recognizable to all as a pure sadist. His 'scientific' staff member, who was also a speaker of that session, was scientifically outlawed from this day forward. Three of those present declared that such experiments are completely meaningless and unscientific and should therefore be omitted. That this was presented in a ´double secret´ meeting seems not to be clear to the author Mitscherlich. It is important that in the conference documents there is a letter from Himmler where he stated: 'People who refuse even today to perform these human experiments, would rather let brave German soldiers die from the effects of hypothermia, I see this as high treason (Hoch- und Landesverrat) and I will not be afraid to call the names of these gentlemen at the appropriate locations.´ The fact that the official record of this memorable session contains nothing about it, only proves how they worked and that no one dared, in such attempts, to inaugurate the real representatives of the science. "The conference speaker, Buechner, accused Holzloehner of the "ethical impossibility" of his human experiments and thought that he had broken with the tradition of medical ethics to only perform dangerous investigations with self-experiments or experiments using human volunteers. Buechner expressed his "indignation and horror" over the human trials that he discussed with Weltz, "even when it was communicated that the test subjects were volunteering because they were criminals with a death penalty and having the choice to rehabilitation" (16). Dr. Hippke (Luftwaffe Surgeon General) explained the attitude of the participants after the second conference in Berlin (6): "Holzloehner reported again about hypothermia treatment, I was present at this lecture as a listener and can recall, that the Luftwaffe doctors, including Rein and Buechner, disapproved experiments on prisoners, even though the occurrence of deaths in the trials of the lecture was not evident. One of these doctors, it was probably Professor Buechner, came later in my office to talk to me and was disaproving of these experiments. I did not consider that as a formal objection, especially as such it would have been to be written down and to be answered officially in a printed letter. According to Rein, German scientists and physiologists terminated their collegial relationship with Holzloehner after these experiments came to their knowledge.

Buechner stated in his 1965 book, "Plans and Coincedence. Memoirs of a German University Teacher" *(Plaene und Fuegungen. Lebenserinnerungen eines deutschen Hochschullehrers)*, that three senior doctors *(Beratende Aerzte)* were unanimous in their rejection of the mentioned human trials (17): "In the foyer Hermann Rein, Hubertus Strughold, and myself [Buechner] and also other doctors one after another objected to the senior medical officer of the Luftwaffe emphatic objection to Luftwaffe doctors participating in such experiments in cooperation with SS officers."

On the basis of the Nuremberg congress findings (not only on the Holzloehner presentation) the Luftwaffe ordered that the operational flight surgeons should use the warm bath therapy to rewarm as part of the resuscitation procedure for cases of hypothermia (18):

> The method of rapid and intensive rewarming in a hot water bath of
> 45°C (40°C-50°C) of people in shock from exposure to cold,
> especially in water, should be immediately adopted as the treatment
> of choice by the Air-Sea Rescue Services of the United States Armed
> Forces. The victims should be undressed, immersed in this bath for
> 10 minutes, and then rubbed dry with towels, and placed in heated
> blankets. If the body temperature does than not continue to rise, the
> hat water treatment should be repeated, until the curve of
> rewarming ascends uniformly by at least one degree every two
> minutes. Collapsible bathing facilities for this purpose should be
> provided so as to be available even in small ships; the necessary hot
> water should be available on all engine driven craft. If large number
> of victims are rescued at once and overtax existing bathing facilities,
> hot water of 50°C – 60°C should be poured at intervals over those
> waiting for the definitive hot water treatment.

U.S. psychiatrist Major Leo Alexander reported in "The Treatment of Shock from Prolonged Exposure to Cold, - Especially in Water" of a meeting with Strughold and Rein at the Physiological Institute in Goetingen in June 1945. This report (called the "Alexander Report") was over 220 pages long and detailed his two year investigation into the Dachau experiments as part of the prosecution team for the post war medical war crimes trials at Nuremburg (Robert S. Pozos, Military Medical Ethics). The Alexander Report is very detailed in exactly who was involved in Dachau and the abundant evidence that was collected from Himmler's cave depository of SS materials captured in

Hallein, Germany. When asked about human hypothermia experiments, Strughold admitted that he knew of this from the Nuremberg winter meeting (19).

Strughold stated to Alexander, that he rejected these experiments on non- volunteers (20): "I've even forbidden thoughts about such experiments at my Institute for moral and medically ethical reasons. For experiments, we used only on a voluntary basis institute members and interested students for our trials."

The Dept. of Justice interviewed Dr. Alexander in 1978 as part of an investigation of Dr. Strughold. Dr. Alexander stated, "He was never involved in any war crimes. No allegations were made against Dr. Strughold from any source." He emphasized that he would testify favorably in behalf of Dr. Strughold if requested (Dept of Justice memo dated 10/16/78).

Appendix 3. Salt Water Drinking Experiments

The sea water experiments were conducted by Dr. Becker-Freyseng (a former assistant of Dr. Strughold's several years before the experiments took place) and Dr. Beiglboeck (from the Department of Aviation Medicine in the Surgeon General's Office of the Luftwaffe) (1). Both were not from Dr. Strughold's Institute at the time of the experiments. Dr. Schaefer (from the Medical Experimental and Instructional Division in Jueterbog) was under Dr. Strughold earlier in the war, but was detached by order of the Surgeon General of the Air Force (Dr. Schroeder, who had replaced Dr. Hippke) to work on the sea water experiments because of his expertise in making sea water drinkable using silver (2).

Dr. K. Schaefer was appointed by the Luftwaffe in the spring of 1942 to investigate the development of thirst and its control, when he was a deputy assistant researcher (*Unterassistent*) at the AMRI (3). In November 1943 he already developed a desalination method, called the Schaefer-agent. At the same time the Berka agent was being tested at the Luftwaffe hospital in Vienna, which only neutralized the taste of sea water. The Luftwaffe´s medical inspection (*Sanitaetsinspektion*) preferred the use of the Schaefer-agent, and pointed out the ineffectiveness and dangers of the Berka-agent. On the other hand, the Technical Department of the Air Force (*Technisches Amt*), which was responsible for the compilation of aircraft equipment, preferred the distribution of the Berka -agent due to the scarcity of raw materials needed for the Schaefer-agent. Since both of the Luftwaffe´s departments could not agree, in late May 1944 a clinical examination of the Berka-agent was initiated on its effectiveness. Professor Eppinger had previously presented the thesis that the Berka-agent could possibly affect the concentration ability of the kidneys in a positive way, which would allow the ingestion of larger quantities of sea water without damage to the organism (4).

Schaefer attended a planning meeting on the experiments in May 1944 at the German Air Ministry. At the Nuremburg Trials, Dr. Schaefer testified that he opposed the experiments, but was threatened that his behavior would be considered an act of sabotage (5).

The 40 designated test-subjects were brought specifically for this experiment from the Buchenwald concentration camp. They were transferred to Dachau with the prospect of an improvement in their conditions. The tests were designed to last for 12 days, but were canceled in many instances when health problems occurred in test subjects after less than a week. The reason why test subjects were chosen from concentration camp inmates was justified by the Luftwaffe, as they claimed that they did not have a sufficient number of volunteers from the German Air Force in 1944 to support for several weeks the scientific research that was needed (6).

There were no deaths in the prolonged exposure to salt water experiments, but serious complications and injuries did occur. Because of the torturous, unethical character of these experiments, Dr. Schroeder was convicted and sentenced to life imprisonment at the Nuremburg Trials, Dr. Becker-Freyseng was convicted and sentenced to 20 years, Dr. Beiglboeck was convicted and sentenced to 15 years, and Dr. Schaefer was acquitted (7). After the verdict documents were found with voluntary statements from some of the participants of the seawater experiments (8).

Appendix 4. The Hypoxia-experiments on Children at AMRI- Berlin.

In 1993, Koch reported that six children aged 11-13 from the psychiatry clinic in Brandenburg-Goerden were tested in an altitude chamber using oxygen-reduced gas mixtures (mild hypoxia). We can assume that there was no informed consent. These tests were carried out at the Strughold directed Aeromedical Research Institute (AMRI) in Berlin on September 17, 1943 (1). The altitude was up to 6,000 m. The trial managers were in the chamber with the youths and they could add oxygen if required at any time. Seizures were not observed (2).

The biologist, Dr. Hans Nachtsheim, performed research during the war on epilepsy in cooperation with Dr. Ruhenstroth-Bauer from the KWI (Kaiser Wilhelm Institute) for Biochemistry. The director of this institute was Dr. Adolf Butenand, a Nobel Prize winner from 1939. About 150 experiments were performed on rabbits beginning in the spring of 1943 (3). This research was sponsored by the *"Reichsforschungsrat"* (German Reich Research Council) and prioritized with the third highest urgency level. (4). Use of the AMRI altitude chamber inducing epileptic seizures in animals (rabbits) had started in June 1943. Ruhenstroth-Bauer liaised with Wuhlgarten, who suggested to use children for the hypoxia experiments from the Goerden psychiatric clinic with its so-called *"Forschungs- und Beobachtungsstation"* (research and observation ward), connected close to Nazi´s euthanasia-program (5). OMR (*Obermedizinalrat*) Dr. Karl Brockhausen made 6 epileptic children available for the experiments at an altitude chamber of the AMRI on September 17, 1943 (6). The children were 11 to 13 years old and were exposed to an altitude up to 4,000 to 6,000 m. The experiments "failed", as no seizure occurred (7): Therefore, the researchers expressed a desire to use younger children (5-6 years old), an age not presently "available" in Goerden. There is no evidence that other human experiments were ever carried out.

The introduction of the 1944 article of Ruhenstroth-Bauer and Nachtsheim on animal experiments stated (8): "For the experimentally working clinicians treating patients the methodological possibilities are always limited, as they should take the patients well-being into consideration. Only in exceptional cases, a researcher could dare in one patient a trial in the interests of future patients, whereof he cannot predict anything certain."

Dr. Gerhard Ruhenstroth-Bauer stated in 2000 (9): "Together with Professor Hans Nachtsheim, I carried out experiments with epileptic adolescents. I would like to stress that in every case Dr. Nachtsheim, a Luftwaffe doctor, and I went up into the vacuum chamber with the children. For each participant with nausea, immediately a supply of oxygen could be applied or the exam could be canceled. This did not occur in any case: on the contrary, the children talked almost cheerfully among themselves and also with

Dr. Nachtsheim. Since no seizure occurred, we finished these experiments and had the impression that the problem concerning "oxygen deficiency in epileptic adolescents" was finished. Now, after more than 60 years, this assumption turned out to be wrong. In my correspondence with Mr. Klee I was made aware of the fact that the institution in Goerden represented an "euthanasia" institution. Understandably, this revelation shook me hard." However, the psychiatric wards were quite well known as questionable treating facilities. Though it is mentioned that no test subject was hurt, Beddies reports that in one test subject a facial cyanosis of the mucous membranes is mentioned as well as a mild dizziness (10).

The medical historian, Von Schwerin, concludes: The experiments with the children from Goerden are not comparable with those of criminal medical experiments that are known mainly from the concentration camps where the death of the subjects participated was anticipated. These experimemts are rather an example of biomedical experimental practice on a daily basis. But the limits of this practice were being exceeded in National Socialism and the boundries stretched (11). Weindling named them *"fremdnuetzige Forschung an nicht einwilligungsfaehigen Patienten"* (research for the benefit of others on patients, who could not give an informed consent) (12).

Dr. Strughold was the head of the institute providing the infrastructure (the AMRI altitude chamber) on September 17, 1943. He was not part of the experiments and did not use its results to our knowledge. The children were not harmed or seriously endangered according to the literature. However, these kinds of experiments were against the medical ethical understanding in Germany as published in 1931. There is no evidence that Strughold knew of, approved of or allowed the children experiments to take place at the AMRI, but it has been assumed. For this reason the termination of the scientific prize of the German Society for Aviation and Space Medicine (DGLRM) was a decision made in Germany in 2004 (13).

Dr. Werner Noell wrote about the special physiology of the brain during anoxia in "German Aviation Medicine in World War II", that was prepared under the auspices of the Surgeon General, U.S. Air Force in 1950. Based upon animal experiments, the state of recognition of anoxia physiology was written in the first article (14). His second article dealt with the human EEG during anoxia (15). Gremmler's experiments on epileptic patients were also mentioned (16). They "showed that their altitude tolerance did not differ markedly from that of normal people." (17). Kornmueller, Palme and Strughold had already performed investigations of anoxia at altitudes up to 7.500 m and published their results in 1941 (18). Notes on problematic human experiments on adults or children are not found in any of these sources.

Appendix 5. Internet Links.

Factual Internet Sites

Nuremberg Attachment 7
http://www.gwu.edu/~nsarchiv/radiation/dir/mstreet/commeet/meet13/brief13/tab_f/br13f3g.txt

Advisory Committee on Human Radiation Experiments
http://www.gwu.edu/~nsarchiv/radiation/dir/mstreet/commeet/meet13/brief13/tab_f/br13f3.txt

Nuremberg
http://www.ushmm.org/research/doctors/indiptx.htm

Encyclopedia of Astrobiology
http://www.daviddarling.info/encyclopedia/S/Strughold.html

International Space Hall of Fame
http://www.spacefame.org/strughold.html

NASA - Beginnings of Space Medicine
http://www.hq.nasa.gov/office/pao/History/SP-4201/ch2-2.htm

Today in Science
http://www.todayinsci.com/cgi-bin/indexpage.pl?http://www.todayinsci.com/6/6_15.htm

Nuremberg Doctor Trials
http://www.gpc.edu/~shale/humanities/composition/assignments/experiment/nazi.html

Brooks AFB History with Oral History Links
http://www.brooks.af.mil/history/people.html

Appear Factual, But Distortions Present

Wikipedia
en.wikipedia.org/wiki/Hubertus_Strughold
-Minor distortion in that Dr. Strughold worked for NASA and trained the flight surgeons for Apollo
Operation Paperclip
http://www.daviddarling.info/encyclopedia/P/Paperclip.html
-Dr. Strughold was a Nazi and in charge at Dachau

Probert Encyclopaedia
http://www.probertencyclopaedia.com/C6D.HTM
-Dr. Strughold was a Nazi, in charge at Dachau, was knowingly protected at Nuremberg Trials, and
performed unethical and erroneous research in the U.S.

Jews Protest Nazi Portrait Among Medical Heroes at Ohio Stat University
http://www.fscwv.edu/users/pedwards/jews_protest_nazi_portrait_among.htm
-Minor distortion as it claims that Dr. Strughold was a Nazi

Anti Defamation League Press Release Concerning New Mexico Space Hall of Fame
http://www.adl.org/PresRele/HolNa_52/4918_52.htm
-Dr. Strughold was a Nazi, directed the Dachau experiments

Anti Defamation League Press Release Concerning Brooks AFB Aeromedical Library
http://www.adl.org/presrele/HolNa_52/2533_52.asp
-Minor distortion in that it quotes the Air Force as a making a statement (that was really coming from the ADL)

Several sites state that Dr. Strughold was a Nazi, directed the Dachau experiments and was involved in Mind Control experiments in Dachau and the U.S. (Obvious Gross Distortions):

Drug (Mind Control) Experiments in Dachau and the U.S. by Strughold
http://www.beyondweird.com/ufos/Bruce_Walton_The_Underground_Nazi_Invasion_52.html

Dachau and US Drug Experiments
http://coat.ncf.ca/our_magazine/links/issue43/articles/mkultra.htm

In Charge at Dachau and Involved in Mind Control Research
http://www.perspectives.com/forums/forum71/29700.html

Mind Control Experiments in Dachau and US
http://www.deepblacklies.co.uk/some_aspects_of_a-pem_weapons.htm

Mind Control Experiments in Dachau and US
www.sonic.net/sentinel/gvcon8.html

Nazi Scientist Involved in Mind Control
http://coat.ncf.ca/our_magazine/links/issue43/articles/mkultra.htm#strughold

Michael E. Kresa Article
http://www.lewrockwell.com/orig/kreca1.html

Mind Control Experiments
http://www.paranormalnews.com/textfiles/ufos/Bruce_Walton_The_Underground_Nazi_Invasion_52.txt

Additional Gross Distortions:

Project Paperclip
http://news.bbc.co.uk/1/hi/magazine/4443934.stm
-Dr. Strughold in charge at Dachau

Sought for at Nuremberg but Released
http://www.jewishsf.com/content/2-0-
/module/displaystory/story_id/2123/edition_id/34/format/html/displaystory.html
-Dr. Strughold was a Nazi and secretly brought to the U.S.

Discarded Lies
http://discardedlies.com/entries/2005/04/wooing_the_nazis.php
-Dr. Strughold was a Nazi, involved in Dachau, and protected at the Nuremberg Trials

UFO Examining MD 1947
http://www.majesticdocuments.com/personnel/benson.php
-Dr. Strughold was present when aliens landed in Roswell, NM in 1947

Roswell 1947
http://home.fuse.net/arcsite/paperclip.htm
-Dr. Strughold was present when aliens landed in Roswell, NM in 1947

Radiation Experiments in Houston
http://members.tripod.com/~cactus_ian/bayou_body_snatchers.html
- Dr Strughold was involved in unethical radiation experiments in Houston in the 1950's

Documents

1. Offices and service positions (1927-1968)

1927 Habilitation and (private) Lecturer at the University of Wuerzburg.

1928/9 Research activity in the United States on a scholarship from the Rockefeller Foundation/Fellowship.

1930 Lecturer for aviation physiology in Wuerzburg (7th July 1930).

1933 Associate Professor of Physiology in Wuerzburg (13th March 1933).

1935 Head of Research Institute of Aviation Medicine of the Air Ministry (RLM) in Berlin, Professor of physiology and lecturer in aviation medicine at the University of Berlin. Regierungsrat, 1936 promotion to Oberregierungsrat (senior executive officer).

1938 Promotion to the rank of a Assistant Physician of Luftwaffe Reserve Corps Awarding of a seat and vote in the Medical Faculty of the University of Berlin.

1939 Associate Professor of Physiology (20th Nov.1939).

1942 Director of the Aviation Medical Research Institute of the RLM (Jan. 15, 1942).

1945 Promoted to Colonel M.C. of Luftwaffe (30th Jan.1945).

1945/6 Senior Scientist at Heidelberg Aero Medical Center of USAAF

1946-9 Professor of Physiology and Director of the Physiological Institute of the University of Heidelberg.

1947-9 Scientific Advisor to the Commander of the USAF School of Aviation Medicine at Randolph Field (Texas).

1949-57 Head of the Department of Space Medicine at the USAF School of Aviation Medicine at Randolph Field (Texas).

1951 Appointed professor of aerospace medicine at the USAF Air University, School of Aviation Medicine, Randolph AFB (Texas).

1958 Appointed Professor of Space Medicine at the Air University USAF, School of Aviation Medicine, Randolph AFB (Texas).

1959 President of the Space Medicine Branch of the Aero Medical Association.

1959-61 Advisor for biomedical research at the USAF Aerospace Medical Center, Air Training Command, Brooks AFB (Texas).

1960 Chairman of the Advanced Studies Group at the Aerospace Medical Center Brooks AFB (Texas).

1962-8 Chief Scientist of the Aerospace Medical Division (AFSC), Brooks AFB (Texas).

2. Honors and Awards

1939 Royal Yugoslavian Order of St. Sava Class IV.
1941 War Merit Cross 2nd Class with swords.
1942 War Merit Cross, 1st Class with swords.
    2nd Commander of the Order Class of the Royal Swedish Order of Vasa.
1943 Middle Cross of the Order of the Hungarian Holy Crown.
1952 "Fellow" of the American Association for the Advancement of Science.
1954 Hermann-Oberth Medal of the German Rocket Society.
1958 Air Force Exceptional Civilian Service Award for his research in space medicine.
1958 Theodore C. Lyster Award of the Aerospace Medical Association "for outstanding
    achievement in the general field of Aerospace Medicine.
1958 John J. Jeffries Award from the Institute of Aeronautical Science "for
    outstanding contributions to the advancement of aero-medical research. "
1958 "Fellow" of the Aerospace Medical Association (later the ASMS), "who have made
    outstanding contributions to aerospace medicine, aeronautics, astronautics,
    undersea medicine or either in research, in the practical usage of research,
    or by precept and example."
1958 Federal Civil Servant of the Year, awarded by the Society for Personnel
    Administration, San Antonio Chapter for Outstanding Service (Texas).
1958 Named Alcalde (Mayor) of La Villita of San Antonio (Texas).
1960 Appointed Honorary Admiral of the Texas Navy.
1963 Air Force Scientific Achievement Award.
1964 Melbourne W. Boynton Award from the American Astronautical Society
    "for distinguished contributing research for the safety of aerospace flight. "
1964 "Bronze Plaque" of the USAF School of Aerospace Medicine (Texas) for 15-year
    aerospace-medical activities.
1964 "Golden Plate" of the American Academy of Achievement, "representing the
    many who excel in the great fields of endeavor."
1965 Louis H. Bauer Award from the Aerospace Medical Association "for the most
    significant contribution in aerospace medicine."
1965 The House of Representatives of the State of Texas adopted a resolution (No. 539
    HSR) citing Strughold for his numerous and significant contributions to space
    medicine and for the role he has played in making possible United States
    Achievements in Space.
1966 Outstanding Scientific Award of the Peace and International Ambassadors'
    Council.
1968 Exceptional Service Decoration for the USAF "extraordinary creative thinking,
    unusual keen perception and analysis of scientific development Which Significantly
    contributed to the advancement of knowledge in the field of aerospace medicine.
1970 "A Grand Knight of Mark Twain" Mark Twain Journal in recognition of his
    Outstanding Contribution to Modern Medical Science.
1972 Louis W. Hill Transportation Award from the American Institute of Aeronautics
    and Astronautics for significant contributions of American enterprise and ingenuity
    indicative in the art and science of space travel.
1973 Americanism Medal of the San Antonio Chapter, Daughters of the American
    Revolution "for outstanding contributions to the advancement of the American
    principles of freedom, justice and equality by a naturalized citizen."

1977 renaming of the Medical Library at the flight Brooks AFB (Texas) in
"Hubertus Strughold Aerospace Medical Library."
1978 recording Strughold name in the "International Space Hall of Fame" in
Alamogordo (New Mexico).
1983 Great Cross of Merit of the Federal Republic of Germany on the occasion of the
85th Birthday.

3. Memberships in scientific societies

Scientific Society for Aeronautics (WGL) since 1927.
German Physiological Society since 1935.
(German) Society for Cardiovascular Research since 1935.
Lilienthal Society 1936-45 (no representative post).
German Academy of Aeronautical Research 1936-45 (since April 1937 corresponding
member and deputy chairman for Aviation Medicine).
German Society for Aerospace Medicine (1943-45).
German Academy of Natural Scientists Leopoldina in Halle (Saale) in 1941.
Academy of Sciences of the University of Heidelberg since 1946.
Honorary Member of the German Society for Aviation and Space Medicine
(DGLRM) 1962.
Honorary Member of the German Society for Space Research.
Aero(space) Medical Association (USA), 1937 Honorary Member, 1958 Fellow.
Space Medicine Branch of Aerospace Medical Association, Charter Member,
1958-1959 President-Elect, 1959-1960 President.
Aerospace Medical Division, Advanced Studies Planning Group, Chairman.
American Association for the Advancement of Science Fellow.
American Astronautical Society.
American Institute of Aeronautics and Astronautics, Fellow.
American Rocket Society, Fellow (Senior Member).
American Rocket Society Space Flight Technical Committee.
American Physiological Society.
Pan American Medical Association (PAMA): North American vice president in the
Section of Space Medicine and Biology.
International Astronautical Federation (IAF).
Bioastronautics Committee of the International Astronautical Federation (IAF).
International Academy of Astronautics (IAA), corresponding member.
Lunar International Laboratory (LIL) Committee of the International Academy
of Astronautics (IAA).
International Academy of Aviation and Space Medicine.
International Mars Committee.
Royal Aero Club of Spain, an honorary member since 1964.
Sociedade Brasileira Interplanetaria, Life Member.
The Torch Club, San Antonio (Texas).
AC Cheruskia Munster (a.o.).

4. Hubertus Strughold Award from the Space Medicine Branch of the AsMA

The "Hubertus Strughold Award" was established by the Space Medicine Branch
(now Association), a constituent organization of the Aerospace Medical Association,
in honor of Dr. Hubertus Strughold, the "Father of Space Medicine", in 1962. It is
bestowed annually since 1963 to a member of the Space Medicine Branch awarded for an
outstanding contribution in the field of space-related medical research and application.
There are the following receipients of the award:

1963 Cpt. Ashton Graybiel, Cpt. M.D., USN
1964 Maj.Gen. Otis O. Benson, Jr., USAF, M.C.
1965 Hans-Georg Clamann, M.D.
1966 Hermann J. Schaefer, Ph.D.
1967 Charles A. Berry, M.D.
1968 David G. Simons, M.D.
1969 Col. Stanley C. White, USAF, M.C.
1970 RearAdm Frank B. Voris, MC, USN
1971 Dr. Don Fickinger
1972 Paul Campbell, M.D.
1971 Don Fickering, M.D.
1972 Col. Paul A. Campbell, USAF (Ret.)
1973 I. Andres Karstens, M.D.
1974 Cdr. Joseph P. Kerwin, MC, USN
1975 Lawrence F. Dietlein, M.D.
1976 Harald J. von Beckh
1977 William K. Douglas
1978 Walton L. Jones, Jr., M.D.
1979 Col. John E. Pickering, USAF (Ret.)
1980 Rufus R. Hessberg, M.D.
1981 MajGen Heinz S. Fuchs, GAF, MC (Ret.)
1982 Sidney D. Leverett, Jr., Ph.D.
1983 Sherman Vonograd P., M.D.
1984 Arnauld E. Nicogossian, M.D.
1985 Philip C. Johnson, Jr., M.D.
1986 S. Carolyn Leach Huntoon, Ph.D.

1987 Karl E. Klein, M.D.
1988 Anatoly I. Grigoriev, M.D.
1989 Brig.Gen. Eduard C. Burchard, GAF, MC
1990 Joan Vernikos-Danellis, M.D.
1991 Stanley R. Mohler, M.D.
1992 Roberta L. Bondar, M.D.
1993 Wyckliffe G. Hoffler, M.D.
1994 Emmett B. Ferguson, M.D.
1995 Mary Anne Basset Frey, Ph.D.
1996 Norman E. Thagard, M.D.
1997 Shannon W. Lucid, Ph.D.
1998 Valery V. Polyakov, M. D.
1999 Sam L. Pool, M.D.
2000 Story Musgrave, M.D.
2001 John B. Charles, Ph.D.
2002 Earl H. Wood, MD, Ph.D.
2003 Jonathan Clark (for STS 107 crew)
2005 William S. Augerson, M.D.
2006 Jeff Davis, M.D.
2007 Clarence Jernigan, M.D.
2008 Richard Jennings, M.D.
2009 Jim Vanderploeg, M.D.
2010 Irene Long, M.D.
2011 Michael Barratt, M.D.
2012 Smith Johnston, M.D.

5. Hubertus Strughold prizee of the German Society for Aviation and Space Medicine DGLRM (Deutsche Gesellschaft fuerLuft- und Raumfahrtmedizin)

The Board and Advisory Committee of the German Society for Aviation and Space Medicine (DGLRM) adopt by statute, the awarding of the Hubertus Strughold Award in recognition of outstanding scientific achievements in research and teaching in the field of aviation and space medicine. The previous winners were (since 1997 the price was discontinued due to political and media pressure):

Rudolf von Baumgarten 1994
Harald von Beckh 1985
Horst Buecker 1995
Hans G. Clamann 1977
Heinz Diringshofen of 1976 (posthumously)
Heinz S. Fuchs 1989
Otto H. Gauer 1978
Siegfried J. Gerathewohl 1982
Henning E. von Gierke, 1980
Emil Heinz Graul 1988
Heinz Haber 1987
James P. Henry 1990
Siegmund Jaehn 1993
Karl-Egon Klein 1996
Erwin A. Lauschner 1983
Bruno H. C. Mueller 1984
Siegfried Ruff 1978

6. List of lectures and courses of Hubertus Strughold (1927-1947)

Julius-Maximilians-University Wuerzburg, 1927-1935.

Summer term 1927 (assistant):
The physiology of reproduction, growth, and the restitution of the people in the light of th doctrine of internal secretion.
General Physiology (Introduction to basic concepts of physiology).

Winter term 1927/28:
Physiology of the central nervous system and sensory organs in humans.
Neurophysiological work in the laboratory.

Summer term 1928 (Associate Professor):
Flight physiology of humans for medical practitioners, scientists and pilots.
Neurophysiological work in the laboratory.

Winter term 1928/29 and summer term 1929:
On leave to U.S.A.

Winter term 1929/30:
Physiology of the central nervous system.
Physiological exercises along with walking. Advice of Professor Frey and Dr. H. Schriever
Physiological studies.

Summer term 1930:
Physiology of circulation and respiration.
Flight physiology of the human with special emphasis on air and seasickness for
physicians, scientists and flight engineers.
Physiological exercises along with walking. Advice of Professor Frey and Dr. H. Schriever
Physiological exercises for students of dentistry together with walking. Advice of Professor
Frey and Dr. H. Schriever.
Physiological studies.

Winter term 1930/31:
Physiology of the sense organs.
Flight physiology of the human with special emphasis on air and sea sickness.
Physiological exercises along with walking. Advice of Professor Frey and Dr. H. Schriever
Physiological studies.

Summer term 1931:
Physiology of circulation and respiration, with demonstrations.
Flight physiology of the human with special emphasis on air-and sea-sickness (with
demonstration at the airport) for physicians, scientists and flight engineers.
Physiological exercises along with walking. Advice of Professor Frey and Dr. H. Schriever
Physiological exercises for students of dentistry together with walking. Advice of Professor
Frey and Privatdoz. Dr. H. Schriever.
Physiological studies.

Winter term 1931/32:
Physiology of the central nervous system.
Flight physiology of the human with special emphasis on air and sea sickness.
Physiological exercises along with walking. Advice of Professor Frey and Dr. H. Schriever.
Physiological studies.

Summer term 1932:
Physiology of circulation and respiration.
Flight physiology of the human with special emphasis on air and seasickness
(With demonstration at the airport) for physicians, scientists and flight engineers.
Physiological exercises along with walking. Advice of Professor Frey and Dr. H. Schriever.

Winter term 1932/33:
Physiology of the central nervous system.
Physiology for Dentists Part I (blood circulation, nutrition, metabolism, excretion).
Physiological exercises together with Prof. Dr. Woehlisch and Dr. H. Schriever.
Physiological training for dental professionals together with Dr. H. Schriever.

Summer term 1933:
Physical exercises, physical part together with Prof. Dr. Woehlisch
Physiology of the vitamins and hormones.
Physiology for students of dentistry. Animal part (muscle, nerve, electrophysiology and
sensory organs).

Winter term 1933/34 (AONB professor of physiology, with tenure of Flight Physiology):
Physiology of the sense organs.
Physiological exercises together with Prof. Dr. Woehlisch and Privatdoz. Dr. H. Schriever.
Physiology for Dentists Part I (blood circulation, nutrition, metabolism, excretion).

Summer term 1934:
Physiological exercises together with Prof. Dr. Woehlisch and Dr. H. Schriever.
Flight physiology.
Physiology for students of dentistry. Animal part (muscle, nerve, electrophysiology and
sensory organs).

Winter term 1934/35:
Physiology of the sense organs.
Flight physiology of man.

Friedrich-Wilhelms-University of Berlin (1935 -1945).

Winter term 1935/36:
No information.

Summer term 1936 and winter term 1937/38:
Aviation Medicine (at Military Medical Academy).

Summer term 1938 until winter term 1939/40:
No information; (Aviation Medicine Course - held by Strughold as part of experimental physiology lecture at the Physiological Institute of Trendelenburg - No. 318).

Summer term 1940:
1st Aviation Medicine (Physiological Institute).
2nd Aviation Medical exercises with S Ruff (DVL) and HG Clamann (AMRI)

Winter term 1940/41 and summer term 1941:
No information; Aviation Medicine in May 1941. Guest lectures in Hungary:
Budapest and Debrezcen.

Winter term 1941/42
Aviation medical training (No. 217)

Summer term 1942 until winter term 1944/45:
No information in university archives, in April 1942, guest lecturer in aviation medicine in Rome, Italy as well as questionable in the winter half of 1943 in Sofia, Bulgaria.

University of Heidelberg (1946 – 1949).

Summer term 1946 until winter term 1946/7:
No information in University archives.

Summer term 1947:
Physiological internship with H. Gauer.

Winter term 1947/48 until summer term 1949:
Leave to the USA.

7.   Adress by J. F. Kennedy on 21th Nov. 1963 at Brooks AFB, Tx.

ADDRESS BY
THE PRESIDENT OF THE UNITED STATES
JOHN F. KENNEDY

at

DEDICATION CEREMONY
BROOKS AIR FORCE BASE, TEXAS
November 21, 1963

Mr. Secretary, Governor, Mr. Vice President, Senator, Members of the Congress, members of the military, ladies and gentlemen.

For more than three years, I have spoken about the New Frontier. This is not a partisan term, and it is not the exclusive property of Republicans or Democrats. It refers instead to this nation's place in history, to the fact that we do stand on the edge of a great new era filled with both crises and opportunity, an era to be characterized by achievements and by challenge. It is an era which calls for action, and for the best efforts of all those who would test the unknown and the uncertain in every phase of human endeavor. It is a time for pathfinders and pioneers.

I have come to Texas today to salute an outstanding group of pioneers—the men who man the Brooks Air Force Base School of Aerospace Medicine and the Aerospace Medical Center. It is fitting that San Antonio should be the site of this Center and this School as we gather to dedicate this complex of buildings. For this city has long been the home of the pioneers in the air; it was here that Sidney Brooks, whose memory we honor today, was born and raised. It was here that Charles Lindbergh and Claire Chennault and a host of others who in World War I and World War II and Korea, and even today, have helped demonstrate American mastery of the sky, trained at Kelly Field and Randolph Field, which form a major part of aviation history. And in the new frontier of outer space, while headlines may be made by others in other places, history is being made every day by the men and women of the Aerospace Medical Center without whom there could be no history.

Many Americans make the mistake of assuming that space research has no value here on earth. Nothing could be further from the truth. Just as the wartime development of radar gave us the transistor and all that it made possible, so research in space medicine holds the promise of substantial benefit to those of us who are earthbound. For our effort in space is not, as some have suggested, a competitor for the natural resources that we need to develop the earth, it is a working partner and a coproducer of these resources. And nothing makes this clearer than the fact that medicine in space is going to make our lives healthier, and happier here on earth. I give you three examples.

First, medical space research may open up new understanding of man's relation to his environment. Examination of the astronauts' physical and mental and emotional reactions can teach us more about the differences between normal and abnormal, about the causes and effects of disorientation, in metabolism which could result in extending the life span. When you study effects on our astronauts of exhaust gases which can contaminate their environment, and seek ways to alter these gases so to reduce their toxicity, you are working on problems similar to those we face in our great urban centers which themselves are being corrupted by gases and which must be cleared.

Second, medical space research may revolutionize the technology and the techniques of modern medicine. Whatever new devices are created, for example, to monitor our astronauts—to measure their heart activity, their breathing, their brain waves, and their eye motions at great distances and under difficult conditions, will also represent a major advance in general medical instrumentation.

Heart patients may even be able to wear a light monitor which will sound a warning if their activity exceeds certain limits. An instrument recently developed to record automatically the impact of acceleration upon an astronaut's eyes, will also be of help to small children who are suffering miserably from eye defects, but are unable to describe their impairment. And also by the use of instruments similar to those used in Project MERCURY, this nation's private as well as public nursing services are being improved, enabling one nurse now to give more critically ill patients greater attention than they ever could in the past.

Third, medical space research may lead to new safeguards against hazards common to many environments. Specifically, our astronauts will need fundamentally new devices to protect them from the ill effects of radiation, which can have a profound influence upon medicine and man's relation to our present environment.

Here at this Center we have the laboratories, the talent, the resources to give new impetus to vital research in the life sciences. I am not suggesting that the entire space program is justified alone by what is done in medicine. The space program stands on its own as a contribution to national strength. And last Saturday at Cape Canaveral I saw our new Saturn C-1 rocket booster which, with its payload when it rises in December of this year, will be for the first time the largest booster in the world carrying into space the largest payload that any country in the world has ever sent into space. That's what I consider.

I think the United States should be a leader. A country as rich and powerful as this, which bears so many burdens and responsibilities, which has so many opportunities, should be second to none. And in December, while I do not regard our mastery of space as anywhere near complete, while I recognize that there are still areas where we are behind, at least in one area—in the size of the booster—this year I hope the United States will be ahead. I'm for it.

We have a long way to go; many weeks, and months and years of long tedious work lie ahead. There will be setbacks and frustrations and disappointments. There will be, as there always are, pressures in this country to do less in this area as in so many others, and temptations to do something else that is perhaps easier. But this research here must go on, this space effort must go on, the conquest of space must and will go ahead. That much we know—that much we can say with confidence and conviction.

Frank O'Connor, the Irish writer, tells in one of his books how, as a boy, he and his friends would make their way across the countryside, and when they came to an orchard wall that seemed too high, and too doubtful to try, and too difficult to permit their voyage to continue, they took off their hats and tossed them over the wall—and then they had no choice but to follow them.

This nation has tossed its cap over the wall of space—and we have no choice but to follow it. Whatever the difficulties, they will be overcome; whatever the hazards, they must be guarded against. With the vital help of this Aerospace Medical Center, with the help of all those who labor in the space endeavor, with the help and support of all Americans, we will climb this wall with safety and with speed—and we shall then explore the wonders on the other side.

8. Hubertus Strughold's questionaire submitted to the Military Government in Germany, in the autumn of 1945 (4 pages) (A23-17).

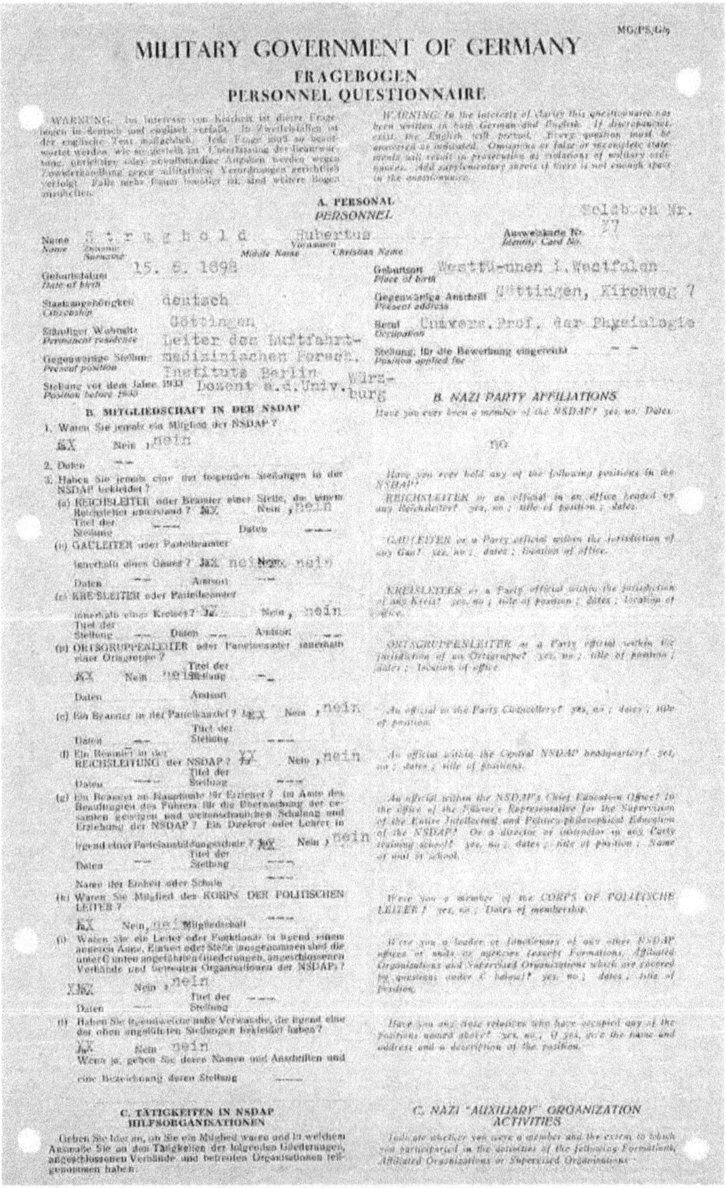

MG/PS/G/9

MILITARY GOVERNMENT OF GERMANY

FRAGEBOGEN

PERSONNEL QUESTIONNAIRE

WARNUNG: Im Interesse von Klarheit ist dieser Fragebogen in deutsch und englisch verfaßt. In Zweifelsfällen ist der englische Text maßgebend. Jede Frage muß so beantwortet werden, wie sie gestellt ist. Unterlassung der Beantwortung, unrichtige oder unvollständige Angaben werden wegen Zuwiderhandlung gegen militärische Verordnungen gerichtlich verfolgt. Falls mehr Raum benötigt ist, sind weitere Bogen anzuheften.

WARNING: In the interests of clarity this questionnaire has been written in both German and English. If discrepancies exist, the English will prevail. Every question must be answered as indicated. Omissions or false or incomplete statements will result in prosecution as violations of military ordinances. Add supplementary sheets if there is not enough space in the questionnaire.

A. PERSONAL
PERSONNEL

Soldbuch Nr. 27

Name / *Name*: Zuname / *Surname*: S t r u g h o l d — Vornamen / *Middle Name* / *Christian Name*: Hubertus

Ausweiskarte Nr. / *Identity Card No.*

Geburtsdatum / *Date of birth*: 15. 6. 1898

Geburtsort / *Place of birth*: Westtünnen i. Westfalen

Staatsangehörigkeit / *Citizenship*: deutsch

Gegenwärtige Anschrift / *Present address*: Göttingen, Kirchweg 7

Ständiger Wohnsitz / *Permanent residence*: Göttingen

Beruf / *Occupation*: Univers. Prof. der Physiologie

Gegenwärtige Stellung / *Present position*: Leiter des Luftfahrtmedizinischen Forsch. Instituts Berlin

Stellung, für die Bewerbung eingereicht / *Position applied for*: – –

Stellung vor dem Jahre 1933 / *Position before 1933*: Dozent a.d. Univ. Würzburg

B. MITGLIEDSCHAFT IN DER NSDAP

B. NAZI PARTY AFFILIATIONS

1. Waren Sie jemals ein Mitglied der NSDAP?
   ~~Ja~~ Nein, nein
   Have you ever been a member of the NSDAP? yes, no. Dates — no
2. Daten — –
3. Haben Sie jemals eine der folgenden Stellungen in der NSDAP bekleidet?
   Have you ever held any of the following positions in the NSDAP?
   (a) REICHSLEITER oder Beamter einer Stelle, die einem Reichsleiter untersteht? ~~Ja~~ Nein, nein
   Titel der Stellung — –– Daten — ––
   REICHSLEITER or an official in an office headed by any Reichsleiter? yes, no; title of position; dates.
   (b) GAULEITER oder Parteibeamter innerhalb eines Gaues? ~~Ja~~ nein ~~Nein~~ nein
   Daten — – Amtsort — –
   GAULEITER or a Party official within the jurisdiction of any Gau? yes, no; dates; location of office.
   (c) KREISLEITER oder Parteibeamter innerhalb eines Kreises? ~~Ja~~ Nein, nein
   Titel der Stellung — – Daten — – Amtsort — –
   KREISLEITER or a Party official within the jurisdiction of any Kreis? yes, no; title of position; dates; location of office.
   (d) ORTSGRUPPENLEITER oder Parteibeamter innerhalb einer Ortsgruppe?
   ~~Ja~~ Nein nein Titel der Stellung — –
   Daten — Amtsort
   ORTSGRUPPENLEITER or a Party official within the jurisdiction of an Ortsgruppe? yes, no; title of position; dates; location of office.
   (e) Ein Beamter in der Parteikanzlei? ~~Ja~~ Nein, nein
   Daten — – Titel der Stellung — ––
   An official in the Party Chancellery? yes, no; dates; title of position.
   (f) Ein Beamter in der REICHSLEITUNG der NSDAP? ~~Ja~~ Nein, nein
   Daten — –– Titel der Stellung — ––
   An official within the Central NSDAP headquarters? yes, no; dates; title of positions.
   (g) Ein Beamter im Hauptamt für Erzieher? Im Amte des Beauftragten des Führers für die Überwachung der gesamten geistigen und weltanschaulichen Schulung und Erziehung der NSDAP? Ein Direktor oder Lehrer in irgend einer Parteiausbildungsschule? ~~Ja~~ Nein, nein
   Daten — – Titel der Stellung — ––
   Name der Einheit oder Schule — ––
   An official within the NSDAP's Chief Education Office? In the office of the Führer's Representative for the Supervision of the Entire Intellectual and Politico-philosophical Education of the NSDAP? Or a director or instructor in any Party training school? yes, no; dates; title of position; Name of unit or school.
   (h) Waren Sie Mitglied des KORPS DER POLITISCHEN LEITER?
   ~~Ja~~ Nein, nein Mitgliedschaft — ––
   Were you a member of the CORPS OF POLITISCHE LEITER? yes, no; Dates of membership.
   (i) Waren Sie ein Leiter oder Funktionär in irgend einem anderen Amte, Einheit oder Stelle (ausgenommen sind die unter C unten angeführten Gliederungen, angeschlossenen Verbände und betreuten Organisationen der NSDAP)?
   ~~Ja~~ Nein, nein
   Daten — – Titel der Stellung — ––
   Were you a leader or functionary of any other NSDAP offices or units or agencies (except Formations, Affiliated Organizations and Supervised Organizations which are covered by questions under C below)? yes, no; dates, title of position.
   (j) Haben Sie irgendwelche nahe Verwandte, die irgend eine der oben angeführten Stellungen bekleidet haben?
   ~~Ja~~ Nein nein
   Wenn ja, geben Sie deren Namen und Anschriften und eine Bezeichnung deren Stellung — ––
   Have you any close relatives who have occupied any of the positions named above? yes, no; if yes, give the name and address and a description of the position.

C. TÄTIGKEITEN IN NSDAP HILFSORGANISATIONEN

Geben Sie hier an, ob Sie ein Mitglied waren und in welchem Ausmaße Sie an den Tätigkeiten der folgenden Gliederungen, angeschlossenen Verbände und betreuten Organisationen teilgenommen haben:

C. NAZI "AUXILIARY" ORGANIZATION ACTIVITIES

Indicate whether you were a member and the extent to which you participated in the activities of the following Formations, Affiliated Organizations or Supervised Organizations:

	Mitglied *Member*		Dauer der Mitgliedschaft *Period of Membership*	Amter bekleidet *Offices Held* Welcher Rang *And Title*	Dauer *Period*
	Ja *Yes*	Nein *No*			
1. Gliederungen *Formations*					
(a) SS		Nein			
(b) SA		Nein			
(c) HJ		Nein			
(d) NSDStB		Nein			
(e) NSD		Nein			
(f) NSF		Nein			
(g) NSKK		Nein			
(h) NSFK	Ja		v.Dtsch.Luft- sportverband übernommen, bis Ende d.Krieges.	---	---
2. Angeschlossene Verbände *Affiliated Organisations*					
(a) Reichsbund d. deutsch. Beamten	Ja				
(b) DAF einschl.		Nein			
KdF		Nein			
(c) NSV	Ja				
(d) NSKOV		Nein			
(e) NS Bund deutsch. Technik		Nein			
(f) NSD Ärztebund		Nein			
(g) NS Lehrerbund		Nein			
(h) NS Rechtswahrerbund		Nein			
3. Betreute Organisationen *Supervised Organisations*					
(a) VDA		Nein			
(b) Deutsches Frauenwerk		Nein			
(c) Reichskolonialbund		Nein			
(d) Reichsbund deutsch. Familie		Nein			
(e) NS Reichsbund f. Leibesübungen		Nein			
(f) NS Reichsbund deutsch. Schwestern		Nein			
(g) NS Altherrenbund		Nein			
4. Andere Organisationen *Other Organisations*					
(a) RAD		Nein			
(b) Deutscher Gemeindetag		nein			
(c) NS Reichskriegerbund		Nein			
(d) Deutsche Studentenschaft		Nein			
(e) Reichsdozentenschaft		Nein			
(f) DRK		Nein			
(g) „Deutsche Christen"-Bewegung		Nein			
(h) „Deutsche Glaubensbewegung"		Nein			

5. Waren Sie jemals Mitglied einer nationalsozialistischen Organisation, die vorstehend nicht aufgeführt ist? *Were you ever a member of any NS organisation not listed above? yes, no; name of organisation; dates; title of position; location.*
XXX Nein Nein
Name der Organisation – – – Daten –––
Titel der Stellung – – – Ort –––

6. Haben Sie jemals das Amt von Jugendwalter in einer Schule bekleidet? XXX Nein Nein *Did you ever hold the position of Jugendwalter in a school? yes, no.*

7. Wurden Ihnen jemals irgendwelche Titel, Rang, Auszeichnungen oder Urkunden von einer der oben genannten Organisationen ehrenhalber verliehen oder seitens dieser andere Ehren zuteil? Ja Nein Nein *Have you ever been the recipient of any titles, rank, medals testimonials or other honors from any of the above organizations? yes, no. If so, state the nature of the honor, the date conferred, and the reason and occasion for its bestowal.*
Falls ja, geben Sie an, was Ihnen verliehen wurde (Titel usw.) das Datum, den Grund und Anlaß für die Verleihung.

H. AUSLANDSREISEN		H. TRAVEL ABROAD
Verzeichnen Sie hier alle Reisen, die Sie außerhalb Deutschlands seit 1931 unternommen haben.		List all journeys outside of Germany since 1931.

Besuchte Länder *Countries visited*	Daten *Dates*	Zweck der Reise *Purpose of Journey*
USA	Sept. 1937	Congress Aero-Medical Association i.New-Yor
Ungarn	April 1937	Internat.Akademie f.ärztl.Fortbildung i. Budapest.
Schweiz	Aug. 1938	Internat.Physiolog.Kongress in Zurich.
Belgien	Juli 1939	Internat.Sportärztekongress in Brüssel.
Ungarn	Mai 1941	Vorlesungen d.Luftfahrtmedizin i.Budapest u. (Debrezen
Italien	April 1942	Vortrag ü.Luftfahrtmedizin i.Rom.
Rumänien	Sept. 1942	Rumänischer Räderkongress in Buharest.

Haben Sie die Reise auf eigene Kosten unternommen? Nein nein
Falls nicht, unter wessen Beistand wurde die Reise unternommen? Saniti..tsinspektion

der Luftwaffe
Beuchte Personen oder Organisationen siehe Zweck der Reise

Haben Sie in irgend einer Eigenschaft an der Zivilverwaltung eines von Deutschland besetzten oder angeschlossenen Gebietes teilgenommen? Nein ne in Falls ja, geben Sie die Einzelheiten über besetzten Amtes, Art Ihrer Tätigkeit, Gebiet

und Dauer des Dienstes an ——

Was journey made on your own account? yes, no. If not, under whose auspices was the journey made? Persons or organisations visited.

Did you ever serve in any capacity as part of the civil administration of any territory annexed to or occupied by the Reich? yes, no. If so, give particulars of offices held, duties performed, territory and period of service.

I. POLITISCHE MITGLIEDSCHAFT.	I. POLITICAL AFFILIATIONS.
(a) Welcher politischen Partei haben Sie als Mitglied vor 1933 angehört? keiner	Of what political party were you a member before 1933?
(b) Waren Sie Mitglied irgend einer verbotenen Oppositionspartei oder -gruppe seit 1933? Nein nein Welcher? —— Seit wann? ——	Have you ever been a member of any anti-Nazi underground party or group since 1933? yes, no. Which one? Since when?
(c) Waren Sie jemals ein Mitglied einer Gewerkschaft, Berufs-, Gewerblichen- oder Handelsorganisation, die nach dem Jahre 1933 aufgelöst und verboten wurde? Nein nein	Have you ever been a member of any trade union or professional or business organisation suppressed by the Nazis? yes, no.
(d) Wurden Sie jemals aus dem öffentlichen Dienste, einer Lehrtätigkeit oder einem kirchlichen Amte entlassen, weil Sie in irgend einer Form ein Nationalsozialisten Widerstand leisteten oder gegen deren Lehren und Theorien auftraten? Nein nein	Have you ever been dismissed from the civil service, the teaching profession or ecclesiastical positions for active or passive resistance to the Nazis or their ideology? yes, no.
(e) Wurden Sie jemals aus rassischen oder religiösen Gründen, oder weil Sie aktiv oder passiv dem Nationalsozialisten Widerstand leisteten, in Haft genommen oder in Ihrer Freizügigkeit, Niederlassungsfreiheit oder sonstwie in Ihrer gewerblichen oder beruflichen Freiheit beeinträchtigt? Nein nein Falls ja, dann geben Sie Einzelheiten sowie die Namen und Anschriften zweier Personen an, die die Wahrheit Ihrer Angaben bestätigen können ——	Have you ever been imprisoned, or have restrictions of movement, residence or freedom to practise your trade or profession been imposed on you for racial or religious reasons or because of active or passive resistance to the Nazis? yes, no. If the answer to any of the above questions is yes, give particulars, and the names and addresses of two persons who can attest to the truth of your statement.

I. ANMERKUNGEN	I. REMARKS

Die Angaben auf diesem Formular sind wahr.

The statements on this form are true.

Gezeichnet *Signed* Prof. H. Strughold

Datum *Date* 4. Sept. 1945

Zeuge *Witness* Prof. H. ...

3200) Wi. 31602 ...

D. SCHRIFTWERKE UND REDEN.

Verzeichnen Sie auf einem besonderen Bogen alle Veröffentlichungen von 1923 bis zum heutigen Tage, die ganz oder teilweise von Ihnen geschrieben, gesammelt oder herausgegeben wurden und alle Ansprachen und Vorlesungen, die Sie gehalten haben; der Titel, das Datum und die Verbreitung oder Zuhörerschaft sind anzugeben. Ausgenommen sind Berichten, die ausschließlich technische, künstlerische, oder unpolitische Themen zum Inhalt hatten. Wenn Sie dies in Zusammenarbeit mit einer Organisation geschrieben haben, so ist deren Name anzugeben. Falls keine, schreiben Sie "Keine Reden oder Veröffentlichungen."

D. WRITINGS AND SPEECHES

Listing a separate sheet publication from 1923 to the present which were written in whole or in part, or compiled, or edited by you, and, all addresses or lectures made by you, except those of a strictly technical or artistic and non-political character; giving title, date and circulation or audience. If they were sponsored by any organization, give its name. If none, write "No speeches or publications."

Keine Reden oder Veröffentlichungen.

E. DIENSTVERHÄLTNIS

Alle Ihre Dienstverhältnisse mit 1. Januar 1939 bis zum heutigen Tage sind anzugeben. Alle Ihre Stellungen, die Art Ihrer Tätigkeit, der Name und die Anschrift Ihrer öffentlichen und privaten Arbeitgeber sind zu vergleichen. Fernge Sie ausführen; Dauer der Dienstverhältnisse, Grund deren Beendigung, Dauer etwaiger Arbeitslosigkeit, einschließlich der durch Schulausbildung oder Militärdienst verursachten Posteslosigkeit.

E. EMPLOYMENT

Give a history of your employment beginning with January 1, 1933 and continuing to date, listing all positions held by you, your duties and the name and address of your employers or the governmental department or agency in which you were employed, the period of service, and the reasons for cessation of service, accounting for all periods of unemployment, including attendance at educational institutions and military service.

Von Front	Bis To	Anstellung Position	Art der Tätigkeit Duties	Arbeitgeber Employer	Grund für die Beendigung des Dienstverhältnisses Reason for Cessation of Service
1927	1933	Universitäts-assistent	Dozent	Universität Würzburg	
8.5.1933	1935	"	Professor	"	
1935	1945	Wehrmachts-amter	Professor Leiter des Luftfahrtmedizinischen Forschungsinstitutes Berlin	Universität Sanitäts-inspektion der Luftwaffe	
30.1.45. Jetzt Oberstarzt			"		

F. EINKOMMEN

Verzeichnen Sie hier die Quellen und die Höhe Ihres Einkommens von dem 1. Januar 1933.

F. INCOME

Shop the sources and amount of your annual income since January 1, 1933.

Jahr Year	Einkommensquellen Sources of Income	Betrag Amount
1933	Gehalt und Vorlesungen Universität Würzburg	5-6 000
1934	Gehalt und Vorlesungen Universität Würzburg	5-6 000
1935	Gehalt von Luftwaffe und Vorlesungen Universität Berlin	4-5 000
1936	" " " " "	5 000
1937	" " " " "	5 000
1938	" " " " "	5-6 000
1939	" " " " "	5-6 000
1940	" " " " "	6 000
1941	" " " " "	6 000
1942	" " " " "	7-8 000
1943	" " " " "	8 000
1944	" " " " "	8 000
1945	als Oberarzt d. Luftwaffe	956 M pr Monat

G. MILITÄRDIENST

Haben Sie seit 1919 Militärdienst geleistet? Ja Nein
In welcher Waffengattung? Luftwaffe Daten Wocnen 1937
Wo haben Sie gedient? Berlin-Sch... Dienstrang Oberstarzt
Haben Sie in militärähnlichen Organisationen Dienst geleistet? Ja Nein
In welchen? Wo? Daten
Sind Sie vom Militärdienste zurückgestellt worden? Ja Nein
Wann? Warum?
Haben Sie an der Militärregierung in irgend einem von Deutschland besetzten Lande, einschließlich Österreich und Sudetenland teilgenommen? Ja Nein Wenn ja, geben Sie Einzelheiten über bekleidete Ämter, Art Ihrer Tätigkeit, Gebiet und Dauer des Dienstes an

G. MILITARY SERVICE

Have you rendered military service since 1919? yes, no. In which arm? Dates. Where did you serve? Grade or rank. Have you rendered service in para-military organizations? yes, no. In which ones? Where? Dates. Were you deferred from military service? yes, no. When? Why?

Did you serve as a part of the Military Government in any country occupied by Germany including Austria and the Sudetenland; yes, no. If so, give particulars of offices held, duties performed, territory and period of service.

148

9. Hubertus Strughold's charge´s comment

Charge Idiotic, Strughold Says

By Jerry Deal

Dr. Hubertus Strughold, known as "the father of space medicine," Thursday said an investigation of whether he was a Nazi war criminal was "idiotic."

Strughold, 75, added that it was "nonsense and false to even think I have ever been a Nazi."

Dr. Strughold was chief scientist in the Aerospace Medical Division at Brooks AFB until his 1971 retirement.

The German native is on a list of 37 persons the Immigration and Naturalization Service in Washington says it is investigating as alleged Nazi war criminals.

'100 Years'

"I guess there will be people investigating and accusing persons as being Nazi war criminals for 100 years," Dr. Strughold said late Thursday. "It appears to be particularly popular for German scientists to be accused of being war

DR. HUBERTUS STRUGHOLD
... "nonsense, false"

Related story, Page 31

criminals these days," he added.

"This investigation is completely news to me," Strughold said. "It is so fantastic, I always have allied myself with enemies of Hitler in those days in Germany."

U.S. Citizen

Strughold, who became a naturalized U.S. citizen in 1956, noted he came to the United States for study in 1928 and 1929.

"I was against Hitler and his beliefs, but I really learned about freedom while I was here in those days," Strughold said.

He said he never had any connection with the party, although he was director of Germany's most prominent institute of aviation medicine from 1935 to 1945.

That institute was the Aeromedical Research in Berlin. "I sometimes had to

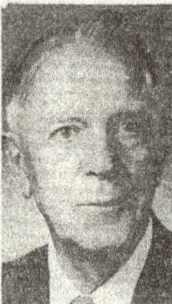

hide myself because my life was in danger from the Nazis," he declared.

He held the rank of colonel at the institute but said those connected with the air force were not forced to become Nazis.

He said all his research involved aviation medicine and there never were any prisoners involved in experiments.

Strughold noted his later close relationship with the late President Lyndon B. Johnson. "I briefed him about what was coming in space and what needed to be done and he used this to push the space program," Strughold said.

The report by the Immigration and Naturalization Service, was released through the Justice Department, its parent agency.

It said Strughold was cleared by all federal agencies before occupying the "highly sensitive position in the United States program."

But, it also stated that inves-

See STRUGHOLD, Page 2

13. Notes

Introduction
1 - Gartmann, H. 1958; Prologue - Dreamer, Researcher and Constructer. The adventures of Space Travel. *Träumer, Forscher, Konstrukteure. Die Abenteuer der Weltraumfahrt.* 4th edition, Econ-Publishing, Duesseldorf 1958.

Chapter one
1 - Birth certificate No. 162 dated 18th June 1898. Birth of Hubert Strughold on June 15th 1898 in Westtuennen, son of the teacher Ferdinand Strughold and Anna Strughold, born Tillmann, both of catholic religion. Private Archive of Mary Strughold, Mico (Texas).

2 - Oral history by Ida Oberdorf, 1996 and documents of the parish of Rhynern, Westfalia.

3- Oral history by Ida Oberdorf, 1996. Additional documents are at the archives of the catholic churches in Elspe and Erwitte. Documents also held by Ferdinande Ueter as presented on interview in 1997.

4 - Oral history by Thomas, 1996, Luelf 1996 and Ueter, 1997. The Strughold family did live in the apartment provided by the school of Westtuennen No. 102.

5 - Oral history Ida Oberdorf, 1996.

6 - The school was destroyed in WWII. School certificates of Hubertus Strughold were not retained. Only one school certificate remains at his sisters Mathilda Strughold's archive.

7 - Glasgow T. A.: 'Father of Space Medicine.' Halley's comet launched his career. Aerospace Historian 1970, 17: 6-9.

8 - Lytle S.: Space Doctor. While NASA was thinking about Earth Orbits, he was planning for Mars. 198: 48-50.

9 - See Strughold H.: Eye Hazards. Aerospace Med 1960, 61: 671.

10 - Death certificate of Strugholds father is held at the parish in Rhynern, dated 19th July 1912.

11 - Thomas S.: Hubertus Strughold. The Father of Space Medicine whose Dramatic Advanced Planning Encompasses the Universe. In: Men of Space, Vol. 4, p. 233-72. Chilton Company - Book Div., Philadelphia 1962. See also Fuchs, 1987: From Aviation to Space Medicine. Astronautik 1987, 1: 5-7.

12 - See Thomas, 1962. The Strughold's at that time lived in house No. 181 and later on in the Church Street in Westtuennen. The Strugholds had to move out of the teachers' residence No. 102 after his father's death. Strughold's mother was buried by her husband's grave in Rhynern. Oral history Luelf, 1996 and Oberdorf, 1996. Strugholds wifes death certificate is held by Hubert Oberdorf, a nephew of Hubert in Iserlohn dated 28th July 1931.

13 - Siegmund, W. 300th anniversary of the Grammar School Hammonense (*Das Gymnasium Hammonense 1657-1957*). In: *325 Jahre Gymnasium Hammonense*). Edited by the society of the friends of the grammar school Hammonense, Griebsch Priting Company, Hamm 1982: 31-156.

14 - See Thomas, 1962.

15 - Oral history Mary Strughold, 1996.

16 - See Siegmund, 1982.

17 - Document dated 30th September 1916 is held by Ferdinande Ueter in Rheda-Wiedenbrueck (see oral history).

18 - Field letter by sergeant Klug, 2nd company of the 94th Regiment dated 13th August regarding splinter injury of Josef Strughold.

19 – Diploma is held by the archives of the German Air Force Institute of Aviation Medicine in Fuerstenfeldbruck.

Chapter two

1 – Documents at Muenster University Archives (Matriculation book, beginning summer term 1917). Strugholds matriculation number was 112, matriculation date for medicine was 26th April 1918. Another document state the 25th as the entry date: Strughold is listed as 73rd person in the Album of the Philosophical and Natural Science Faculty of the Royal University of Muenster. For background informations on the Muenster University while the Weimar Republic see Poeppinghege, 1994.

2 – Oral history by Mai, 1996. The religious oriented CV Cheruskia-Muenster was one of the most important ones in the university town and politically close to the democratic Centre Party. See Poeppinghege, 1994.

3 – Questionnaire of Military Government in Germany, AAF Aeromedical Research Center, 21st October 1945, 8 pages. Private archive Mary Strughold, Mico, Texas.

4 – Courses attended while medical study are documented in the Bibliobography by Harsch, 2004: 173-4. For the last preclinical term Strughold applied on November 26th, 1918, what was slightly too late. Assumingly this was due to his continued reserve military service in Muenster while War years.

5 – Documents and certificates from his study years are preserved by Ferdinande Ueter, born Strughold in Rheda-Wiedenbrueck. See Harsch, 2004: 121-2.

6 – See Thomas, 1962.

7 – Oral history by Haenel, 1996 and Ueter, 1997. For documents see also Harsch, 2004: 122. Strughold joined the student association "AC Palatia Goettingen". Oral history by Mai, 1996.

8 – See Harsch, 2004: 138 ref. 8 and oral history Karlheim 1996, Oberdorf, 1996 and Ueter, 1997.

9 – See Harsch, 2004: 174.

10 – See Thomas, 1962 and oral history by Kilwing, 1996.

11 – Archive of LMU Munich, book of enrollment summer term 1921, No. 9120. He had to pay 382,- German marks tuition for 38 hours of lectures per week.

12 – Oral history by Mary Strughold, 1996, Mai 1996, Harsch, 2004: 8 and Thomas, 1962.

13 – Documents held by Mary Strughold, Mico, Texas.

14 – See also Ebert, 1971 and references in Harsch, 2004: 138.

15 – On oral examination on 4th of november, 1922 Rosemann asked about physiology, anatomy. Ballowitz examined anatomy topics and Feuerborn questioned zoology. The test results were both "good". Rosemann highlighted Strughold´s performance and commitment: "The author has carried out the investigation with great energy, diligent care and thoughtful criticism, and has acted independently in different places on the suggestions given to him also. I suggest that as a predicate, 'an elaborate work with valuable results.' See document in Harsch, 2004: 111.

16 – See references and documents in Harsch, 2004: 108, 111, 112 and 124.

17 – See Strughold, 1923: Density of the points of pain and swelling of the epidermis in different body regions (*Ueber die Dichte und Schwellen der Schmerzpunkte der Epidermis in den verschiedenen Koerperregionen*). Medical theses, Wuerzburg - Documents also at GAFIAM, Fuerstenfeldbruck. See Harsch, 2004: 108 and 138. The citation is re-translated by Thoams, 1962: 238f. At this time Strughold was member of the student corps „KDStV Markommannia" as stated by Mai, 1996. His scar on the left mandible is testifying his "active" membership in a fighting student association.

18 – See reference part in Harsch, 2004: 112 and 122.

Chapter three

1 - Beside Strughold famous assistants to Dr. von Frey were Paul Hoffmann, Hans Schriever, Edgar Woehlisch and Hermann Rein. See Ebert, 1971 and Bretschneider, 1997.

2 - See Lytle, 1985: "Being a family doctor was not my cup of tea."

3 – See Thomas, 1962.

4 – Document in Historical Archive of the German Research Centre for Air and Space Travel (DLR), Berlin: Assessment on Strughold and permission of absence by Max von Frey, Wuerzburg dating 25th June 1925. Adressee Paul Hoffmann, head of Freiburg Physiological Institute, duration of Strugholds delegation 1st October, 1925 to 31st March. 1926.

5 - Strughold lived in Freiburg in the Breisgau from 14th October 1925 to 31st March 1926. Oral history by Griesbaum, 1996. See also document in private archive of Ferdinande Ueter, Rheda-Wiedenbrueck: Certificate of good conduct by the City of Freiburg, 31st July, 1928 regarding Strugholds residence for duration of 14th October, 1925 to 31st march, 1926. During this time a lively exchange of letters between Strughold and Frey existed, for the most part concerning their joint scientific publications at the Historical Archive of the German Research Centre for Air and Space Travel (DLR), Berlin.

6 - The importance of his work may be seen by the fact that a popular German textbook of Physiology of the 1990s was still referencing Strughold's work. There is one figure that shows pain and pressure points on the human skin, whose determination was made with barbed bristles. This 23rd Edition published in 1987 by Schmidt and Thews was first edited by H. Rein (1st - 10th edition 1936-48) and later edited by M. Schneider (11th - 16th edition 1955-71). It shows a figure from Strughold's medical theses (dissertation) on the pressure points and the Ruff-Strughold-Atlas of the physiological hypoxia zones.

7- See documents at University Archives of LMU in Munich: List of lectures and personal inventory for summer term 1927 until summer term 1934 at the Julius Maximilians Univ. Wuerzburg.

8 - See Lytle, 1985. CA Lindbergh started in May 1927 from New York (NY) for direct flight to Paris. Here he flew non-stop 3610 miles in 33 ½ hours. See also Beamish, 1927.

9 - See Thomas, 1962

10 – See Thomas, 1962 and list of lectures and personal inventory for summer term 1927 until summer term 1934 at the Julius Maximilians Univ. Wuerzburg.

11 - In the literature, 1927 is mentioned as the year of the first aeromedical lecture by Strughold, but this could not be verified by the documents. It could have been aeromedical topics within his physiological lecture, but a separate lecture was not offered for the first time until 1928.

12 – See Engle and Lott, 1979. See also list of lectures and personal inventory for summer term 1927 until summer term 1934 at the Julius Maximilians Univ. Wuerzburg.

13 – The airplane "Udet Flamingo" was produced by Ernst Udet in the years after the first World War I in Munich. Oral history Fuchs, 1997.

14 – Newspaper article "Scientific demonstration flight at the airport for the students" in the *Wuerzburg General Anzeiger* of 1928 is deposit at the private archive of Ueter, Rheda-Wiedenbrueck.

15 - The Bárány pointing test (according to Robert Bárány) is a step in the clinical examination of the nervous system, with the focus on the movements of the upper extremities as part of coordination tests. The examiner investigates using the pointing finger of the test person with the eyes open. The hand should be in the supine position and the finger pointing to the plane of the examiner. The test is then repeated with the

eyes closed. Deviation in the vertical is considered abnormal and this indicates a malfunction of the equilateral cerebellar or of the brain stem.

16 – Oral history Oberdorf, 1996.

17 - See Jungk R: The Space professor. News paper article, in Harsch 2004.

18 – Strughold flew in a balloon in Germany. In the United States he added to his flight experience for physiological studies by observations in a small airship. See Strughold H.: Flight Physiological studies. The sense of touch (pressure sense of the skin) at low oxygen pressure. (A contribution to determining the physiological performance limits at high altitudes). He expressed thanks to Dr. Karl Strughold Goelge, vice president of the Zeppelin Corporation. in Ahren (Ohio) for making possible his observations in the blimp. He was also grateful to Wuerzburg architect Hack Stetter for the free balloon flights in Germany.

19 - See Thomas, 1962 and newspaper article by Jungk (in Harsch, 2004) "I held my recording instruments, and a champagne bottle tightly, I was desperate to give up just as we came over the wires and immediately landed in a corn field."

20 - See newspaper article: Space scientists from Westphalia, 1960 (in Harsch, 2004). A statement of the local German Aviation Company (Deutsche Luftfahrt GmbH Wuerzburg) from 1930 confirmed Strughold's physiological test flights on light and aerobatic aircraft. Letter dated 10th March 1930. Included the bill for local physiological experimental flights, total flight time 2 hrs. 10 min., 260.- RM (*Reichsmark*).

21 - See Thomas, 1962. In the Biography of Robert Ritter von Greim (1892-1945) it can be read, that this flying school was the first after World War I. He was the director of the Wuerzburg Flying School and in 1933 was a major in the "stealth" air force and then the establisment of the first fighter squadron to participate in the build-up to World War II. See F. King: Illustrated history of aviation and military pilots from 1910 to 1945. VPM Verlagsunion Pabel Moewig KG, p. 18.

22 - Per interviews with witnesses: they had the impression that his motives were of a more complex nature than from "fear of flying." Health reasons, the fact that Strughold was less strained on a boat trip, and that he liked to have more time to prepare for the visit (of the country, congress, etc.). Dr. John Roadman said: "Strughold really liked to keep his feet on the ground." See Lytle, 1985: 48. See also Graul, 1970. Under the influence of a local anaesthetic, the sensations are usually affected in the following order: pain, cold / heat, touch, pressure, and then they return to function in the reverse order. See also Thomas, 1965 and Baerwolf, 1969, 1994 and 1995.

23 - Rockefeller Foundation, 2179, 16th march, 1923: Prof. Dr. Paul Hoffmann, Prof. Dr. Frey, and Dr. Rein from the Physiol. Institute in Wuerzburg were each given regular monthly cash subsidies of $ 5. National Archives, Koblenz, sign. 5 - R 73 217: Rockefeller Foundation: Log of the Committee meeting for selection of the Rockefeller scholarships. Document of the German Science Emergency Association (*Notgemeinschaft d. deutschen Wissenschaft*), Berlin 7th. March, 1925. Stock R 73: Emergency Association of German Business / German Research Foundation (*Notgemeinschaft der Deutschen Wirtschaft/Deutsche Forschungsgemeinschaft*).

24 – Letter dating 5th November, 1952. Wiggers noted that his success was based in large part to the stimulating contact with men like Strughold, and not in the least to their loyalty and faithfulness. Letter was enclosed in writing to Dr. Loeser, Vice president of the scientific magazine Space Research (*Weltraumforschung*), 28th october, 1952 regarding possible German publication of his book „The Green and Red Planet".

25 - Strughold held a seminar on aviation medicine during this period. A Chicago newspaper then ran the headline "New Field of Science in Aviation Medicine, Educator Says". See Glasgow, 1970: 7. Also in Minneapolis (Minnesota), he was a part of a Physiol. Symposium in 1929, presenting a flight physiologic lecture (Sensory Mechanics Involved in Aircraft Control.). See Flight Physiological studies II (1930: 226).
26 - See Harsch, 2004: 140 ref. 26.
27 - See Certificate No. 345 of Bavarian State Ministry of Education and Culture, 13th march, 1933 regarding his nomination as associate Professor at the medical Faculty. Copy No. V 8828th. Certificate at the archive of GAFIAM, Fuerstenfeldbruck. In the Yearbook of the Scientific Aeronautical Soc. WGL of 1934 it is found on p. 58 that Strughold recently received the first dedication to teach Aviation Physiology in Wuerzburg by the Bavarian Minister of Culture. He was referring to the appointment of Strughold as an "*ausserordentliche*", a Professor with special teaching of Flight Physiology on 13th March 1933 by the old German government before the takeover by the Nazi party. See National Archives, Washington, (D. C.). Joint Intelligence Objectives Agency (J.I.O.A.) File Copy, Record Group 330, 89 pages.
28 - See this report on the Medical Committee. In: Yearbook of the WGL e. V. (1929), p. 35/36, published by R. Oldenbourg, Munich and Berlin.
29 - The financial resources of the governmental transport ministry were mainly funneled to support the work of Dr. Koschel and Dr. Gillert, who worked with the German Aviation Society (*Luftsportverband*) and other flying organizations. See archives of Wuerzburg University, report of 20th june, 1931. Harsch, 2004: 140 ref. 30. Founded in 1912, the Scientific Society for Air Ship Travel (WGF) two years later was renamed the Scientific Society for Aeronautics (WGL).
30 - See archives of Wuerzburg University, various reports from summer 1931. Harsch, 2004: 140.
31 - See archives of Wuerzburg University, report of 20th June, 1931. Harsch, 2004: 140.
32 - During this state of emergency it was impossible for the "Ministry of Finance" to support the creation of a new professorship - an extraordinary act as it would have been an additional financial burden. Harsch, 2004: 140.
33 - Loeffler, the mayor of Wuerzburg wrote to the rectorate of the university on 8th July, 1931 regarding the sought professorate of Strughold.
34 - National Archives, Washington, (D. C.), Joint Intelligence Objectives Agency (J.I.O.A.) File Copy, Record Group 330: Special contract for employment with the German citizen of the United States Department of WAR, 14th February, 1947, (effective date of employment: July 12th, 1947), pp. 67-74.
35 - See Ward, 1959.
36 - See Thomas, 1962 and National Archives, Washington, (D. C.), Joint Intelligence Objectives Agency (J.I.O.A.) File Copy, Record Group 330.
37 - See archives of Julius-Maximilians-University, Wuerzburg: 16th, 18th and 20th July regarding aviation medical professorate in Wuerzburg. See Harsch, 2004: 124.
38 - See archive of GAFIAM, Fuerstenfeldbruck: Certificate of Bavarian state ministry (V 8828), see above.
39 - See Strughold statement at the Nuremberg medical trials, 10th January 1947 regarding Dr. Oscar Schroeder, former chief Luftwaffe´s Medical Corps. State archive Nuremberg, exhibit No. 7. Harsch, 2004: 112. The medical officer Anton Waldmann (1878-1941) was appointed by the President as the Army Medical Inspector in 1932. Oral history Fuchs, 1998.
40 - See private archive Mary Strughold, Mico, Texas: Bavarian AME Guide 1935 (*Bestimmung zum Sachverständigen für die ärztliche Untersuchung der Segelflugzeug-*

und Freiballonführer im Bereich des Luftamtes Nürnberg, 15th *Feb. 1935*). See also private
archive of Ferdinannde Ueter, Rheda-Wiedenbrueck: references 38 and 39 in Harsch,
2004: 124. At the annual meeting of the WGL in Kiel 1931 the agreement between the
Minister of Transport and the medical committee of the WGL was mentioned to
implement an AME course to be held in Braunschweig. Strughold was planned to be one
of the lecturers.

Chapter four

1 – See Harsch,1994 and 2004.
2 - Diringshofen had only been there for one year. His next assignment was at the
aeromedical laboratory in Jueterbog, Altes Lager (old camp) south of Berlin. He had
begun his aeromedical activities in the early 1930s serving at the Wuerzburg Institute of
Physiology on a command basis dealing with acceleration experiments at the local
airfield. Further information on the interaction between Diringshofen and Strughold
could not be found. Also, the Marburg Professor, Dr. Graul, who was the godson of
Diringshofen, stated that Strughold had allegedly pushed him out of the Berlin office. See
Pers. Mitt Graul, 1998. The Luftwaffe Surgeon General, E. Hippke, put this point clearly: "
It would have been obvious to me to keep von Diringshofen as the appointed director of
the Aviation Medical Research Institute; but such confinement in one institution was
against his temperament. He needed the freedom of the skies." See Hippke, 1967: 311.
3 – See Harsch, 2004: 104, 105, 107 and 124.
4 – Harsch, 2004: 108 and 124. 1th Apr. 1936 his RLM household post was pay graded
as "A 2 b". See Harsch, 2004: 104, 113 and 122. The course catalog of the Berlin
University showed Strughold for the first time in the summer term 1936 until the winter
term 1940-41. In the winter term 1939-40 it is noted, that Strughold's experimental
physiological lecture would be held by Trendelenburg (Harsch, 2004: 104 and 124). See
also: Catalogue of the faculty of the University of Berlin I, 1810-1945, rev. J. v. Asen, ed. v.
O. Harrasowitz, Leipzig 1955.
5 - According to the instructions given to him teach, he was still committed to the
Medical Faculty of the Univ. Berlin to represent the subject "Physiology" in lectures and
exercises. See Harsch, 2004: 104. In the question about who should succeed
Trendelenburg on the Physiology chair there have been some difficulties to finding the
best solution. After Achelis and Wagner rejected, the dean of the Friedrich-Wilhelms-
University of Berlin proposed in his letter dating 6th December 1944 Prof. Wetzler
(Frankfurt), Strughold (Berlin) and Schütz (Münster) for the occupation of the chair. See
Harsch, 2004: 105 and 122.
6 - see Harsch, 2004 and oral history Karlheim, 1996. Strughold´s Secret Service
"GeStaPo"-File No. 15720. In English:

Police Department of Würzburg, Bavaria 7th of September 1936.
No. 2171 WZBG 7006; II/IC Munich.
Regarding: confidential inquiry (to telex no. 27205 of 4th Sept. 1936 B.No. 70233).
Strughold, Hubert, professor, born 15th June 98 in Westtuennen, department of
Hamm/Westfalia, son of + teacher Ferdinand Strughold and of Anna, born Tillmann, single,
Catholic, citizen of the empire (Reich), was living from 1921 until 1st of April 1935 in Wuerzburg
with interruption. He finished his medical studies at the university with the state exam and
received there a doctorate (Dr. med.). After his habilitation in 1927 he concentrated mainly on
aviation medical tasks. In 1935 he was appointed to Berlin, where he became the head of the
Aeromedical Research Institute on 1st of April 1935.
During his stay in Wuerzburg no disadvantagious information in political, criminal or other
respects was noticed. He was a member there of the group of German National University
Teachers (Deutschnationale Hochschullehrer), but was more old fashioned German orientated

and stood close to the monarchist idea. It is not known if he was a member of any political party before the radical change (by the Nazi party).
He is not registered as NSDAP-member (Nazi party member) in the local office. Also there is no information of membership in any Nazi subdivision.
We did report about Strughold already on 11th April 1935 (telex no. 781 of 11th april 1935 to the book no. 9012/35 of RPP).
Wuerzburg 6th September 1935; Police department, outpost of RPP

Wuerzburg Police department 781 of 11th April 1935 (1847).
No. 2537, department 9: telex to the Bavarian political police, Munich.
Regarding: confidential inquiry to telex no. 4897 of 18th march 1935 Z.St.B.No. 9012/II/IC
Strughold, Hubert, Dr. phil. et. cand.med. , single, lecturer, born 15th June 98 in Westtuennen, department of Hamm/Westfalia, Catholic, citizen of the empire (Reich), son of deceased teacher Ferdinand Strughold and of Anna, born Tillmann, was living here from 1921 until 6th of April 1935. From 16.10.29 until 1.4.35 he was lecturing at the university. His last monthly salary was (gross) about 395-400 RM (Reichsmark). In the circles of the university teachres he is reported as being unobjectionable. As we know there he belongs to the group of German National University Teachers (Deutschnationale Hochschullehrer). On 6.4.35 he moved from Wuewrzburg to Berlin. Closer comments could not be provided even on a more confidential way.
Policedepartment, Würzburg 11th April 1935.

Bavarian Political Police – Munich telex mue 4867 of 18th March 1935 (1859).
To the political police outpost in Wuerzburg regarding confidential enquiry.
Professor Strughold, born 15.6.98 Westtuennen, resident Rountgenring 9 is in touch with a central authority (meaning the Reichsluftfahrtministry). I request information about reputation, family and financial situation, etc. and correct particulars to be reported in a confidential way. There is no criminal background regarding this request.
Bavarian political police b.no. G 9012/35 Roem.2/1 C AK (Z.St.) I.A. B…

7 - Files from the GeStaPo-archives (secret service) from Wuerzburg (*Geheime Staatspolizei* GESTAPO) of Nazi-Germany from 1934 and 1935. The files are located in the Stete-Archives in Munich (Staatsarchiv München, Gestapo-Akte Strughold_hubert, Nr. 15720), and were released on 30 th May 1980 to the prosecution office (*Staatsanwaltschaft*) Wuerzburg.
8 – This radiokinematographic method was applied under the direction of Gauer. See report of Strughold on 7 th Aug. 1942 at the German Academy of Aeronautical Research. See also Gauer, 1939 and Strughold H.: The tasks of the aviation medicine in the light of the technical developments of aviation. German military doctor, 1936: 35. See also review by Harsch: German Acceleration Research from the Very Beginnings. In: Aviat Space Environ Med 2000, 8 : 854-6.
9 - Sixteen people lost their lives in an snow avalanche before reaching the 8125 m high summit, including Hartmann and the expedition leader, Vienna. Luft survived due to his stay in the base camp and led the expedition again in 1938 with two other participants. Investigation results were published in 1941 in the journal "Aviation Medicine". Another research victim at AMRI was the WWI fight pilot Friedrich Noltenius, who worked on high altitude issues since 1935. He was killed in March 1936 in a flying accident at Berlin-Adlershof. See Strughold, 1936.
10 - See Strughold, 1950 (Aviation Medicine World War II).
11 - See BA-MA 20/306 H: 2 Conference on Mountain Physiology held 23.-24. Sept. 1943. See also Unger 1991 and Harsch, 2004: 117. Strughold gave a presentation on Hypoxidosis.
12 - The stratosphere flight by Piccard in 1931 to 15,000 m was achieved in a hermetically sealed cabin. This technique was used to achieve great heights in air and spacecraft. See Piccard, 1954.

13 - See Strughold, 1950 (German Aviation Medicine in World War II).
14 - See Harsch, 2004: 117 and 119.
15 - In 1944 Lutz was assigned to the German Research Institute for Glider Aircraft in Ainring in order to study animal experiments concerning the rescue capabilities at high altitude (15,000 m to 25,000 m).
16 - The amount of educational studies were divided into four tests. Test No. 4 had to be carried out every day by the medical officer himself. The time reserve was first tested with an oxygen-nitrogen mixture (7 + / - 0.1% O^2 corresponding to an altitude of 7,500 m). Following that, climbs up to 12,000 m with 100% O^2 breathing were performed. Rapid (Blitz) ascents up to and over 12,000 m with 100% O^2 breathing and rapid decompression to 15,000 m were performed in the next exercise. The pressure reduction was followed by a stay to the level reached up to the appearance of symptoms of altitude sickness (hypoxia) and then a subsequent "descent", in some cases without additional O2 breathing. See Strughold, 1950.
17 - This is documented in the methodologies of the studies that were published.
18 - See H. Strughold: the animal nervous system at high altitudes. German military doctor 1937, 2: 77.
19 - Strughold presented his scientific and ethical point of view concerning these relevant trials: "The interest for scientific research was present in Becker-Freyseng so deep that he did not shrink from complex self-experiments. He performed at least 100 self-tests concerning oxygen deficiency, which frequently led to his loss of consciousness and this speaks to the daily hardships of my co-workers. They were not forced, but they often did projects against my recommendations at their own risk, such as this one by Becker-Freyseng: a self-experiment of almost three days' duration in 1938 in a chamber, which was filled with nearly pure [100%] oxygen. In this experiment, in which my first assistant, H.G. Clamann, attended, there were some animals, including rabbits, in the chamber. Although on the second day B.F. raised complaints, but they didn't gave up. Only a few hours before the end of the third day, the experiment was stopped because of life threatening symptoms by B.F. (vegetative state, irritation and paralysis). B.F. was transferred with severe symptoms to the clinic of Prof. Denning, (...), after 8 days, his condition improved somewhat again. His appearance was the same as those that had occurred in the experimental animals. The rabbit died, B. F. recovered. Following a similar, shorter intermediate trial, several months later Becker-Freyseng performed a three-day trial with nearly pure oxygen at an altitude of 9000 m. By these two tests, he definitively provided the first evidence that breathing pure oxygen for a sufficiently long time in high altitudes could be well tolerated. Since that time the aviation world knew that oxygen breathing above 4.000 m for a prolonged time was not dangerous. On the other hand, below this altitude there could only be a temporary dose of pure oxygen breathing acceptable. It was a heroic self-experiment, which will claim its place in literature. " See Harsch, 2004: 112 (A19-1: State Archive Nuremberg, Doc. No. 401).
20 - See Hippke, 1937: 150. General Prof. Dr. Erich Hippke was the first Head of the Luftwaffes Medical Corps in April 1935 until the end of 1943. He was suceeded by General Prof. Dr. Oskar Schroeder, who was tried at Nuremberg in 1947. The Medical Corp Air Force Academy was installed in 1941 in Berlin-Wittenau. Its faculty members were "Consulting Specialists" with the AMRI. See (Harsch, 2004: 106). Strughold was an "Advisor in aviation medicine" from 1935 to early 1945. The leading Reich's military physiologist Dr. Otto F. Ranke, a former Strughold assistant at the AMRI, listed the two different career types of aeromedical specialists: State employees (Strughold, Ruff and Benzinger) and Medical Officers (Major M.C. von Diringshofen). The first group was scientifically on the top and in close connection with the development and testing centers

(Adlershof and Rechlin). The military types were only former doctor assistants and were operational medical officers with the troops. Conversely, the test site under Dr. von Diringshofen was without sufficient contact with the university level. See Unger, 1991, documents (Harsch, 2004: 106).

21 - See Harsch, 1994.

22 - See Harsch, 2004: 104. Since 1934, the lecturer in aerospace medicine at the universities were: H. von Diringshofen (1934) with a teaching assignment for aerospace medicine, followed by S. Ruff and H. Strughold (1935), H. Lottig (1938), and U.C. Luft (1943). See Harsch, 2004: 113.

23 - See Harsch, 2004: 113. In Year book of the German Academy of Aeronautical Research, 1th Jan. 1942. Strughold's deputy at AMRI from 1943-1945 was H.G. Clamann, before that the deputy is unknown.

24 - This is based on the organizational plan from the summer of 1945 (Harsch, 2004: 106), written by the Luftwaffe's Surgeon General Schroeder. This list was supplemented by information in the literature cited. It is a comprehensive compilation. The grade designations, academic degrees and affiliations troops not be resolved in all cases. The grade equivalents were: Under physician = Cadet, Physician assistant = Lieutenant, Senior physician = Lieutenant, Surgeon = Captain, etc. Doz. means Dozent, a lecturer grade at the university.

25 - See Fuchs, 1986. See also Harsch, 2004: 110, 111 and 117. See also Reimer, 1979.

26 - See Cubers, 1938 in Wien Med weekly Journal 1938, 34: 902.

27 - See Thomas, 1962: 246

28 - Oral history Gibson, 1999: "He [Wing Commander (later Air Marshal) Sir Philip Livingston] was a pilot-flight surgeon who specialized in ophthalmology. The photograph must have been taken in May 1937. It was reported that on his visit to Germany, Livingston was received with courtesy and openness and was given a comprehensive tour of all of the establishments. He found them all well-equipped and staffed with scientists of high reputation. He was thoroughly alarmed because German aviation medicine was so much more advanced than British aviation medicine. His report, on his return to the UK, led indirectly to the setting up of what was become the RAF Institute of Aviation Medicine."

29 - Visiting scientists were employed at the AMRI. One of them was the Chinese physician Tsu-Te Chang, who graduated at the Univ. Berlin with experimental animal work to obtain his Physiology PhD. Oral history Chang 1996. Chang visited his "doctor-father" Strughold on several occasions. Strughold preferred classical music and was an avid piano player. His favorite composers were Mozart, Schubert, Beethoven and Chopin. He preferred the literature by Shakespeare, Goethe and Schiller. When they visited the different Chinese establishments in Berlin Strughold liked the Nanking Restaurant best. Chang came to Berlin on a Chinese aviation medical scholarship from the Humboldt Foundation in 1936, led by Woehlisch from Wuerzburg Physiological Institute. They had advised him to take up a research position at the Strughold Institute, where he worked from 1937- 1938. Chang received his doctorate in 1938 with the animal experimental work "Age and level of resistance in animal experiments". During this time the Institute hosted over 10 foreign scientists who were very active." See Fig. 10 with Chang and Strughold accompanied by a Yugoslav scientist. Chang returned to his native country, to help in the development of Chinese aviation medicine during the fight against the Empire of Japan, and thereafter was a lifelong victim of the Communist Chinese regime. See Harsch V.: In Memoriam. Aviat Travel Med (Flug- und Reisemedizin) 1996, 2: 50.

30 - See Harsch, 2004: 113.

31 – See Harsch, 2004: 104. Instructions for performing the journey can be found, however.

32 - See Harsch, 2004: 106. The congratulatory letter from the President on July 12, 1941 ended with "Heil Hitler," Strughold ´replied "By respectfully greeting, always yours, H. Strughold".

33 - The "News from the Center for Scientific Reporting", which were reports of an official character and was provided to the relevant authorities, complemented the spectrum. Publications had to be approved by the Air Force Chief of Medical Services through the Head of the Training Division "Science and Research" (WUF). The same person also had a veto in the publications of inaugural dissertations (medical theses) with an aeromedical background. See Strughold, 1950: Aviation Medicine World War II), (Harsch, 2004: 107). The AMRI bibliographer and ophthalmologist, Dr. Ingeborg Schmidt, published the "Bibliography of Aviation Medicine" in 1938. The systematic classification of publications was carried out in collaboration with Strughold. Schmidt published the "radiographic cinematographic-acceleration in the service of physiological research" in 1943. In the report by the chairman of the working group "Aviation Medicine", Rein pointed out the special importance of aviation physiological research as the contributing science for altitude resistance. War-related themes such as "death in detonations" (Benzinger) and "air blast effect on the organism" (Roessle) were presented in the first scientific meeting on March 1, 1943. Strughold drew the conclusion that the USAF should also create a similar institution: "Of great value was the close exchange of experience between aviation medicine and technical sciences in the 'Lilienthal Society'. About every three months engineers, university professors, pilots and Lufwaffe officers met and discussed selected topics that were of mutual interest, such as oxygen equipment, ejection seat development, and instrument flight. Two or three papers covered the area around each of the selected themes. The remaining time was used to discuss issues and to give proposals and recommendations to all relevant institutions." See Harsch, 2004: 117-21. Important aeromedical publications were made by G. Schubert, W. Schnell, H. von Diringshofen. The handbook "Aviation Medicine" was edited by Ruff and Strughold and published in a further two editions in 1944 and 1957. See Aviat Med (Luftfahrtmed) 1940, 4: 166. In a review by the Goettingen physiologist, Rein: "In this book at no point is just theory or 'laboratory-aviation medicine' offered. Though written with thoroughness, you always feel the passion of the authors for flying. The great and important task of flight safety as well as preserving the aviator's health were major points in this book. It presents a tremendous amount of scientific facts, that readers would have had to otherwise search for in numerous publications. " In 1942 the "Atlas of aviation medicine" was edited by Ruff and Strughold. About 100 plates intended for display on normal projection devices (epidiascope) gave the state of science regarding altitude and accelaration physiology. See Aviat Med (Luftfahrtmed) 1942, 6: 357.

34 - In 1936 the "Lilienthal Society" for aeronautical research succeeded the WGL. Strughold reported concerning the Committee on aeromedical research. See Yearbook of 1936 Lilienthal Society for Aeronautical Research. R. Oldenbourg Verlag, Munich. See also Radinger and Schick, 1991. Strughold was a corresponding member of the "German Academy for Aeronautical Research" since April 1937. Other members in that society were Benzinger, Buechner and Ruff. He was the deputy chairman of the "Aviation Medicine Working Group" of the Academy. Scientific meetings and conferences were also conducted with the Lilienthal-Society. See Harsch, 2004. The Academy had 45 ordinary and 87 corresponding members in 1943, including Otto Hahn, Ludwig Prandtl, Carl Bosch, and Strughold. Livingston was alarmed because it was obvious that German

aviation medicine was so much more advanced than British aviation medicine. His report, on his return to the UK, led indirectly to the setting up of what would become the RAF Institute of Aviation Medicine."

35 - See Harsch, 2001 and 2004: 106.

36 - See Schott, 1993 and oral history Hollmann, 1996 and 1999: Hollmann W. Sportmed 1998, 49: 358-9.

37 - See Strughold 1936: 212-5.

38 - See Fuchs, 1987: From aviation to space medicine. In Memoriam Hubertus Strughold - "Father of Space Medicine". Astronautics 1987, 1: 5-7. The fire disaster of the "Hindenburg" of 6 May 1937 in Lakehurst (New Jersey) led to an abrupt end to the Zeppelin era.

39 – Harsch, 2004.

40 – See Harsch, 2004: 112. At AMRI color and night-vision research was of military driven priority while the nightly air raids became more frequent. In July 1943 a scientific meeting for night vision took place at AMRI, in which 58 participants were present. See Unger, 1991.

41 - See Taddey, 1979 and Schwabe, 1989. Waldmann in Harsch, 2004: 122.

42 - See Harsch, 2004: 112, 113, 123. See also Thomas, 1962 and oral history Lauschner, 1992. Professor Spatz said: "Prof. Strughold did not have NS-party relationships and would state that he opposed the National Socialist ideas." See Harsch, 2004: 112 and 123, see Thomas, 1962: 247.

43 - See Harsch, 2004: 123.

44 - See Thomas, 1962 and Harsch, 2004: 112 regarding interference with SS.

45 - See Harsch, 2004: 123.

46 – Oral history with relatives Hanke, 2009 in Neubrandneburg and Karlheim, 1996 in Stadthagen.

47 - See Harsch, 2004: 123.

48 – See Strughold´s personnel file JIOA in Harsch, 2004: 123.

49 - A front organization of the German Air Force called the DLV was a "sports organization." Strughold served as a physician at the equivalent rank of a Captain. His membership card (No. 10 711) was the first issued in October of 1933. See Harsch, 2004: 122. The organization for sport aviation, the "German Air Sports Association", was disbanded and was succeeded by the National Socialist Flying Corps (NSFK), founded on 20th April 1937. The record sheet at the University of Berlin noted that Strughold belonged to the organization as a physician member since 1934, specifically to subgroup 6, Lower Franconia.

50 - See Thomas, 1962: 248. Strughold lived from 1935 to 1942 in Berlin-Charlottenburg (Wielandstraße 16 c/o Schultz) and moved to Berlin-Wendeschloss in 1942, where he remained until 1943. Strughold followed his institute to Silesia and stayed at the invitation of a baroness in Silesia. Strughold weekly traveled to Berlin to perform the duties and local correspondence. See also Harsch, 2004: 104.

51 - See also Williams, 2000: 70.

52 - See Harsch, 2004: 123.

Chapter five

1 – See Harsch, 2004: 113 and Bretschneider, 1997. In Harsch, 2004 123 (A26-3), however, it is noted that he had already been in Niedernjesa at Goettingen during 1944/45. A material transfer from AMRI would follow shortly after. There is an important document from the Luftwaffe´s command (OKL Chief of Medical Services) (Az

11 B 38), addressed to the AMRI in Goettingen, dated March 6th, 1945 on the relocation of the library and the devices to Prague and Goettingen. See Harsch, 2004: 122.

2 – Oral history Bretschneider, 1996.

3 - See Thomas, 1962 and Harsch, 2004.

4 – See Kirsch and Winau, 1986, and Harsch, 2004: 117.

5 - See Bower, 1987 and 1988; see Benford, 1955; see newspaper article of. Justice B. 3rd October 1961: Russia Hunted for Space Age Medicine; U.S. Got Him.

6 - The CIOS (Combined Intelligence Objectives Subcommittee) was a secret service committee of the U.S. Congress to define the post-war aims. See Freeman, 1995. They described the German scientific results as being outdated already. See Hunt, 1991: 17 and Bower, 1988: 288

7 - See Fuchs, 1986.

8 - Quoted in Bower, 1987: 16

9 – See Harsch, 2004: 105 and 113.

10 - See Gauer and Haber, 1950. Oral history Kirsch, 1997 and 1999.

11 - See Benford, 1947: 9

12 - Col. Harry G. Armstrong, Col. Otis B. Schreuder, Col. Wilford F. Hall, and Lt. Col. Woodrow B. Estes were assigned to the first group, who were entrusted with the selection of facilities and staff. The second group was responsible for the procurement of supplies and equipment, with Col. Newton C. Spencer, Col. George L. Ball, Lt. Col. Estes, Maj. Howard B. Burchell, and Capt. Anthony N. Domonkos. See Benford, 1947.

13 - The forerunner of the OMGUS (Office of Military Government of Germany) was the U.S. Group Control Council (USGCC). See Henke and Oldenhage, 1994. See also Harsch, 2004: 117 and Benford, 1947.

14 - Among the first was O. Gauer, followed by T. Benzinger on Sept. 20th, 1945, and shortly after S. Ruff. On October 16, 1945, H. Rose, E. and A. Opitz Kornmueller were added. See Benford, 1947 Col. Robert J. Benford was named as head of the Third Central medical facility of the U.S. Armed Forces in Heidelberg on Nov. 9th, 1945.

15 – He tersely wrote to his childhood friend, Hubert Oberndorf, in Westphalia on Jan. 24, 1946: "I am the head of a research group here with more than 30 people with their necks on the line" See Harsch, 2004: 109, 112 and 123. Strughold stated in "Report from Heidelberg", that Nov. 1st, 1945 and not Oct. 16th was the date of his arrival in Heidelberg.

16 - Document image kindly provided by Mary Strughold, Mico (Texas).

17 - The working research group headed by Strughold, which dealt primarily with questions of sensory physiology, includued the electronics engineer John Prast, Strughold's assistant, Dr. Ingeborg Schmidt, Dr. Henry Rose, the physicist, Dr. Heinz Haber, and the psychologist, Dr Siegfried. In a second research group led by Dr. Siegfried Ruff and concentrated on acceleration research, there was Dr. Hermann Becker-Freyseng, Dr. Otto Gauer, Dr. Konrad Schaefer and an engineer, Karl Hausser. Concerned with the development of new oxygen equipment for aircraft and methods of measurement CO_2, was the research group headed by Dr. Theodore Benzinger. His staff included Dr. Heinz Maier-Leibnitz, Dr. Charlotte Kitzinger, Dr. Helmut Beinert and an engineer, Henry Seeler. Led by Dr. Ulrich Henschke was a fourth research group which studied aeronautical matters. Working with Henschke were John Polte, Willi Buehring, Sepp Zott, William Schaffhauser and an engineer, Hans Mauch. Henschke, formerly at the Institute of Radiology at the University of Berlin and Munich, was the medical director of the Munich Institute for Aviation Research (Medical Research Institute of Aviation Establishment) during the last two years of the war.

18 - The majority of these reports were not published as were other secret special

reports from various research facilities in the Air Force. Important aeromedical literature was translated at the AMC into English. See Harsch, 2004: 117.

19 - The impetus for the creation of the monograph comes from a visit to the AMC by Gen. Grow and Lt. Col. O. O. Benson, Jr. in February 1946. This acknowledged the research done so far and suggested that a summary be published in the United States.

20 - See Harsch, 2004: 117 and Benford, 1947.

21 - Link and Coleman (1955) According to the AMC, the organization was desolved on March 15, 1947, but the USAF states April 1947 was the date of deactivation of the Center. See Harsch, 2004: 117.

22 - See Fuchs, 1986 and J Aviat Med 1950, 21: 361 "German Aviation Medicine World War II."

23 - See Harsch, 2004: 110.

24 - Originally 81 papers from 59 authors contributed to the monograph. The contributors to the final version were: Hans Autrum, Heinz Beauvais, Hermann Becker-Freyseng, Theodor Benzinger, Abraham G.A. Bingel, Franz Buechner, Konrad Buettner, Hans Desaga, Hans W. Denzer, William Ernsthausen, Henry Freise, Hermann Frenzel, Otto Gauer, Siegfried Gerathewohl, Otto Graf, Franz Grosse-Brockhoff, Heinz Haber, Horst Hanson Immo von Hattingberg, Ulrich K. Henschke, Wolfgang Heubner, William Hornberger, Heinz Kensche, Frederick A. Kipp, Kurt Kramer, K. Kreipe, Henry Kuhn, Gunther Lehmann, Werner E. Loeckle, Ulrich C. Luft, Max Matthes, Hans A. Mauch, Werner Noell, Erich Opitz, Franz Palm, Joseph Pichotka, Erich Regener, Hermann F. Rein, Henry W. Rose, Robert Rössle , Siegfried Ruff, Hans Schaefer, Konrad Schaefer, Hubert Schardin, Francis N. Scheubel, Ingeborg Schmidt, Oskar Schroeder, Justus Schneider, Erich Schuetz, Herbert Schwiegk, Henry Seeler, Herbert Siegmund, Hugo Spatz, Hubertus Strughold, Wolf von Wittern and Karl Wezler. See USAF, 1950: "German Aviation Medicine World War II." USAF SAM, Randolph Field (Texas) Apr. 1950. John B. West stated in his book, "High Life. A History of High-Altitude Physiology and Medicine "(1998) that the German physiologists had the best research in the 1930's and 1940's (pp. 246-53).

25 - See Strughold, 1950 (German Aviation Medicine World War II).

26 - The Berlin Helmholtz Institute in 1944 was located south of Mount Wendelstein, in Munich. It was evacuated and relocated in the spring of 1946 and the 25-member working group of the laboratory were based at the Nussdorfam Inn. In early 1947, they were transported to Wright Field AFB, Ohio. In the book "Vanishing Paper Clips", the German "Paper Clip" physicist, Ernst Franke, stated that more than 70 scientists and engineers were sent to Wright Field. Their research activity was primarily in the field of sensory physiology and supersonic research, therefore they were mentioned in the AMC monthly reports ("Monthly Status Report"). See Benford, 1947.

28 - The diary of the AMC records a visit to a German University in the British and U.S. zone by Dr. Hall and Capt. Victor. See Harsch, 2004: 117. In addition to visiting Berlin and Hamburg, they also went to Kiel, but they had the worst impressions due to the conditions experienced. There was no heating, virtually no equipment and the scientists they encountered appeared to be half-starved. Under these unfavourable conditions there was no attempt to perform valuable research. In addition, an inspection trip to the German universities in the Soviet zone of occupation was planned for Feb. 1947. Whether or not this took place is not apparent from the available material.

29 - The importance of the AMC in the scientific area is demonstrated by the number of high level visits from both civilian and military leaders. In addition to the "Air Surgeon," Gen. Grow, there were also visits by the head of USAF research, Col. Benson, and the commander of the School of Aviation Medicine at Randolph Field, Texas. Col. H.G.

Armstrong was also among the visitors and scholars that appeared at the Heidelberg AMC. Others included Dr. F.G. Hall (physiology professor at Duke University), Dr. E.H. Wood (Mayo Aero Medical Unit), Dr. H.B. Burchell and Dr. E.I. Baldes (both Mayo Clinic), and Dr. John W. Heim and Capt. Horrace O. Parrack (both at Aero Medical Laboratories, Wright Field). The recruitment of German scientists for American business was one of the reasons for the visit by Col. Armstrong. 326 visitors were counted to appear at AMC in Nov. 1946. See Benford, 1947. As a background it should be noted that in July 1945, project "Overcast" went into effect, which was directed at shortening the war in the Pacific. See Harsch, 2004: 110. Over 350 German specialists were identified for possible support in conducting U.S. military research after the war. See Harsch, 2004: 111. The successor to this project was Project "Paper Clip". A specially appointed Project Alsos mission (there were three secret service Project Alsos missions in Post-World-War II by the US in conjunction with the Manhattan project) was entrusted with the implementation of the projects "Overcast" and "Paper Clip". See Kurowski, 1982. The Project Alsos group was originally founded in 1943, to obtain information concerning German developmental research in the field of nuclear energy. Walter Bothe was at the KWI for Medical Research at Heidelberg during the war. Here was the only German cyclotron located. See Hoffmann, 1993. The mid-sized device was located on the premises of the AMC. In a post-war document "Report from Heidelberg," it is stated (Benford, 1947: 16): "They always insisted that this German cyclotron was used for pure medical research and had never been a real part of their effort to develop an atomic bomb." In the book review of "Dr. Ox's Experiment" (Jules Verne) by Mary Lou Mulch in 1966 it is mentioned, that Strughold, who had the reputation of being a "mad scientist", told the Americans at the end of World War II, that the Potsdam Conference was prolonged because of a dispute over a valley in eastern Germany. He said that they thought that his brain had deteriorated from malnutrition and started sending him food packages. After the first atomic bomb exploded in Japan, they learned that the valley had the richest known deposit of uranium in Europe and they returned to speak to him in penance. German scientists, engineers and technicians were detected in the Soviet Union and the three Western occupation zones and deported to the USSR or recruited to Western countries, particularly the USA. In the case of the U.S., the armed forces were not always coordinated and the different services were partly competing in the recruitment contest. See Albring, 1991, Kurowski, 1982; Magnus, 1993; Stuhlinger and Ordway, 1992. According to Kurowski (1982), in October 1946 over 20,000 German specialists and family members were covertly deported to the Soviet Union. At a U.S. Pentagon meeting on May 24th, 1945 the entry of 100 nuclear and missile experts to the United States was approved. A list of 869 scientists and engineers was developed in late June 1946. President Truman signed a Declaration of Principles on the status of German scientists to be brought to the U.S. on Sept. 13, 1946. See Harsch, 2004: 110-1. This process of "scientist exports" to the United States. was slowed as the persons concerned had to be approved by a tribunal review under the "Law for Liberation from National Socialism and Militarism". See Harsch, 2004: 110 and 123. Persistent Nazis should not be considered for "Paperclip". See Freeman, 1995. A divergent view, however, was proposed by Bower (1987) and (1988) and Hunt (1991), who believed that "Paper Clip" was a "conspiracy" by U.S. authorities to employ "Nazi" scientists in the U.S. Their entry into the USA had to be done under certain security protections. Between May 1945 and December 1952 under the framework of project "Paper Clip", 573 German scientists, engineers and technicians were brought to the United States. See Freeman, 1995. Lasby, 1975. Other sources speak of 642 foreign specialists. See also Freeman, 1995.
30 – See Harsch, 2004: 111. In the AMC diary entry for Dec. 16th, 1946 there is a list of

the names of 20 German scientists for possible jobs at the SAM in the U.S. submitted at the request of the "Air Surgeon". Strughold traveled during the summer of 1947 to the U.S. At the turn of 1946-47, T. Benzinger, K. Buettner, U.C. Luft, H. Haber and H.G. Clamann had already left the Heidelberg AMC to go to the SAM in the United States. U.K. Henschke, O. Gauer, and H. Giercke signed contracts to work at the Aeromedical Laboratory at Wright Field AFB, Ohio. H. Schaefer and D. Beischer went to the Naval School of Aviation Medicine in Pensacola, Florida. See also Harsch, 2004: 117.

31 - At the Nuremberg Trial of the Major War Criminals (Oct. 18th, 1945 – Oct. 1st 1946), medical crimes were mentioned only in passing. This was followed by 12 subsequent processes, including the so-called "Doctors' Trial" that was under under U.S. jurisdiction. See Taylor, 1996. These medical experiments during the war had been made possible by the special position of the Foundation "Ancestral Heritage" (*Ahnenerbe*) of the "protective squadron" (Schutzstaffel, SS), which initiated these horrific human experiments in concentration camps under their responsibility.

32 - See Gerst, 1997 and Jurgen, 1994. T. Taylor was the chief prosecutor, the psychiatrist, L. Alexander, was the medical advisor for the prosecution, and Dr. A.C. Ivy of the University of Illinois was an expert witness concerning ethical questions. See German, 1997. See also Nuremberg Code of 1947. In: German Med J (Dtsch Aerztebl) 1996, 93: C-1021st See also Kudlien, 1985.

33 - The leading German physiologist, Hermann Rein, criticized in his article in the Goettingen university newspaper, "Science and Inhumanity", the publication of this paper by Mitscherlich and Mielke in a very harsh way. His point was that some outstanding scientists that were known for their complete ethical uprightness were brought to the terrible suspicion that they gave approval to or that they even participated in these crimes. Rein judged that these medical experiments were unscientific and unnecessary. He criticized Mitscherlich for having established the "propagandistic assertion" that "German science" was being judged in court and would be by its very nature be the cause of the crimes and the inhumanity See Harsch, 2004: 108.

34 - "Case No. 1: U.S. against Karl Brandt et. al." lasted from November 1946 to August 1947. Indicted were 20 doctors and three non-physicians. See Maser, 1988; Kanovitch, 1997; Benzenhoefer, 1996; Mitscherlich and Mielke, 1989, Taylor, 1996 and Harsch, 2004: 110-1. Seven defendants were sentenced to death and executed, five defendants were sentenced to life imprisonment (including G. Rose and O. Schroeder) and four were sentenced to long prison terms (including H. Becker-Freyseng). Seven defendants were acquitted, including H.W. Romberg, P. Rostock, S. Ruff, K. Schaefer and G.A. Weltz. Benzinger was arrested in Heidelberg, but released after interrogation. Strughold gave sworn statements for the accused - Becker Freyseng, Schroeder, Ruff and Schaefer. In a fifth statement, he highlighted the research atmosphere at the AMRI and the RLM. See Harsch, 2004: 112. Despite Ruff's request, American and German colleagues from the USAF AMC in Heidelberg were not allowed as witnesses, but their affidavits were used. See also Roth, 2001.

35 – See Harsch, 2004.

Chapter six

1 - See Harsch, 2004: 108. Rein also suggested Schoedel, Opitz, Kramer, and Thauer.

2 - See Harsch, 2004: 108.

3 - See Harsch, 2004: 108. Lt. Col. Leon P. Irvin, director of the Office of Military Government at the Univ. Heidelberg.

4 - See Harsch, 2004: 108.

5 - See Harsch, 2004: 110.
6 - See Harsch, 2004: 109.
7 - See Harsch, 2004: 113. U.S. officials requested from the faculty of medicine at the University of Heidelberg in a letter dated Feb. 18, 1947, whether or not Strughold could be available for a few months in the U.S. This was answered in a positive way.
8 - See Peter, 1994
9 – Harsch, 2004: 108.
10 – Harsch, 2004: 108. Hahn and Rein wrote the critical article „Invitation to USA" and highlighted the problems for German universities.
11 - See Harsch, 2004: 120: "... the medical specialists were somewhat more reluctant."
12 – Oral history Alcott, 1997.
13 – See Campbell, 1959.
14 – See Harsch, 2004: 108-10. There are just a very few documents left from 1947. Just before his departure to the USA he wrote a letter dated 18th July to the rector of Heidelberg University, Prof. Dr. Freiherr von Camphausen (Harsch, 2004: 109): "I leave Heidelberg with a heavy heart, but on the other hand, with a certain amount of optimism in regard to my responsibilities. Although when I arrive in the United States many people will probably be on vacation, but I still hope to send to your Magnificence a report as soon as possible." He further noted that the U.S. authorities intended to give a daily supply of food to the Heidelberg students if the German authorities would agree to this. The head of medical research in the U.S. Navy questioned Dr. Strughold and received information on the food situation of the Heidelberg students: "He invited me to Washington to be his guest and asked me to elaborate on a report that I made for him on the cruise with detailed medical data and maybe to write an essay for the journal 'Science'. He also promised me that he would do anything to help me and the situation here in Heidelberg to improve the student living situation."
15 – See Harsch, 2004: 109 and 124.
16 - Dornberger was the military leader of the Army Research Institute for rocket development in Peenemuende-East during the war years. Strughold and Dornberger met together repeatedly in the U.S. See Harsch, 2004.
17 - See Thomas, 1962.
18 - See Harsch, 2004: 123; J.I.O.A.-file: Statement of reasons why he desires immigration.
19 – See Harsch, 2004: 123.
20 – See Harsch, 2004: 108-110 and 114.
22 – See Harsch, 2004: 109. When Strughold visited the Washington office, which administered the food aid to the occupied territories, the delivery of a protein-wheat-soy combination for the Heidelberg University was agreed to. Strughold regarded this composition as very suitable particularly for "surgical convalescents". At Harvard University in Boston, Strughold held a lecture on this nutritional topic. See Harsch, 2004: 108. In 1948 Hoepke thanked him for his support: "We extend to you the greatest thanks for you have provided material not only for so very many of our colleagues, but you have also done a lot for the students. Your seed is now going on."
23 – See Harsch, 2004: 109. The administrative director of the University of Heidelberg wrote after a food delivery, to the U.S. side in his acknowledgments: "We all are grateful to the unknown American donors who helped with their high-hearted actions not only to alleviate material poverty, but to bridge understanding between people and the belief in the progress of humanity." .
24 – See Harsch, 2004: 109. A "small air bridge" was tested on April 1948 and 200 tones were transported in the first air lift to Berlin-Tegel. The subsequent actual air lift

lasted from June 26th, 1948 to the end of the Berlin blockade by the Soviet Union on May 12th, 1949. See Scherff, 1998.

25 – See Harsch, 2004: 109 and 113. His return was also expected among the students. In October 1947 four medical students demanded in the name of the Heidelberg students that Strughold return at the earliest possible time.

26 - See Harsch, 2004: 109.

27 - In the document of April 16, 1949, Strughold mentioned that he is still involved in Washington on nutritional issues for Germany. See Harsch, 2004: 109.

28 - See Harsch, 2004: 109-10.

29 – See Harsch, 2004: 109: "The question to ask Mr. Street is why name him as an honorary professor since the faculty found it difficult to understand why Strughold left the chair, which he had only recently held, for 1 ¾ years without specifying his precise reasons for his non-return and not keeping to his deadlines without a leave of absence."

30 - See Harsch, 2004: 110.

31 - See Goyer, 1997. The AAF School of Aviation Medicine, Randolph Field, Texas had already been transferred a year earlier from the "Air Training Command" to the "Air University". See Office of History, 1995: A Short History of Air University.

32 - The reorganization of the U.S. Army Air Force found its expression in the founding of the U.S. Air Force as an independent part of the forces on Sept. 18th, 1947. See Goyer, 1997. Reintegrating U.S. scientists in their civilian work created gaps. See Armstrong, 1959. Already in December 1946 the assistant to Strughold, Imgeborg Schmidt, arrived at SAM, followed by Clamann, Luft, Balke, Rose, Noell and Tonndorf in January 1947. Later Buettner, H. Haber and others followed. In June 1947 the three German translators met at AMC Heidelberg, Erwin Buechel, Tatjana Schmidt - sister of Dr. Ingeborg Schmidt - and Hildegard Weiss. To support the work on the aeromedical handbook other specialists followed. The Department of Library Services was reinforced by Dr. Helmut Sieg of the Aero Medical Laboratories, Wright Field, Ohio in January 1948. Ms. Schmidt left the SAM after a year of work and completion of the manuscript, "German Aviation Medicine World War II" in June 1948. In addition to the handbook at the Department of Library Services, more than 50 publications were published on aeromedical subjects. See Harsch, 2004. In the archives of the USAFSAM in San Antonio, Texas several working papers of Strughold were available in German language.

33 – Oral history Alcott, 1997. In addition, the electronic specialists J.W. Freytag and E. Prast came to the SAM. See also Lasby, 1971: 258 and Harsch, 2004: 120. They were "wards" as they were referred to - that is, "without official status of the state department."

34 - SAM began in 1918 as "Medical Research Laboratory" in Hazlehurst Field, Mineola, Long Iceland (New York). See USAF, 1992 and Schafer, 1968.

35 – See Harsch, 2004: 123.

36 - See H. Strughold: Hypoxia, Hypoxidosis, Hypoxidation, Hybernation, Apparent Death and Suspended Animation. In: J Aviat Med 1954, 25: 113-22. Strughold was initially assigned to the Department of Physiology. According to DeHart (1985) it was actually the Department of Ophthalmology. The Department of Physiology in 1948 had the following employees: R.F. Adler, A.W. Heterington, H.W. Dorris, Jr., L. Burkhardt, H. Strughold, U.C. Luft, K. Kramer and H.G. Clamann.

37 - See DeHart, 1985 and Beckh, 1979.

38 - See H. Armstrong, H. Haber, H. Strughold: Aeromedical Problems of Space Travel. J Aviat Med 1949, 20: 383-417. Discussion contributions came from Dr. AC Ivy, Harry G. Armstrong, Heinz Haber, Com. Charles F. Gell, Dr. John C. Flanagan, Dr. Behrens, Dr. Hall, Com. Goodwin, Dr. Buettner and Dr. Dill.

39 - See Harsch, 2004: 110.

40 - See Armstrong, 1959. Predictions for the next few years, they have already made well in advance. See McGinnis, 1998: 1108: "Strughold and his modest SAM staff in 1949 estimated that the main medical problems could be formulated for spaceflight and the majority of the questions fully answered within 10-15 years. Hardware could be developed within 15 to 20 years. The first manned space flights that would become feasible between 1964 and 1969. "

41 - Strughold stated: "The fact that my stay here finally led to the loss of the Physiology assignment in Heidelberg, I greatly regret. But I have the feeling that the tasks brought to me, stand above this things. Facts, which are also in the interest of Germany, now and later." Armstrong supported Heinz Haber and Strughold to establish the department of space medicine. In May 1949 Strughold was determined as the first head of the Department of Aerospace Medicine, USAF SAM. A short time later K. Buettner and F. Haber joined the department. See, Armstrong, 1959. Strughold headed the department until 1957, and was replaced by G.R. Steinkamp. In 1958 the Department of Space Medicine expanded to a Division of the USAF SAM. See also Harsch, 2004: 110 and 116.

42 - See Harsch, 2004: 109.

43 - See Ward, 1959. A 12-year-old applied in 1949 for a flight to Mars. See Astro Medic 9th Nov. 1961. The young writer from New Hyde Park, New York wrote in 1949: "Dear Sirs, I would like to volunteer to go with the Mars expedition. I think I am qualified both physically and mentally, though I am only 12 years old. "

44 - See Thomas, 1962.

45 - See Preface by C.H. Roadman, p. 13-14, in H. Strughold: Your Body Clock, 1971. Another is not found on this trip. When the AMA Congress of was held in New York in 1949, he was not present because of his Euro-stay. His return flight from Frankfurt was on Nov. 26, 1949 and scheduled to arrive in Westover Field on Nov. 27th, 1949.

46 – See Marbarger, 1992: 2.

47 – See von Beckh, 1979.

48 - See J Aviat Med 1951, 22: 163 and J Aviat Med 1950, 21: 359-60.

49 - The first international astronautical congress took place in Paris early in October 1950. As the Korean airlift diminished the capacities for the transatlantic routes, Strugholds presence was doubtful up until September. See Harsch, 2004: 110. In 1951 he was the treasurer of the Space Medicine Branch, in 1958 he was the President-elect and in 1959 he was named as President. See J Aviat Med, oral history Rayman and Fuchs 1997.

Chapter seven

1 – In the glossary part of the journal a definition of space medicine was first introduced. See J Aviat Med 1950, 21: 359-60.

2 –See J Aviat Med 1958, 29: 705, and J Aviat Med 1958, 29: 408. Also "Space Medicine Bibliography". This bibliography of space medicine by Charles A. Roos published in 1958 already contained 282 articles. See Marbarger (ed.): Space Medicine - The Human Factor in Flights Beyond the Earth. In: J Aviat Med 1952, 23: 526-7.

3 - See Berry, 1986: A63.

4 - See Strughold H.: Space Medicine and it's Relation to Space Law. USAFSAM paper, no date. In: Harsch, 2004.

5 - See Harsch, 2004: 117.

6 – The author A. C. Fischer, Jr. visited what he considered to be all of the important national aviation research centers: Pensacola, Dayton, Randolph, Johnsville and Holloman. See Fischer, 1955.

7 - See Stuhlinger and Ordway, 1992.

8 – See Harsch, 2004: 119. "Doctors in Space" was produced at the WUHT-TV-studios at the University of Houston, Texas from 1956-1957. It was financed by the Ford foundation and broadcasted nationwide by the National Educational TV Center in Ann Arbor, Michigan. See J Aviat Med 1958, 29: 483. Vol. 12 of 13 was titled "Satellites and Missiles" (G. Peyton). See Thomas, 1962. In the archives there is an additional request by R. F. Schenkkan, director of Radio Television at the Univ. of Texas in Austin, asking Strughold to record a presentation at the Space Age Forum in Dallas, Texas on Apr. 14th, 1959 to be used for a TV documentary by the National Education Television and Radio Center. Strughold also prepared a paper entitled "The Trip to the Moon. Medical Problems." for a presentation at the Denver Public Schools for the National Educational Television Network, KRMA-TV, Channel 6. A report about the proposed "Twentieth Century" production of CBS-TV "Man on the Moon" can be found in Astro Medic 23th Nov. 1961. T. C. Bedwell, John E. Pickering, Billy E. Welch and H. Strughold are mentioned as co-editors.

9 – The Air University was active in the field of aeromedical education (postgraduate medical college). Aeromedical lectures by Strughold are documented. See Harsch, 2004: 117 and 120.

10 - See Baerwolf , 1978 and 1994: 180.

11 - See Glasgow, 1977.

12 - See Roadman, 1968 und Marbarger, 1992.

13 - See Strughold H.: Suggestions Concerning the Proposed Program for the "Symposium on the Upper Atmosphere", 1951.

14 – The former superior to von Braun, W. Dornberger, who was employed by the Bell-Aircraft-Corporation, could not attend this meeting because he was traveling in Germany. He congratulated Strughold in 1952 regarding his contribution to space medicine and to aeronatical development, saying that Strughold and the Space Medicine Division's activities broke up the frozen thinking of many people in the American aviation industry. See Harsch, 2004: 115.

15 - See Marbarger, 1992.

16 - See J Aviat Med 1954, 25: 323.

17 - See Berry, 1986, Marbarger, 1992 and Harsch, 2004: 117.

18 - In the German magazine "Weltraumfahrt" (Space Travel, Vol. 4, 1951, p. 81f.) the behaviour of organisms in zero gravity was discussed. Strughold, H. v. Diringshofen, GfW, Univ. Frankfurt a. M.; O. Ranke, Physiolog. Institute of the Univ. Erlangen; H. Schaefer: Physiolog. Institute of the Univ. Heidelberg; J. Schneider, GfW, Fulda; G. Schubert, Physiolog. Institute of the Univ. Wuerzburg and Dr. E. Langer, GfW, Wiesbaden.

19 - See Harsch, 2004: 117.

20 - See Strughold H.: Mechanoreceptor, Gravireceptor, 1957.

21 - The flight surgeon H.D. Stallings stated that more than 4,000 parabolic flights were performed at USAF SAM with a total duration of approximately 37 hours. See Harsch, 2004: 117, 118 and 120.

22 - Bruno Balke of the Department of Physiology and Biophysics at the USAF SAM spent six weeks at an altitude of 14,800 ft. in the Peruvian Morococco. Then at the school he tolerated a cabin altitude height of 58,000 ft. with 100%-oxygen-ventilation for three minutes. See Strughold, 1954: Hypoxia, Hypoxidosis, Hypoxidation, Hibernation, Apparent Death and Suspended Animation.

23 – See Strughold, 1953: XVI and von Braun, 1969.

24 - See Harsch, 2004: 115. In his of 28th Oct. 1952 there are also personal notes: „This summer I did a trip to the West again. Unfortunately, the trips are 2000 and up to 3000 km. For two years now I have had a car, it´s a Plymouth. On the weekends I often drive to

the Gulf of Mexico. This is a rather uninhabited and wild region. (...) Right now I still live in a small cute house."

25 – See Ward, 1959.

26 - U. C. Luft left SAM for an appointment at the Lovelace Foundation in Albuquerque, New Mexico to become the research director. F. Haber obtained a job at the Arco Corporation in Connecticut. An appointment at the University of Washington in Seattle was given to K. Buettner, at the University of Missouri in St. Louis to P. Cibis, at the University of California in Los Angeles to H. Haber, at the University of Buffalo in New York, New York to W. K. Noell, at the University of Indiana in Bloomington to I. Schmidt, and at the Iowa State University Hospital to J. Tonndorf. In 1960, Dr. Bruno Balke and several other colleagues from USAF SAM left to go to the FAA "Civil Aeronautical Research Institute" (CARI). See: Historical Report of the SAM, Vol. 17 in: Harsch, 2004: 117.

27 – Many US-scientists left military service. Major G. T. Hauty left his appointment as a psychologist to continue work as a civil servant at SAM at Randolh AFB, Texas. In the space program he did research in biological rhythms and long term isolation. He continued to work at the FAA CARI in the late 1950´s as the chief scientist of the Aviation Psychology Branch. Oral history Mohler, 1996.

28 – See Harsch, 2004: 117, 118 and 123.

29 – The first nominee was Wernher von Braun, the second was A. V. Cleaver, chairman of the British Interplanetary Society. See. J Aviat Med 1954, 25: 439.

30 - See. Strughold H.: General and Medical Observations During a Recent European Trip (1954). See also newspaper report by Kendricks, 1954. At the IAF-Congress in Stockholm 1960 there were already 1/3 of the attendees from biomedical sciences. See newspaper report by Sonnenborn, 1959.

31 – Strughold kept in close communication to his sister Mathilda (Harsch, 2004: 123): "Dear Mathilda! Enclosed is a cheque and a letter by bishop E. Spiess from Afrika! You see, I am not that stingy as other people seem. Kind regards, Your brother Hubert." In a newspaper report Strughold stated ironically: "In Texas I do not feel far away from my home in Westfalia. (...) Texans are called the ´Westfalians of Amerika´ because of their love to their country. These cultures are comparable." See Weiss, 1954.

32 - See Strughold H.: Space Medicine. Speech on May 25, 1956. At SAM there was a space medical symposium on Jan. 19-20, 1956. Strughold was the chairman. Among the guests was Krafft Ehricke, a specialist in rocket and cruise missile design from the Convair Aircraft Corp. in San Diego, California.

33 – See newspaper report by Hense, 1957.

34 - See Aviat Space Environ Med 1986, 67: 1220: Hubertus Strughold.

35 - See Baerwolf, 1995 and Moritz, 1967. The first geophysical year was announced by scientists in the early 1950s to promote international research of the Earth (1st July 1957 – 31st Dec. 1958). See. Gartmann, 1958. The launch of Sputnik on 4th Oct. 1957 shattered the western hemisphere.

36 – See Strughold H.: My European Trip to the International Astronautical Federation Congress in Barcelona 1957.

37 – Oral history Voß, 1996; Ueter, 1997 and Kolander, 1996.

38 – See Thomas, 1962: 265. See J Aviat Med 1958, 29: 1-14. The balloon flight took place at space-equivalent conditions (10 mbar, space radiation, temperature control, psychological reactions). Simons as a precaution wore a partial pressure suit. At the meeting 23 out of the 44 papers came from America and only five from Soviet scientists. Seven papers were of space medical or astrobiological background. Strughold regarded Simons lecture as the one with the highest impact at this meeting. For political reasons,

the anticipated lectures by D. E. Okhotsimskii , T. M. Eneev and V. A. Egorov, all from the Soviet Academy of Sciences did not occur, as they did not arrive. They were supposed to speak about satellite issues and "Some Considerations of the Dynamics of a Flight to the Moon"! See Strughold H.: My European Trip to the International Astronautical Federation Congress in Barcelona 1957.

39 - See Engle und Lott, 1979: 128.

40 – See newspaper report by Feiden, 1957.

41 – See newspaper report by Zimmermann, 1957.

42 - See Strughold H.: My European Trip to the International Astronautical Federation Congres in Barcelona 1957

43 – USAF SAM history in Harsch, 2004: 117.

44 – Based on the results of this experiment, Strughold was already convinced in 1959, that a moon mission was possible from a medical standpoint. See newspaper report by Sonnenborn, 1959.

45 – See Thomas, 1962 and newspaper reports in Harsch, 2004.

46 - See Glasgow, 1970: 8.

47 - See Stuhlinger und Ordway, 1992: 466.

48 - See Strughold H.: Compendium of Aerospace Medicine. Vol. 2.; 1979, p. 14. 1958 Strughold stated: "We are at the threshold to manned space flight." See also J Aviat Med 1959, 30: 217. Strughold said about President Johnson, that he was the first statesman who had expressed an interest in the possibilities of manned space travel. He showed foresight in the importance of further development in this area and therefore a political activist behind the successful moon landing. See Thomas, 1962. The following statements by President Johnson confirm this assessment by Strughold (1965): "We expect to explore the moon, not just visit it or photograph it"; 'We plan to explore and chart planets as well"; "We shall expand our earth laboratories into space laboratories and extend our national strengths into the space dimension." See private archive of Mary Strughold in Harsch, 2004: 112 f.

49 - See Strughold H.: Building a Living Room in Space. Paper. See also The U.S. Air Force Experimental Sealed Cabin, Aviat Med 1956, 27: 50.

50 - Strughold gave the following example: Dr. Dornberger was at Randolph AFB, Texas several times beginning in 1954 to discuss medical issues concerning his aviation projects. Strughold had the impression that he could have launched a space craft in 1957. Strughold guessed that this did not happen due to the fact that there were to many commitees involved. See Strughold H.: Space Medicine and Astrobiology. Paper, 5 p. Report to be submitted to House Select Committee on Astronautics and Space Exploration, Room 214, New House Office Building, Washington (D. C.) 5. May 1958 p. 2508. Walter Dornberger, former vice president of Bell Aircraft Corp. in Buffalo (New York) visisted Strughold in 1968 (not for the first time) at SAM. In Astro Medic 1968, 7: 13: Distinguished Visitor.

51 - International Symposium on the Physics and Medicine of the Atmosphere and Space. In: Tomorrow through research, Vol. XII, No. 182, Southwest Research Institute 1958. See also J Aviat Med 29 (1958) 485-92. See also Journal Space Travel - "Weltraumfahrt" 1958, 9: 94.

52 - See Roadman, 1968: XIII.

54 - See Harsch, 2004: 115.

55 – See newspaper report by Jungk R.: The space professor. See also Baerwolf, 1969 and Aerospace Med 1971, 42: 1244. NASA assigned USAF SAM to construct a space capsule for a rhesus monkey, "Sam", who flew in 1959 in a Little Joe test rocket to demonstrate the rescue abort system of the Mercury astronauts.

56 – See Harsch, 2004: 115.

57 - See J Aviat Med 1959, 30. H. G. Armstrong: The Origin of Space Medicine; H. Strughold: Space Medicine of the next decade as viewed by a Physician and Physiologist; H. Haber: Space Medicine of the next decade as viewed by an Astrophysicist; K. J. K. Buettner: Space Medicine of the next decade as viewed by an Environmental Physicist; F. Haber: Space Medicine of the next decade as viewed by the Engineer.

58 - See Thomas, 1962.

59 – In 1953, the Department of Space Medicine consisted of Strughold, Cpt. J. E. Keator and two civil servants. One year later the financial resources were even cut further. Strughold was left alone with one part time civil servant. See Berry, 1986. However, after the Sputnik shock in 1957 the attention for space related research drastically changed.

Chapter eight

1 – The committee members met again Apr. 24th – 29th at the historic building No. 70 at USAF SAM at Brooks AFB, Texas. See Harsch, 2004: 118.

2 - Strughold was the scientific advisor to the school's commander and was a member of the Advanced Studies Group. His assignment instructions determined the following: "The advisor for Research serves as a member of the immediate staff of the Commandant of the Aerospace Medical Center. It is his responsibility to keep the Commandant informed on new scientific and technological developments on the national and international scene. He must analyze these developments and evaluate them as to their importance for manned flight of both of the atmospheric and space type. He has to make recommendations for the direction and recurring re-orientation of the over-all research program of the Center and of its various portions in order to always keep the program in consonance with the requirements of a modern Aerospace power of the United States. The Advisor for Research is also an ex-officio member of the newly established Advanced Studies Group. The mission of this Group is to study the present state and future potentialities in aeronautics and astronautic technology, propulsion systems, etc., and new developments in the medical and biological sciences, and to develop new theories and to search for new avenues of approach in the perfection of manned flight. In addition to the ex-officio members and one permanent staff member, this Group, which is under the immediate authority of the Commandant, may include experts of international reputation in pertinent fields for a temporary time for the purpose of exploring new methods, new power systems, new protective devices and new possibilities in the expansion of the vertical frontier of the Air Force." See Harsch, 2004.

3 - See J Aviat Med 1963, 34: 89.

4 – See Harsch, 2004: 120.

5 – The following five installations networked in this organisational structure: Aerospace Medical Research Laboratory, Wright Patterson AFB (Ohio); Aeromedical Research Laboratory, Holloman AFB (New Mexico); The Arctic Aeromedical Laboratory, Ft. Wainwright (Alaska); Epidemiological Laboratory, Wilford Hall USAF Hospital, Lackland AFB (Texas) and the School of Aerospace Medicine, Brooks AFB (Texas). See Harsch, 2004.

6 - See J Aviat Med. 1962, 63: 497-8 and 1024. In a letter of the US Foreign Service from 1962, official requests were made at the Universities of Heidelberg and Wuerzburg regarding Strughold's person, as he applied for a government job in the US. See Harsch, 2004: 110 and 124.

7 - Individual Request for Attendance at Meeting of Technical, Scientific, Prof. and other similar Organizations dated 22. July 1963.
8 – See newspaper article: Whats Up? Dr. Strughold says, Russians May be Soon. 1961.
9 - The successful launch of the Saturn rocket was celebrated by Wernher von Braun together with Hubertus Strughold and Mary Webb Dalehite in the "Old Town Inn" in San Antonio, Texas. See Fig. 35.
10 - See Thomas, 1962.
11 – See Harsch, 2004: 115.
12 - It was also planned to attend the annual meeting of the German Rocket Society of 20-22. Sept. 1963 in Hamburg. More information on this could not be found.
13 – See Harsch, 2004: 115.
14 – At the Rome Congress, the German ´Flight surgeon and Gynecologist G. Mutke gave a presentation on aerospace medical aspects of gynecology. Before the lecture Strughold came up to him and asked: "Tell me Mr. Mutke, I've seen in the program the talk about gynecological problems in aviation and space medicine. What's that? Mutke replied: That's for sure! How long can a flight attendant fly from Frankfurt to New York in the pregnant state? Is that still in the eighth month? And what about the menstruational periodicity during time zone travel, under the influence of stress and climatical factors? And how long can a flight instructor fly when pregnant? Ah, said Strughold, I didn´t think about this so far." Oral history G. Mutke, 1999.
15 - See Harsch, 2004: 115. See also the Main-Post 12th Oct. 1963. Pope Pius XII was "space-minded": He already gave a speech to the delegates of the 7th International Astronautical Congress in Rome in 1956.
16 - Strughold gave a lecture "Basic Medical Research in the adaptation of Man and Machine in Aviation and Space Travel". See Harsch, 2004: 115. The German DGLRM was founded on 1st Dec. 1961. The 1963 meeting was chaired by Heinz von Diringshofen. The first session was titled "Medical Research of the adaptation of humans and machines in the aerospace industry." See Aviat Space Environ Med 1979, 50: 529-30: The German Aerospace Medical Association was founded by HJ Grunhof. Besides Strughold, several other former "Paperclip" specialists were early society members. See list of Members of the DGLRM of 1963: 4 - H. von Beckh, Holloman AFB (New Mexico), 5 - D. Beischer, SAM Pensacola (Florida) 6 - T. Benzinger (Maryland), 30 - S. Gerathewohl, Air Univ. USAF, NASA Armes Research Center, Mountain View (California); 31 - H. von Giercke, Wright Air Development Center, Dayton (Ohio); 75 - H. W. Rose, Space Medicine Research Laboratory, Lockheed MSC, Palo Alto (California); 77 - H. Seeler, Aeromedical Laboratory, Wright Air Development Center, Dayton (Ohio); 83 - I. Schmidt, Div. Optometry, Indiana University, Bloomington (Indiana).
17 - See Harsch, 2004: 119.
18 - See J Aviat Med 1963, 34: 1084 and J Aviat Med 1964, 35: 407
19 - Five years later, Strughold wrote a report to Lauschner for the Technical University of Munich concerning his honorary professorship. See Harsch, 2004: 116.
20. See Aerospace Med 1964, 35: 86-8: "I have come to Texas to salute an outstanding group of pioneers - the men who man the Brooks Air Force Base School of Aerospace Medicine and the Aerospace Medical Center."
21 - See Baerwolf, 1969 and Aerospace Med 1964, 35: 86-8.
22 - See Roadman, 1968. The meeting was held from Nov. 16-18, 1964, and 500 scientists, engineers and physicists were expected for the event.
23 – See Harsch, 2004: 116. W. von Braun, Director of NASA-George C. Marshall Flight Center in Alabama thanked Strughold for his work in a letter dating 7th Dec. 1963:

"Please know that we are always mindful of the great and many contributions that you have made to spaceflight and medical research."

24 - See Baerwolf, 1965 and the newspaper article Westfaelische Nachrichten of 29th Aug. 1965: "The path to week-long space flights is free. I am convinced that we can send astronauts safely to travel for over several weeks. This space flight is a milestone in the development of manned space flight. We can go from an eight-days duration space flight to at least several weeks, if not longer. I think that space flight to the moon without artificial gravity is absolutely possible." See Baerwolf, 1995. 204-5.

25 - See Harsch, 2004: 116.

26 - See Thomas, 1962.

27 - See Faust, 1965: Why to the moon?

28 - See Aerospace Med 1968, 39: 219/907. The catalogue "Fourth International Symposium on Bioastronautics and the Exploration of Space" was edited by C. H. Roadman, H. Strughold and R. B. Mitchell. Strughold proclaimed that Arthur C. Clarke was a "Martian Indian Chief" . Clarke was a reknown "Science-Fact-and-Fiction"-author from Columbo, Ceylon. On his movie based on the book, "2001-A Space Odyssey". See Aerospace Med 1968, 39: 1147.

29 - Strughold refereed "The Physiological Clock" and the influence of time zone travel by jet planes and space capsules. See Aerospace Med 1968, 39: 911, 1252.

30 - See Aerospace Med 1968, 39: 1262.

31 - See Harsch, 2004: 116.

32 - See Aerospace Med 1968, 39: 1371.

Chapter nine

1 – Oral history Oberndorf, 1996. More personal impressions arise from the following remarks by Baerwolf: "'The flight to the moon, I might still live to see ... , there will be robots that will be landed in the seventies on Mars and then men will follow in the eighties or nineties ... , then yes, you can read in peace and quote me, but do so very well". See Baerwolf, 1995: 102. In a newspaper interview Strughold was asked, if he would fly on a space flight for the clarification of his scientific work? Strughold answered: "I am now 61 years old. The old design the plans and give the younger generation the tools for such a space flight. That way, they may also contribute their share to the exploration of outer space. "See newspaper report by Sonneborn, 1959. The USAF SAM commander Col. George C. Mohr recalled: "Dr. Strughold's modest office was located in the northwestern end of the second floor of Building 150th The room was crammed with objects that Strughold's collective passion brought together over the years: books, reports, and a selection of objects, some of which were of obscure origin. For the visitor he left little space. Still, I appreciated his kindness and his broad scientific knowledge. " See Harsch, 2004: 120-1. Because of his illness, Strughold came less frequently to his office for "small talk". On occasions he entertained the former employees with selected cartoons. But he also remained open minded to new developments. The former adjutant to the Luftwaffe´s surgeon general during World War II, Erwin A. Lauschner, described Strughold's casual appearance:" He always wore a little rumpled-looking black suit with a white shirt, his tie loosened and slightly crooked. Once engaged in a conversation he suddenly awoke and unfolded an enormous interest in everything with his extensive range of knowledge ". See Lauschner, 1984: 356.

2 - See Baerwolf, 1995: 100

3 - See Thomas, 1962. The indigenous Westphalian said during a speech in front of the Brooks AFB Officer's Wife's Club in 1963 what his favorite foods were: pumpernickel bread, cake and pudding. Furthermore, beer soup, sausage, pea soup with potatoes, fried

sausage, and not least, Westphalian ham. He also recommended baby's food as "the best food in the world". See Baerwolf, 1994.

4 – See Harsch, 2004: 121.

5 - See Aerospace Med 1970, 41: 835, 1971, 42: 919. Much of his correspondence and working papers were at this place, but not always in an orderly manner or archived. A part of his private correspondence and documents were transferred from Ms. Strughold into private ownership after his death. See also Harsch, 2004: 112-17.

6 – See 1977: Strughold does not talk about accomplishments.

7 - See Strughold H.: Compendium of Aerospace Medicine, Vol 2, 1979.

8 – Retranslated from German. See Harsch, 2004: 116.

9 - Oral history Boubel, 1998.

10 - See Harsch, 2004: 120. As early as 1966, Strughold was informed of the project through a letter from M. Calvin who was at NASA.

11 - A group of "Junior ROTC" cadets interviewed Strughold about the role of space in American history. The survey was held in the spring of 1976 at Hangar 9 in which the space museum is housed. See Aerospace Med 1976, 47: 57: "Role of Aerospace in American History."

12 – At this facility there have been catalogued 107,000 volumes, 1,900 periodicals and 127,000 foreign documents, some of these are on microfiche. See Aviat Space Environ Med 1977, 48: 294

13 - Information on the International Space Hall of Fame can be found in the Internet homepages.

14 – See Compendium of Aerospace Medicine Vol 2 1979, p. 12.

15 – See Harsch, 2004: 119 and 123. H. S. Fuchs: Hubertus Strughold - Brief biographies of the aviation and aerospace. Supplement to the Air and Space 1987, 4: 2 p.

16 – Letter was located in the city archives of Hamm. Already in 1967, the city's mayor had honored Strughold as a well-known citizen of the city. See Harsch, 2004: 116. At a reception in honor of Bedwell, Strughold and Ellingson at the 14th year anniversary of the founding of the Space Medicine Department at the SAM, the mayor of San Antonio advertised the motto of the city: "The Road to the Stars Starts Here." See J Aviat Med 1963, 34: 289. In the same year (1963), in honor of Strughold, an annual scientific price was created by the Space Medicine Branch of AsMA. The first award winner was Cpt. Ashton Graybiel, MC. See Aerospace Med 1965, 36: 699

17 - See Aerospace Med 54 (1983) 975: "He is a living example of what an individual can accomplish with ties to two countries."

18 - See Lytle, 1985: 50

19 - See Aerospace Med 1963, 34: 289 and Aerospace Med 1965, 36: 699

20 - The obituary in the San Antonio Express of Sept. 27, 1986 stated: "Strughold, 88, died in his San Antonio home at 11:20 pm Thursday. A rosary is scheduled for 7 p.m. at Porter Loring Funeral Home with services scheduled for 11:00 AM, Tuesday ... ."

Chapter ten

1 - A chronological overview of Strugholds scientific papers, lectures and speeches can be found in the bibliography part on page 185 ff.

2 - See Fuchs, 1987.

3 - See Lytle, 1985.

4 - Strughold essays can be found in The Americana Annual, Annuals of the New York Academy of Science, Advisor for Research, Air University Review, Astronautics and Aeronautics, International Science and Technology, Space Science, Astron, American Journal of Physiology, M. D. Publishers. Inc., Acta Astronautica, Jet Propulsion, Space

Travel, Aeronautical Engineering Review, The New Phys. Areas of Research and Space Medicine and Astrobiology. Strughold advised the editors of "Aerospace Medicine" (1966) and was "Contributing Editor" of "Missiles and Rockets", a member of the new "Editorial Advisory Committee on Space Technology" magazine "Aero / Space Engineering." See J Aviat Med 1958, 29: 478. Jules Vernes "Dr. Koch's" experiment was not published in the United States before 1966. The foreword was written by Willy Ley and the epilogue by H. Strughold.

6 – In the citation Index (ISI), Philadelphia, PA (USA) under Strughold, can be found some 400 literary works for the period from 1945 to 1986: 1945-54 80, 1955-64127, 1965-74137 and 1975-84 54. These numbers were evaluated by me in the late 1990´s and could be higher today.

7 – See Fuchs, 1987. The first Japanese aviation medical textbook "Medicine and the Stars" was dedicated to Strughold. See Aerospace Med 31 (1959) 537

8 - See Section Documents 1 "Offices and service positions (1927-1968)" p. 135.

9 - See Section Documents 2 "Honors and Awards" p. 136.

10 – In the mid 1950s, Strughold was represented in a 3-year period at more than 100 meetings as a guest speaker. A flood of other space-medical invitations to speak and lecture is also documented from this period. See Section Documents " Memberships in scientific societies" p. 137. In the "Curriculum Vitae" by H. Strughold 3rd Oct. 1956 have listed some of the organization and committees to which Strughold was invited as guest speaker. Whether the presentations were actually acted upon by him, the source material is not apparent. Strughold in 1965 was an informal advisor to the Washington "National Air Museum", In 1968 he was a member of the "Board of Directors" at the Texas Academy for Advancement of Life Sciences. See Harsch, 2004: 120.

11 - See archival sources. For example, the correspondence between Strughold and U.S. President Lyndon B. Johnson was cited: "Dear Dr. Strughold. You have the skillful hands of the physician, the cool brain of the scientist, the loyalty of a trusted servant of the people and the warm heart of a friend. Your attention - to remember my birthday - contributes to my growing admiration. With best wishes! Signed: L. B. Johnson. " See Harsch, 2004: 115, 116, 119 and 120.

12 – See the philosophical theses of H. Strughold in Muenster on 13th June 1923. In J Biol 1923, 78: 195-230: "The majority of the tests I made on myself, but I owe it to the kind willingness of Prof. v. Frey, Dr. Webel, and the candidates in medicine Du Mesnil de Rochemont, Palm and Dütemeyer to be able to verify the results of my research by volunteer testings on them."

13 - See Strughold H.: Contributions to the knowledge of the refractory period of human spinal cord. Medical habilitation, Freiburg 1927.

14 – This was also reported in 1931 at a WGL meeting (skin senses and their importance to flight). In 1934 Strughold published with the director of the Wuerzburg Physiological Institute, Edgar Wöhlisch, in another science field: "Is thrombin a proteolytic enzyme? "

15 - He had the feeling as if the aircraft would slip from under his body. Strughold was thereafter glad to stand on his feet on solid ground again.

16 - See Zuntz, 1912: 27.

17 - See J Aviat Med 1956, 27: 158.

18 - See Harsch, 2004: 114.

19 - When human experiments where performed by Strughold or his colleagues, they were self-experiments and experiments with colleagues, volunteers and aviation personnel. See methodology sections of the papers.

20 - See H. Strughold: The altitude effect in the light of neurophysiological considerations. Luftfahrtmed 1938, 3: and 210-22. See also "The symptoms of altitude

effects in the film image". Report of Akad Dtsch Luftfahrtforschung 1940, 3: 22/23.
21 - As the time reserve decreases with increasing altitude, Strughold suggested the mandatory use of altitude resistance tests before flight qualification. See Luftwiss 1940, 7: 269-76 and Mitt Luftfahrtmed 1940, 5: 66-75 and Luftfahrtmed 1938, 3: 55-63.
22 - See Strughold H.: The physiological effect of high altitudes. Luftwiss 1940, 7: 269-76.
23 - See O. Gauer, E. Opitz, F. Palme, H. Strughold: parachute jump and time reserve at high altitudes. Luftfahrtmed 1942, 6: 340-55.
24 - See H. Strughold: The medical problems in the Substratosphere. Dtsch Med Wschr 1939, 8: 281-5: "There is no doubt about it, that the medical problems have to be resolved. Precondition for this is their detailed investigation with quantitative methods."
25 – The ethical aspects of this paper is of tremendous importance, as in other places unethical medical tests were performed without any additional "outcome".
26 – According to Engle and Lott (1979) the term "Aerospace Medicine" was introduced by Strughold. He saw Space Medicine as part of occupational medicine. See Strughold H.: Space Medicine, ed. H. G. Armstrong, 1961.
27 - See H. Strughold: From Aviation Medicine to Space Medicine. In: Air Univ Quart Rev 1958, 10: 15
28 - In the "New York World-Telegram and Sun" of 5th March 1958 he referred to weightlessness as the revolutionary aspect of space medicine, because it was hardly perceptible before. See Moritz, 1966.
29 - See Strughold: From Medicine to Space Aviation Medicine, 1952, p. 318. See also O. Gauer, H. Haber, "Man Under Gravity-Free Conditions" "Aviation Medicine World War II" 1950, p. 641-4. See also Benson, 1951: 316: "A new frontier has now opened - the 'vertical' frontier '.
30 - See Gartman, 1958 (dreamers, scientists, engineers) and Strughold H.: Space Equivalent Conditions. Ast Acta 1955, 1: 32; Strughold et al. Where Does Space Begin. J Aviat Med 1951, 22: 342; Strughold H.: A Simple Classification of the Present and Future Stages of Manned Flight.
31 - The term "Bioastronautics" was first used by Strughold in 1957 at a scientific meeting in San Diego (California). Astrobiology (exobiology) deals with the ecological conditions of other celestial bodies and the question of the possibility of life on these, thus the planetary ecology. See Levitt, 1961: 25-6.
32 - Strughold H.: The importance of oxygen for life. Script of Univ. Heidelberg 1948, 3: 86-95.
33 - The roots of astrobiology date back to 1877, when Italian astronomer GV Schiaparelli in Milan discovered the so called "canali" on Mars what fired peoples' imaginations. A highlight was reached around 1910 when P. Lowell from Observatory in Flagstaff (Arizona) believed to have observed a Martian artificial irrigation system. Subsequent work considered vegetation zones, consisting of primitive mosses and lichens which were quite conceivable. See Strughold H.: From Aviation Medicine to Space Medicine. In: Air Univ Quart Rev 1958, 10: 12
34 - See Avat J Med 1957, 28: 507
35 - See Strughold, 1953 and J Aviat Med 1954, 25: 201 The review in the body of the Aero Medical Association, speaks of a "speculative" study on the possibility of extraterrestrial life. See also H. Strughold: From Aviation Medicine to Space Medicine. In: Air Univ Quart Rev 1958, 10: 12. 1953 G.A. Thikhof from Alma-Ata Observatory published a book on astrobiology. The Space Times 1998, 37: 15-7 list a selected bibliography on Mars exploration, including Strughold Mars-book with the following remark (p. 17): "Strughold was one of the leading authorities of the 1950s on space

medicine and this scientific book suggested that life on Mars was possible."

36 - Findings from spectrographic studies went ahead with space-ecological and medical concepts. See Strughold H.: From Aviation Medicine to Space Medicine. In: Air Univ Quart Rev 1958, 10: 12 Exobiology = study of extraterrestrial life in the solar system. See Kooistra, Mitchell and Strughold: Problems Common to the Fields of Astronomy and Biology: A Symposium. IV The Behavior of Microorganisms under Simulated Martian Environmental Conditions, 1958.

37 - A new approach was needed after the "Mariner IV"-Mars mission, "A New Look at Mars since Mariner IV" (1965). At the 15th International Missile and Space Symposium of the German Rocket Society in Bremen (22nd – 25th Sept. 1966) Strughold's contribution to the space-related medical problems on the flight path to Mars was presented (p. 1 and 14): "With the rapid advances in the field of astronautics there is already the first post-lunar planetary target, a manned Mars landing, in the preparation stage. (...) A minimum time and maximum comfort are the medical prescription for a maximum of success of a manned planetary landing mission. With careful extrapolation of what has been learned so far, the medical response regarding the prospects of a Mars flight, is affirmative and optimistic, if time-saving trajection methods be applied "See Baerwolf, 1995: 105.

38 - See Harsch, 2004: 115 and 120; see also Ch.H. Roadman, in: Strughold, 1971: 13-4.

39 - See Benford, 1947: The AMC Heidelberg was in contact with Prof. Artur Jores, from University of Hamburg, a specialist in this field.

40 – Issue of March 1961. An example of Strughold thoughts on changes in the biorhythm in a sequence of time-zone flights was related by Heinz Haber in 1986 (World on Sunday): "One day Strughold came into the office and said: 'Yesterday was a conference in Moscow that Dean Acheson (former U.S. Secretary of State) took partin. He threw a newspaper on the table and shouted:. My goodness, Acheson departed from Washington yesterday. As he was facing the Russians in Moscow, it was for him like 4 o'clock in the morning. That's not fair! " Strughold was remembered in a contribution of the "San Antonio Express" of 2nd November 1961 about his time as a professor in Heidelberg. A couch in his office was secured, and the time from 12.00 to 14.00 was free time for the teachers: "If the administration had the sofas removed, then certainly the last professor would have left the university."

41 - See Strughold, 1977: 12 (Compendium of Aerospace Medicine, Vol 1).

42 - See Thomas, 1962: 270

43 - An example of its expression at this point is a letter to the astronaut, M. Scott Carpenter, who was involved in the Sea Lab II Project at California's Scripps Institute of Oceanography (cited Harsch, 2004): "From deep in the heart of the presently dry Texas lithosphere , best greetings to you deep in the Pacific Section of Earth's hydrosphere! "

44 - See Strughold H.: On the issue of standardization of terms and methods in aerospace medicine. Aeromed dependence (Luftfahrtmed Abh) 1936/37, 1: 290.

45 - See H. Strughold: Compendium of Aerospace Medicine, Vol 2, 1979.

Chapter eleven
1 – See Harsch, 2004: 77-8.
2 - Nuremburg Trials Document. Doc. 437. Affidavit of Dr. Sigmund Ruff. October 25, 1946.
3 – See Kudlien, 1985; Benz, 1988; Mitscherlich and Mielke, 1989: 20-50 and Harsch, 2004: 74-6 and 162-4.

4 - Nuremburg Trials Doc. 451. Cross Examination of Dr. Wolfgang Lutz. December 12, 1946. Pages 266-74.

5 - Autrum, 1996.

6 – Harsch, 2004: 163-4.

7 – Benzinger, 1946. ATI No. 58275. AAF AMC, Heidelberg 1946.

8 - Ruff S. Rescue Possibilities from High Altitude Flights. Presentation at the 9th Scientific Members Meeting of the German Academy of Aviation Research on 6th November 1942. Pages 3-18.

9 – Benz, 1988; Mitscherliuch and Mielke, 1989; Kanovitch, 1997.

10 – Romberg, 1941: 310-4; Roth, 2001: 110-51; Harsch, 2004: 75.

11 – Benz, 1988: 192, 213-4.

12 – Mitscherlich and Mielke, 1989: 50.

13 – Harsch, 2004: 35; Hunt, 1991: 84.

14 – Military Medical Ethics, Vol. 2: 2003; Berger 1990: 1435-40.

15 – Harsch, 2004: 76-7; Pueschel, 1978; Peter, 1998.

16 – Mitscherlich and Mielke, 1989.

17 - Nuremburg Trials Document. Doc. 451. Cross Examination of Dr. Wolfgang Lutz. December 12, 1946. Pages 266-74.

18 – Harsch, 2004; Buechner, 1965; Pueschel, 1978; Rein, 1946.

19 – Buechner, 1965; Rein, 1946.

20 – Buechner, 1965; Harsch, 2004: 76-7, 164-6; Pueschel, 1978; Rein, 1946.

21 – Mitscherlich, 1946.

22 – Rein, 1946: **3-5.**

23 – Buechner, 1965.

24 - Harsch, 2004: 76-7, 166.

25 – Mitscherlich and Mielke, 1989; Deutsch, 1997.

26 – Bower, 1987: 228.

27 – Weidling, 2004.

28 – Harsch, 2004: 10: 32-5.

29 – Bower, 1987.

30 – Harsch, 2004: 70-3, 160-2.

31 – Schmidt, 2004.

32 – Alexander, 1946: Report # 250.

33 – Bower, 1987: 220.

34 – Bower, 1987: 224.

35 – Hunt, 1991: 16.

36 – Koch, 1993.

37 - Ruhenstroth-Bauer and Nachtsheim, 1944: 18-20.

38 - Ruhenstroth-Bauer, 2000.

39 – Klee, 1997.

40 – Weidling, 2003.

41 - Beddies, 2003: 219-48.

42 – Von Schwerin, 2004.

43 – Schmuhl, 2005

44 – Hunt, 1991: 232.

45 – Harsch, 2004: 70-3.

46 – Blumenthal, 1976.

47 – Hunt, 1991: 232.

48 – Bower, 1987.

49 – Bower, 1987: 214.

50 – Bower, 1987: 224.
51 – Bower, 1987: 228.
52 – Benford, 1948.
53 – Bower, 1987: 221.
54 – Bower, 1987: 218.
55 – Mackowski, 2006.
56 – Eckart, 2012.
57 – Ashman and Wagman, 1988.
58 – Roth, 2001.
59 – Eckart, 2012.
60 – Hunt, 1991.
61 – Hunt, 1991: 86.
62 – Hunt, 1991: 153.
63 – Hunt, 1991: 92.
64 – Hunt, 1991: 259.
65 – Hunt, 1991: 16.
66 – Hunt, 1991: 84.
67 – Hunt, 1991: 85.
68 – Hunt, 1991: 79.
69 – Hunt, 1991: 81.
70 - Doerner, 2000: 314-5.
71 - Doerner, 2000: 314-5, 484-5; Harsch, 2004: 78, 166-7).
72 – Freeman, 1995: 212-3.
73 – Mackowski, 2006.
74 – Kornbluh, 1992.
75 – Harsch, 2004: 164.
76 – Bower, 1987: 205.
77 – Mackowski, 2006.
78 – Harsch, 2004: 32-45.
79 – Mackowski, 2006.
80 - http://nuremberg.law.harvard.edu.
81 – Harsch, 2004: 77; Weindling, 2004.

Appendix 1

1 - Harsch, 2004: 75.
2 - Clamann, 1939; Benzinger, 1946; Harsch, 2007: 907.
3 - Gauer et al., 1941.
4 - Romberg, 1941.
5 - Harsch, 2007: 907. In a memorandum of 23rd October 1941 by the superior institutions a ban on ED experiments on humans was ordered.
6 - Roth, 201: 116-8, 135.
7 - Harsch, 2000: 448 and 855. In a Luftwaffe-report dated October 31 1944 is mentioned, that only the "Spitfires" 6 and 7 as well as the USAAF "Thunderbold" were equipped with a pressure cabin, but only to a limited extent or not at all in use. The altitude bombers "Boeing B-29" were designed for eight-man crew and allowed at an altitude of 13,500 meters a cabin pressure related to 4,500 m. This type was also not widely operated with the pressure cabin to avoid explosive decompression. See Schwerdfeger and Luft, 1944.
8 - Mitscherlich and Mielke, 1989; Doerner et al., 2000; Roth, 2001: 119.

9 - Harsch, 2004: 107-8, 110-1. Dr. S. Rascher was a Luftwaffe reservist and an SS member. He refused to forward information concerning his hypoxia experiments to his 1942 military superior, Luftwaffe's Major Dr. Welz. Rascher explained it was his obligation for secrecy to Himmler.

10 - Kudlien, 1985: 182-3.

11 - Benz, 1988; Harsch, 2004.

12 - The final report of Ruff, Romberg and Rascher that was finished on 28th July 1942 stated that no deaths occurred (Doc. No. 402). The repeated participation of 10 to 15 "exposed subjects" took place on a "voluntary basis". See Kanovitch, 1997. In Rascher's secret report to Himmler from 11th May 1942 on the other hand is stated, that in his so called *terminal experiments* several deaths occurred. See Mitscherlich and Mielke, 1989: Doc. No. 220. Ruff stated later: "Following a series of tests experiments have been performed on prisoners. In these experiments, insofar as they have been with my responsibility, there have been no deaths and no permanent damage to the prisoners. (...) Those persons who were required to carry out our series of experiments, volunteered. They have been considered to be criminal prisoners and not those which were in custody due to persecution on political or racial reasons. These detainees had been promised to receive privileges for participating in the experiments. (...) For the success of our experiments it was largely even required, that the subjects volunteered as it was necessary, that they participated in a particular form. See Harsch, 2004: 107 (A9-10). Prior to the conclusion of the official test series Rascher initiated additional Luftwaffe unauthorized deathly experiments. They took place not under Luftwaffe's responsibility and therefore Romberg, Ruff and Weltz were not charged by the American Military Tribunal in August 1947.

13 - See Harsch, 2004: 107(A9-8) and Doc.No. 269 in Harsch, 2004: 110 (A16-8).

14 - See Harsch, 2004: 163. SS Obergruppenfuehrer Wolff commented in a letter to Field Marshal Milch on this experiments and the lack of support by Luftwaffe doctors: "The problems are still the same. The medical circles of the Luftwaffe keep the position, that a young German pilot has to risk his life, on the other hand the life of a criminal - who is not drafted into the military - is too holy for this and they don't want to make their hands dirty. Furthermore they take the test results of the scientist who made them and ignore him. The Reichsfuehrer-SS has looked at the trials and has - that I can say without exaggeration - at every stage of this research he participated by helping and stimulating. He does not want that you and he worry about this development. He believes that it will take at least another decade, until such narrow-mindedness is brought out of our people. Meanwhile the necessary research to support our young and impeccable soldiers and airmen should not suffer." However, Prof. Hippke denied later, that he was informed about casualties in Dachau. See Kogon, 1995: 200 ref. 25. An Luftwaffe's memorandum confirms it's critical posture towards Rascher: "They were not only glad to get rid of him, because Rascher was regarded of being a 'troublemaker' and they wanted to have nothing to do with the experiments which he had been carried out under the protection of Himmler, but also under the formal responsibility of the Luftwaffe." See Benz, 1988: 196.

15 - Hypothermia and altitude themes were discussed at the Meeting on Mountain Physiological Problems (*Besprechung über gebirgsphysiologische Fragen*). The Meeting was held in fall of 1943 at the Mountain Medical School in St. Johann (Tyrol). Leading aviation medical specialists participated. Luft lectured on altitude adaptation, Opitz on gas exchange in high altitudes, Schwiegk on oxygen deficiency effects on the heart (all from Berlin).

16 - See Roth, 2001: 132, 136 and 146.

17 - Harsch, 2004: 163-164.

18 – See Benzinger, 1946; Harsch, 2007. Beside Theodor Benzinger other doctors attended the presentation: William Bruhl, Heinz Kalk, Paul Wuerfler, but not Strughold. A discussion about the film document did not happen. Also it was not mentioned, where the tests took place. See Benz, 1988.

19 – Roth, 2001, ref. 48 and 63; 131-2; Ruff S. Resue Possibilities from High Altitude Flights. Presentation found at University Library Hannover (ZS 4730 g (1057).

20 - In 1947 Strughold explained, why he chose S. Ruff in 1938 as co-editor of the "Outline of Aerospace Medicine": The main reason was due to his scientific achievements in the field of aviation medicine combined with practical knowledge as a flight captain. As well he valued his political distance to the Nazi regime. See Harsch, 2004: 112 (A19-4). The first edition was published in 1939, the second in 1944. The third edition was newly edited and expanded solely by Ruff. In a letter to the U.S. Surgeon General Harry G. Armstrong from 1954 Strughold stated, that it would not be in his mind to appear again in the literature with Ruff. See Harsch, 2004.

21 - See Ruff and Strughold, 1944: 127ff.

22 - See Harsch, 2004: 112 (A19-4: 4) and 108 (A12-2).

23 - Autrum, 1996: 80-1.

24 - Benz, 1988: 192, 213-214.

25 - Mitscherlich and Mielke, 1989: 50.

26 - Harsch, 2004: 35, Harsch, 2007.

27 - Harsch, 2004.

Appendix 2

1 – See Harsch, 2004: 76-7. 95 participants are listed in the report. These included Air Force members, civilian doctors, university professors, and in the minority SS agents. See (Doc. No. 401).

2 – Oral history Peter, 1998. Pueschel, 1978 is mentioning the other particpants having objected this experiments at the Nuremberg meeting: Captain Knothe (Professor from Jueterbog Flight Test Center), von Werz (Institute for Aviation Medicine, Munich), Capt. Dennecke (Medical Clinic Nuremberg), Hildmann (Army´s Oberarzt). Luftwaffes Captain M.C. J. Doerfler, left the meeting "ostentatiously", which can be interpreted as impotent protest. The meeting was organized and headed by Captain Prof. Dr. A. J. Anthony of the Luftwaffe´s office RLM L.In.14. Buechner, 1965: 81 and Pueschel, 1978:107-8 mention about the meeting: "The afternoon session of the first day seemed to end, as the leader of the discussion announced outside the program that the following presentation was top secret (*geheime Kommandosache*) and who would speak about it outside the meeting and to others than to the conference participants, had to reckon with his execution. Then followed the presentation on hypothermia experiments on humans by the SS-doctor Rascher, as published in the book of Mitscherlich and Mielke. Rascher is cited of having said, that the subjects were criminals with death penalty having the opportunity to earn their lives by participation in the experiments. (...) Immediately after the lecture, the meeting of the day was ended without discussion "

„Die Nachmittagssitzung des ersten Tages schien beendigt, als der Leiter der Diskussion (...) außerhalb des Programms eine Mitteilung mit den Worten ankündigte, der nun folgende Vortrag stände unter geheimer Kommandosache, wer darüber außerhalb der Tagung und über den Kreis der Tagungsteilnehmer hinaus spreche, habe mit seiner Erschießung zu rechnen. Es folgte dann die durch die Bücher von Mitscherlich und Mielke bekannte Mitteilung eines SS-Arztes über Unterkühlungs-Experimente am Menschen, von denen dieser sagte, es habe sich um zum Tode verurteilte Schwerverbrecher gehandelt, die durch

*das Experiment ihr Leben hätten erkaufen können. (...) Sofort nach dem Vortrag wurde die
Sitzung des Tages ohne Diskussion beendigt." Zit. n. Buechner, 1965: 81.*
3 – Institute for Contemporary History in Munich, Letter of Minister of Aviation and
Commander of Luftwaffe (Reichsministers der Luftfahrt und Oberbefehlshabers d. Lw.)
Berlin posted to the Reichsfuehrer-SS (File number 55 No. 5340/secret/42/L.In14, 2 II
B) dating 8th of october 1942 regarding research contract on hypothermia. 2 pages, Doc.
No. 286.
4 - See Benz, 1988 and the Alexander Report, 1946.
5 – See Mitscherlich and Mielke, 1989: 59. Hippke did see the need for this experiments
and stated: "The decision on medical measures to save lives of hypothermia patients in
distress was needed. The first 57 trials by Holzloehner and Rascher were sufficiently.
The volunteers were anesthetised for the tests. Even with these experiments already 13
people were killed, so it was preferred (by the Luftwaffe) to withhold even that part of
the report. All other attempts and victims were caused by and therefore in responsibility
of Dr. Rascher and were completely unnecessary." See Hippkes objection in Kogon, 1995.
Note 25 – 4.
6 – See Kogon, 1995. See also ref. 2.
7 – Holzloehners conference reports (Doc. No. 401) and (Doc. No. 428). The Report of
the second conference EAST of the conculting physicians 30th Nov. – 3rd Dec. 1942 at the
Military Medical Academy in Berlin is hold by Military Medical Library at the Office of
the German Armed Forces (Bundeswehr), Bonn. See also Doc. No. 286. There is no list of
participants of the second conference. It is not documented, if Strughold was present
(Harsch, 2004). Hippke explained the attitude of the participants on this Berlin
conference: "Holzloehner reported again about hypothermia treatment, I was present at
this lecture as a listener and can recall, that the Luftwaffe doctors, including Rein and
Buechner, disapproved experiments on prisoners, even though the occurrence of deaths
in the trials of the lecture was not evident. One of these doctors, it was probably
Professor Buechner came later in my office to talk to me and disaproving this
experiments. I did not consider that as a formal objection, especially as such it would
have been to be written down and to be answered officiallly in a printed letter. See
Mitschrelich and Mielke, 1989: 283, note 12 and Peter, 1994. Strugholds participation at
the 3rd hypothermia conference on 24th May 1943 is also not documented. However he
is listed as invited participant in the preliminary program. At this meeting unethical
experiments on females at the concentration camp in Ravensbrueck came to knowledge
of the attendees (Harsch, 2004).
8 – Holzloehners conference report 7/43 (Doc. No. 401) and (Doc. 428): Report of the
Second Conference of Special Medical Consultants from 30th Nov. to 3rd Dec. 1942 at the
Military Medical Academy, Berlin. See also Archive of USAF School of Aerospace
Medicine, Brooks AFB, San Antonio (Texas): Annex Conference on Problems of Mountain
Physiology 4th to 6th Oct. 1943 in St. Johann, Tyrol. Translat. prep. by: Office of Military
Governm. for Germany (US). Office of Naval Advisor Medical Section March 1948.
9– See Doc. No. 401 as mentioned above. The assistant researcher to Hermann Rein in
Goettingen, Grosse-Brockhoff stated at the discussion („Aussprache") in Nuremberg, that
human experiments in general could be replaced by research on animals and are
therefore unnecesarry. See Bretschneider, 1997: 48, Grosse-Brockhoff, 1954: 51,
Matschke, 1975: 55 and German Aviation Medicine World War II, 1950: 828 f.
10 – The original German text is: „Im Hinblick auf die experimentellen
wissenschaftlichen Versuche, aber auch zur Orientierung für den Seenotdienst ist es von
Interesse zu wissen mit welchen Temperaturen man in den in Frage kommenden
Meeren in den verschiedenen Jahreszeiten zu rechnen hat. Hierüber liegt bereits

wertvolles Literaturmaterial vor mit Beschreibungen und Seekarten. (...) ." In the Wall Street Journal text it is written as: "With regard to the experimental scientific research, but also for the orientation of the
Sea Distress service, it is of interest to know what temperatures are to be counted on in the oceans concerned during the various seasons."
11 - Holzloehners conference reports (Doc. No. 401) and (Doc. No. 428).
12 - See Buechner, 1965; Harsch 2004; Pueschel 1978 and Rein, 1947.
13 - Not only Becker-Freyseng noted that he did not recognize the true nature of the experiments from the lecture. See Mitscherlich and Mielke, 1989: 58; protocol, p 8022f. See also Berger, 1990 and Kudlien, 1985. Becker-Freyseng was at this time assistant (Hilfsreferent) at Anthony's office.
14 - See Buechner, 1965 and the docs of the Institute of Contemporary history in Munich (Harsch, 2004: A16- 1 to 5).
15 - See Mitscherlich, 1947 and Mitscherlich & Mielke, 1989. Buechner had demanded after the publication of the book "The dictate of inhumanity" of the authors Mitscherlich and Mierlke and the publisher to correct the passage concerning the Nuremberg winter meeting because he "repeatedly and explicitly protested against this kind of experiments " (*mehrfach ausdruecklich und entschieden Protest*). Again, in December 1942, he had raised "formally protest" at Hippkes office. See Peter, 1994. Buechner was the Luftwaffes 'Advisory pathologist' and headed the Institute for Aviation Medical Pathology of the RLM in Freiburg. Additional criticism called forth the "false statements" about the Nuremberg Winter Meeting, which Rein put it: "The author of the book was not present at the meeting. He would not have forgotten the bitterness and indignation of the scientists attending this meeting. The initiator of those experiments, an SS doctor, was immediately recognizable to all as a pure sadist. His 'scientific' staff, who was the speaker of that session, was scientifically outlawed with this day. Three of those present declared that such attempts are completely meaningless and unscientific and should therefore be omitted. To declare this in a 'double secret' meeting, seems not to be clear to the author Mitscherlich. It is only good that at the handling documents is a letter from Himmler where he speaks: 'People who refuse even today to perform these human experiments, rather let die brave German soldiers from the effects of hypothermia, I see as high treasoner (Hoch- und Landesverrt) and I will not be afraid to call the names of these gentlemen at the appropriate locations.' The fact that the official record of this memorable session contains nothing about it, only proves how they worked and that no one dared, in such attempts to inaugurate the real representatives of the science. "
„Der Verfasser des Buches war bei der Tagung nicht zugegen. Er würde die Erbitterung und die Entrüstung eben jener von ihm nunmehr in so leichtfertiger Weise abgeurteilten Wissenschaftler nicht vergessen haben. Der Initiator jener Versuche, ein SS-Arzt, war allen sofort als reiner Sadist erkennbar. Sein 'wissenschaftlicher' Mitarbeiter aber, der Vortragende jener Tagung, wurde von diesem Tage an in Acht und Bann getan. Drei der Anwesenden erklärten, dass solche Versuche völlig sinnlos und unwissenschaftlich seien und daher unterlassen werden müssten. Was das in einer 'doppelt geheim' erklärten Sitzung bedeutete, scheint Herrn Mitscherlich nicht klar zu sein. Gut ist nur, dass unter den mitgeteilten Dokumenten sich ein Schreiben Himmlers befindet, in dem er ausspricht: 'Leute, die heute noch diese Menschenversuche ablehnen, lieber dafür tapfere deutsche Soldaten an den Folgen dieser Unterkühlung sterben lassen, sehe ich auch als Hoch- und Landesverräter an und ich werde mich nicht scheuen, die Namen dieser Herren an den in Frage kommenden Stellen zu nennen.' Dass das amtliche Protokoll dieser denkwürdigen Sitzung darüber nichts enthält, beweist nur, wie damals gearbeitet wurde und dass man es nicht wagte, in solche Versuche die wirklichen Vertreter der Wissenschaft einzuweihen. "

See University archives Goettingen (Harsch, 2004: A11-8: 4). Rein F. H. Science and Inhumanity (Wissenschaft und Unmenschlichkeit. Bemerkungen zu drei charakteristischen Veroeffentlichungen). Goettingen University Newspaper 1947, 14: 3-5.
16 – Buechner critizised in 1960 the authors of "Medicine without Humanity" Mitscherlich and Mielke having denigrated Hermann Rein. See Peter, 1994: 215. Buechner showed opposition to the Nazi doctrine, including through his presentation, "The Hippocratic Oath" on 18th Nov. 1941, in which he spoke out publicly against euthanasia. At this occasion he demonstrated his commitment for the principles of medical ethics, regardless of the possibility of self-endangerment. See, Peter, 1994: 179 See also Affidavit of F. Buechner of 24 Apr. 1947 (AMA II 2/26.1 [6]), in: Peter, 1994: 170 and Buechner, 1965.
17 See Buechner, 1965.
18 – In the USA the results of the Nuremberg paved the way for a general recomendation of the warm bath therapy of hypothermia patients in the armed forces. See Alexander-Report, 68: VIII. Conclusions.
19 – According to Rein, German scientists and physiologists quitted their collegial relationship with Holzloehner after this experiments came to their knowledge. Harsch, 2004: 166 ref. 30.
20 – See Alexander report, 1945 and Harsch, 2004.

Appendix 3
1 - See Harsch, 2004: 166 (A19-2: 3-4) and (A16-25: 2257). Strughold was convinced of Becker-Freyseng´s innocence, a former assistant at AMRI.
2 - For the approval of the human trials Luftwaffe´s Surgeon General Dr. Schroeder was jointly responsible and sentenced to prison. Strughold knew Schroeder since 1923, when he was an assistant doctor at the Wuerzburg ENT clinic. In 1947 Strughold gave the following assessment: "His attitude towards experiments was to my knowledge in all these years against using prisoners. He was very interested in the work we performed at my Institute partly by heroic self-experiments of my assistants on hypoxia, hyperbaric oxygen exposition and acceleration. Furthermore, he supported at my institution the planning of animal experiments in a large scale. (...) Professor Schroeder was as professional medical officer and physician and politically not interested. He is a representative of the good old German culture and tradition and a rational patriotism. Hitler and his party were to him not only unappealing, but he hated it in his heart. He has vigorously resisted making the Medical officers to become political officers (NSFO) and kept them strictly to care for sick and wounded. See Harsch, 2004: 166 (A19-3: 2-4).
3 - Dr. Konrad Schaefer was assigned to the AMRI around 1942, where he had also performed research work with Strughold until 1943 at the outsourced Institute in Silesia. His worked thereafter was in the industry, as his university career was not successful, not least because he was an outspoken opponent of Nazism. In addition to his studies on the physiology of thirst, he developed zeolite to make salt water drinkable. Strughold stated in this regard: "He performed in 1942 a three day lasting self-experiment staying thirsty, with the participation of both of his two assistants. This experiment falls into the category of the heroic, self-medical experiments and the 3 people involved can rightly be proud of this effort." See Harsch, 2004: 166 (A19-5: 1-3). In 1942 Schaefer stated to Strughold, that he was against experiments on non-volunteers. Schaefer two years after his acquittal spent a short time working at USAF-SAM at Randolph AFB (Texas), and later he moved to the U.S. Navy (Harsch, 2004: 166).
4 – See Mitscherlich and Mielke, 1989; Harsch, 2004.
5 - Harsch, 2004: 77-8 and 166.

6 - See Mitscherlich and Mielke, 1989: 77. Prot. p. 8147.
7 - Harsch, 2004: 77-8.
8 - Mitscherlich and Mielke, 1989: 285, remark 5; Deutsch, 1997.

Appendix 4
1 - See Koch, 1993: 123.
2 – See Schwerin, 2004.
3 - Schwerin, 2004: 300.
4- Schmuhl, 2005: 429.
5 – Weindling, 2003: 247.
6 – Koch, 1993: 124; Schmuhl, 2005: 432-3.
7 – Schwerin, 2004: 309; Letter of Nachtsheim, in Koch, 1993: 125.
8 - Ruhenstroth-Bauer and Nachtsheim, 1944: 18.
9 – Ruhenstroth-Bauer, 2000.
10 – Beddies, 2003: 240.
11 – See Schwerin von, 2004.
12 – Weindling, 2003: 251.
13 – Harsch and Wirth, 2008: 60 years Aviation Medicine after WWII.
14 – See Noell, 1950: 286-300.
15 – See Noell, 1950: 301 f.
16 – See Gremmler, 1942.
17 – See Noell, 1950: 302.
18 – See Kornmueller, Palme and Strughold, 1941.

List of sources

Archival sources

Archives visited for research, documents outlined in Harsch, 2004: 104-24.

1) Archives of the Humboldt University, Berlin
Personal record Hubertus Strughold, Friedrich-Wilhelms-University, Berlin; starting 31st Aug. 1935, closed 23rd June 1942 / 29rd Oct. 1943. 18 documents (14 pages (23rd June 1942), 26 pages (29th Oct. 1943)).

2) National Archives (Bundesarchiv, BA), outpost department Berlin-Zehlendorf (former Berlin Document Center).
Personal record of Professor Dr. med. et phil. Hubert Strughold; 5 documents, 1941 – 1944.

3) National Archives (Bundesarchiv, BA), outpost department Dahlwitz-Hoppegarten.
Personal record Siegfried Ruff (ZB2 1994); 4 documents from 1938.

4) Historical Archives of German Research institution for Air and Space Travel (DLR), Berlin.
25 documents, 1915 - 1986.

5) National Archives – Military Archives (Bundesarchiv/Militaerarchiv BA-MA), Freiburg i. Brsg.
10 documents, 1939 – 1944.

6) City archives Hamm. 5 documents, 1893 – 1983.

7) Archive of German Academy of natural scientists, Halle (Saale).
10 documents, 1936 – 1983.

8) National Archives (Bundesarchiv BA), Koblenz.
10 documents, 1923 – 1944.

9) Memorial Archive, Dachau.
10 documents, 1942 – 1966.

10) Archive of German Air Force Institute of Aviation Medicine (GAFIAM - FlMedInstLw), Fuerstenfeldbruck.
7 documents, 1916 – 1972.

11) Univ.-Archive Georg-August-University, Goettingen.
8 documents, 1946 – 1947.

12) Lower Saxony State and University Library, Dept. of Manuscripts and rare prints.
2 documents, 1941 - 1947.

13) Univ.-Archive, Heidelberg.
Personal record of Strughold (6024, PA235 und PA 1206, Univ.-File HIII 584/1): 39 documents, 1945 – 1962.

14) Archive of German Society for Aviation and Space Medicine (DGLRM), Cologne.
10 feet of document folders, 1961-2001.

15) Archive of Ludwig-Maximilians-University, Munich.
2 documents, 1921 -1934.

16) Institute of Time History, Munich.
29 records, 1942 – 1982.

17) Univ.-Archive, Muenster.
7 records, 1918 – 1923.

18) Military Medical Library of Bundeswehr Medical Office (Sanitaetsamt), Bonn.
2 documents, 1942 – 1946.

19) State Archive, Nuremberg.
6 documents, 1942 – 1947.

20) Parish, Rhynern.
2 documents, 1898 - 1912.

21) Private archive Hubert Oberdorf, Iserlohn.
3 documents, 1931 – 1960.

22) Archive of the Foundation of the Social History of the 20th century, Bremen.
6 documents, 1942 – 1947.

23) Private archive Frau Mary Strughold, Mico (Texas).
125 documents, 1898 – 1986.

24) Archive USAF School of Aerospace Medicine, Brooks AFB, San Antonio (Texas).
112 documents, 1939 – 1986.

25) Private archive Ferdinande Ueter, born Strughold, Rheda-Wiedenbrueck.
62 documents, 1880 – 1979.

26) National Archives, Washington, (D. C.).
Joint Intelligence Objectives Agency (J.I.O.A.) File Copy, Record Group 330,
9 pages.: 33 documents, 1946 – 1954.

27) Univ.-Archive, Wuerzburg.
19 documents, 1931 – 1962.

Bibliography

List of works and sources of Hubertus Strughold 1923-1979

1923
Strughold H.: Die Wirkung der Kampfstoffe Diphenylarsinchlorid (Blaukreuzstoff) und Aethylarsindichlorid auf die Haut des Menschen (The effect of the agents Diphenylarsinchlorid [Blue Cross agent] and Aethylarsindichlorid to the skin of the human) Phil. Diss. Muenster, 13th June 1923; see also Z Biol 1923, 78: 195-230.

1924
Strughold H.: Ueber die Dichte und Schwellen der Schmerzpunkte der Epidermis in den verschiedenen Koerperregionen. Eine Untersuchung mit v. Frey´schen Stachelbosteln (On the density and thresholds of the sore points of the epidermis in the various parts of the body. A study with the "Stachelbosteln" of von Frey [thorn of a porcupine]. Med. thesis Wuerzburg, 6th November 1923; see also Z Biol 1924, 80: 367-81.
Strughold H.: Ueber Beziehungen zwischen den Raumschwellen und der Verteilung der Druckpunkte auf der Haut des Menschen (Relations between the space thresholds and the distribution of the pressure points on the skin of humans). Z Biol 1924, 2: 249-64.

1925
Frey M. v., Rein H., Strughold H.: Beitraege zur Frage des tiefen Drucksinns (Contributions to the question of the deep sense of pressure). Z Biol 1925, 82: 359-77.
Rein H., Strughold H.: Untersuchungen ueber die Raumschwellen der Warmempfindung (Studies on the threshold of warm feeling). Z Biol 1925, 82: 553-68.
Strughold H., Karbe M: Die Topographie des Kaeltesinnes auf Cornea und Conjunctiva (The topography of the cold sense on the cornea and conjunctiva). Z Biol 1925, 83: 189-200.
Strughold H.: Die Schwellen des Kaeltesinnes am Auge, bestimmt mit Reizen von kleiner Flaeche und geringer Waermekapazitaet (The thresholds of the cold sensation in the eye, measured with stimulus of small areas and low heat capacity). Z Biol 1925, 83: 201-6.
Strughold H., Karbe M: Die Dichte der Kaltpunkte im Lidspaltenbereiche des Auges (The density of the cold points of the eyelid). Z Biol 1925, 83: 207-12.
Strughold H., Karbe M.: Vitale Faerbung des Auges und experimentelle Untersuchung der gefaerbten Nervenelemente (Vital staining of the eye and experimental investigation of the colored nervous elements). Z Biol 1925, 83: 297-308.
Strughold H.: Die Topographie des Kaeltesinnes in der Mundhoehle (topography oft he cold sense of the mouth). Z Biol 1925, 83: 515-34.

1926
Schriever H., Strughold H.: Ueber die der Nasen- und Rachenschleimhaut eigentuemlichen Empfindungsqualitaeten (Sensation qualities peculiar of the nasal and pharyngeal mucosa). Z Biol 1926, 84: 193-206.

Strughold H.: Das Verhalten der Horn- und Bindehaut des menschlichen Auges gegen Waermereize (The behavior of the cornea and conjunctiva of the human eye to thermal stimuli). Z Biol 1926, 84: 311-20.

Frey M. v., Strughold H.: Weitere Untersuchungen über das Verhalten von Hornhaut und Bindehaut des menschlichen Auges gegen Beruehrungsreize (Further studies of the behavior of the cornea and conjunctiva the human eye to moving stimuli). Z Biol 1926, 84: 321-34.

Strughold H.: Der spezifische Empfaenger der Kaltempfindung (The specific recipients of cold sensation). Verh Physik Med Ges Wuerzburg NF 1926, 51: 31-44.

Strughold H.: Zur Kenntnis der Refraktaerphasen des Patellarreflexes (Notes on the refractory periods of the patellar reflex). Verh Phys Med Ges Wuerzburg NF 1926, 51: 94-101.

1927

Strughold H.: Beitraege zur Kenntnis der Refraktaerphasen des menschlichen Rueckenmarkes (Contributions to the knowledge of the refractory periods of the human spinal cord). Med. Habil. Freiburg, 1927; see also Z Biol 1926, 85: 453-69.

Hoffmann P., Strughold H.: Ein Beitrag zur Frage der Oszillationsfrequenz der willkuerlichen Innervation (A Contribution to the question of the oscillation frequency of the arbitrary Innervation). Z Biol 1927, 85: 599-603.

Frey M. v., Strughold H.: Ist der Drucksinn einheitlich oder zwiespaeltig (Is the sense of pressure uniform or mixed)? Z Biol 1927, 86: 181-6.

Frey M. v., Grundig I., Strughold H.: Zur Frage des tiefen Drucksinns (On the question of the deep sense of pressure). Z Biol 1927, 86: 227-30.

Strughold H.: Die Reflexe, betrachtet nach ihrer funktionellen Bedeutung (The reflexes, considered according to their functional significance).
Nervenarzt 1927, 1: 470-8.

1928

Rein H., Strughold H.: Die Simultanschwellen der Kaltempfindung (The simultaneous thresholds of cold sensation). Z Biol 1928, 87: 599-609.

Strughold H.: Die Sensibilitaet der Horn- und Bindehaut des normalen menschlichen Auges (The sensitivity of the cornea and conjunctiva of the normal human eye). Zentralbl Ges Ophth 1928, 19: 353-68.

Muench, Strughold H.: Ueber die von den Zaehnen ausloesbaren Reflexe (About the releasable reflexes from the teeth). Vjschr Zahnheilkde 1928, 44: 472-7.

1929

Strughold H.: Beitraege zur Kenntnis der Refraktaerphasen der Eigenreflexe beim gesunden Menschen. 1. Mitt. Der Einfluss der Atembewegung auf den Patellar- und Achillessehnenreflex (Contributions to the knowledge of the refractory periods of the reflexes in healthy humans. 1. Notification. The influence of respiratory motion on the patellar and Achilles tendon reflex). Z Biol 1929, 88: 346-62.

Strughold H.: Flugphysiologische Studien. 1. Der Tastsinn (Drucksinn der Haut) bei niedrigem Sauerstoffdruck. (Ein Beitrag zur Bestimmung der physiologischen Leistungsgrenzen beim Hoehenflug)(Flight physiological studies. 1. The sense of touch [pressure sense of the skin] at low oxygen pressure. (A contribution to the determination of the physiological capacity limitations at the high altitude flight).
Z Flugtechn 1929, 20: 387-90.

Strughold H.: Der Direkteffekt von temporaerer Anoxaemie auf die systolische und diastolische Herzgroeße bei konstantem Rhythmus (The direct effect of temporary anoxaemia on the systolic and diastolic heart size with a constant rhythm). Amer J Physiol 1929: 1929: 532.

1930
Strughold H.: Flugphysiologische Studien. 2. Sauerstoffmangel und die Feinheit der Wahrnehmung der Gliederbewegung (Flight physiological studies. 2. Oxygen deficiency and the fineness of perception of limb movement). Z Flugtechn 1930, 21: 226-8.
Strughold H.: Flugphysiologische Studien. 3. Kinematographische Studien der Herzgrößen bei Sauerstoffmangel ("Direkteffekt" auf das Herz) (3. Cinematographic studies of heart size in oxygen deficiency ("direct" effect on the heart). Z Flugtechn 1930, 21: 645-8.
Strughold H.: Das Kinokardiogramm (The cinocardiogram). Verh Physik Med Ges Wuerzburg NF 1930, 55: 195-205.
Strughold H.: The Mechanical Threshold of the Cornea-Reflex of the Usual Laboratory Animals. Amer J Physiol 1930, 94: 235-40.
Strughold H.: A Cinematographic Study of Systolic and Diastolic Heart Size with Special Reference to the Effects of Anoxemia. Amer J Physiol 1930, 94: 641-55.

1931
Strughold H., Porz R.: Die Dichte der Kaltpunkte auf der Haut des menschlichen Koerpers (The density of cold spots on the skin of the human body). Z Biol 1931, 91: 563-71.

1933
Strughold H., Joerg H.: Beitraege zur Kenntnis der Eigenreflexe der quergestreiften Muskeln beim gesunden Menschen. 2. Mitt. Der Patellar- und Achillesreflex bei willkuerlicher Hyperventilation der Lungen (Contributions to the knowledge of the reflexes of the striated muscles in healthy humans. 2. notification. The patellar and achilles reflex during voluntary hyperventilation of the lungs).
Z Biol 1933, 94: 150-8.

1934
Strughold H., Hagen F.: Beitraege zur Kenntnis der Eigenreflexe der quergestreiften Muskeln beim gesunden Menschen. 3. Mitt. Der Patellar- und Achillesreflex bei akuter experimenteller Dyspnoe (Contribution to the knowledge of the reflexes of the striated muscles in healthy people. 3. notification. The patellar and achilles reflex in acute experimental dyspnea). Z Biol 1934, 95: 588-98.
Strughold H., Woehlisch E.: Ist das Thrombin ein proteolytisches Ferment (Is thrombin a proteolytic enzyme)? Z Physiol Chem 1934, 223: 267-80.

1935
Strughold H.: Aufgaben der Luftfahrtmedizin innerhalb der deutschen Luftwaffe (Aeromedical tasks in the German Luftwaffe. Med Welt 1935, 9: 1599-1601.

1936

Strughold H.: Friedrich Noltenius. Luftfahrtmed 1936, 1: 49.

Strughold H.: Geschichtliches zur Luftfahrtmedizin (Historical aspects of aviation medicine). Luftfahrtmed Abh 1936/7, 1: 16-22.

Strughold H.: Das Zentralnervensystem und die Sinnesorgane in großen Hoehen (The central nervous system and sense organs at high altitudes). Luftfahrtmed Abh 1936/7, 1: 58-64.

Strughold H.: Zur Frage der Hoehenkraempfe (On the question of altitude convulsions). Luftfahrtmed Abh 1936/7, 1: 181-2.

Strughold H.: Zur Frage der Vereinheitlichung der Benennungen und Methoden in der Luftfahrtmedizin (On the question of standardization of terms and methods in aviation medicine). Luftfahrtmed Abh 1936/7, 1: 286-90.

Strughold H.: Die Aufgaben der Luftfahrtmedizin im Lichte der technischen Entwicklung der Luftfahrt (The tasks of aviation medicine in the light of technical development of aviation). Dtsch Militaerarzt 1936, 1: 29-36.

Strughold H.: Luftfahrtmedizinische Forschung. 2. Internat. Sportaerztekongress in Berlin. Verhandlungsbericht (Aerospace Medical Research. Second Internat. Sports Medicine Congress in Berlin. Conference Report). Thieme, Leipzig 1936: 212-5.

Strughold H.: Luftfahrtmedizin. Festschrift Sportmedizin und Olympische Spiele (Aviation medicine. Celebration report on sports medicine and the Olympic Games. Dtsch Med Wschr 1936, 62: 58-60.

Strughold H.: Ausschuss für flugmedizinische Forschung (Committee for aeromedivcal research). Jb Dtsch Akad Luftfahrtforsch 1936: 635.

1937

Strughold H.: Die Hoehenwirkung im Lichte nervenphysiologischer Betrachtung (Altitude effect in the light of neurophysiological reflection). Luftfahrtmed 1937, 2: 210-22.

Strughold H.: Das animale Nervensystem in großen Hoehen (The animal nervous system at high altitudes). Dtsch Militaerarzt 1937, 2: 71-8.

Strughold H.: Gliederung der biologischen Hoehenwirkung nach praktischen, quantitativen Richtlinien (Outline of the biological altitude reaction regarding practical and quantitative guidelines). Dtsch Militaerarzt 1937, 2: 376-8.

Strughold H.: Zur Frage der Hoehenumstellung (On the question of altitude adaptation). Med Welt 1937, 2: 1712-5.

Strughold H.: Nervenfunktion und Hoehe (Nerve function and height). Jb Dtsch Akad Luftfahrtforsch 1937: 106-10.

1938

Strughold H.: Die Zeitreserve nach Unterbrechung der Sauerstoffatmung in großen Hoehen (The time of useful consciousness after interruption of breathing oxygen at high altitudes). Luftfahrtmed 1938, 3: 55-63.

Strughold H.: Die Hoehenwirkung im Lichte nervenphysiologischer Betrachtung (The effect of altitude in the light of physiological nerve examination). Luftfahrtmed 1938, 3: 210-22.

Strughold H.: Das Herz bei Sauerstoffmangel unter kontrollierten Kreislaufbedingungen (The heart in hypoxia under controlled circulatory conditions). Luftfahrtmed Abh 1938, 2: 36-43.

Strughold H.: Atmung und Wirkstoffe (Respiration and active substances). Luftfahrtmed Abh 1938, 2: 192-7.

Strughold H.: Bericht über die 1. Deutsche Tagung für luftfahrtmed. Forschung v. 25.-28. Okt. 1937 (Report on the first German Conference on aeromedical research in Berlin). Dtsch Militaerarzt 1938, 3: 140-1; also in Klin Wschr 1938, 17: 283-6 and Wien Med Wschr 1938, 88: 902.

1939

Strughold H.: Die chemische und mechanische Seite der Hoehenwirkung; gezeigt am Verhalten der Flamme (The chemical and mechanical side of altitude effect, shown in the behavior oft he flame). Luftfahrtmed 1939, 4: 25-30.

Strughold H.: Die biologische Hoehenwirkung vom Standpunkt der Luftfahrt (The biological effect level from the standpoint of aviation). Wien Klin Wschr 1939, 52: 857-60.

Strughold H.: Zeitreserve nach Unterbrechung der Sauerstoffatmung in großen Hoehen (Time of usefull consciousness after interruption of breathing oxygen at high altitudes). Luftfahrtmed 1939, 3: 55-63; also in Jb Dtsch Akad Luftfahrtforsch 1939, 2: 84-8.

Strughold H.: Die medizinischen Probleme in der Substratosphaere (Medical problems in the substratosphere). Dtsch Med Wschr 1939, 8: 281-5.

Strughold H.: Modellversuch der Hoehenwirkung: die Flamme in großen Hoehen (Model test of the effect of altitude: the flame at high altitudes). Luftwiss 1939, 6: 278-9.

Strughold H.: Luftfahrtmedizinische Fragen (Aviation medical issues). Med Welt 1939, 13: 32.

Ruff S., Strughold H.: Grundriss der Luftfahrtmedizin (Handbook of aviation medicine). J. A. Barth, Leipzig 1939.

Strughold H.: Flugmedizin (Aviation medicine). Jb Dtsch Akad Luftfahrtforsch 1939: 128-31.

1940

Strughold H.: Die physiologische Wirkung grosser Hoehen (The physiological effect of high altitudes). Luftwiss 1940, 7: 269-76.

Strughold H.: Die Zeitreserve nach Unterbrechung der Sauerstoffversorgung in großen Hoehen (The time of useful consciousness reserve after interruption of supply of oxygen at high altitudes). Mitt. Luftfahrtmed 1940, 5: 66-75.

Strughold H.: Die Erscheinungen der Hoehenwirkung im Filmbild (The effects of the altitude effect in the film image). Jb Dtsch Akad Luftfahrtforsch 1939/40: 21-4.

1941

Kornmueller A. E., Palme F., Strughold H.: Ueber Veraenderungen der Gehirnaktionsstroeme im akuten Sauerstoffmangel (EEG-changes due to acute lack of oxygen). Luftfahrtmed 1941, 5: 161-83.

Strughold H.: Luftfahrtmedizinische Forschung (Aeromedical research). Ill Aerztl Zeit 1941: 4967.

Strughold H.: Die Hoehenwirkung nach Unterbrechung der Sauerstoffatmung in großen Hoehen. Analyse und praktische Folgerungen (The effect of height after interruption of breathing oxygen at high altitudes. Analysis and practical implications). Jb Dtsch Akad Luftfahrtforsch 1940/1: 378-80.

1942

Gauer O., Opitz E., Palme F., Strughold H.: Fallschirmabsprung und Zeitreserve in großen Hoehen (Parachute jump and time reserve at high altitudes). Luftfahrtmed 1942, 6: 340-55.

Strughold H.: Neue Ergebnisse und Probleme der medizinischen Stratosphaerenforschung (New results and problems of medical research stratosphere). Luftwiss 1942, 9: 177-81.

Kornmueller A. E., Palme F., Strughold H.: Die Ableitung der Gehirnaktionsstroeme, eine Methode zur Untersuchung der Hoehenkrankheit (Using an EEG as a method to study the altitude sickness). Klin Wschr 1942, 21: 5-8; also in Jb Dtsch Akad Luftfahrtforsch 1941/2: 410.

Ruff S., Strughold H.: Atlas der Luftfahrtmedizin (Atlas of aviation medicine). J. A. Barth, Leipzig 1942.

1943

Gauer O., Strughold H.: Roentgenkinetographie im Dienste der physiologischen Beschleunigungsforschung (X-ray in the service of the physiological acceleration research). Jb Dtsch Akad Luftfahrtforsch 1943: 57-60.

Strughold H.: 250 Zentner Sauerstoff verbraucht ein Menschenleben (250 quintals of oxygen consumed by a human life). Der Adler 1943, 5.

1944

Strughold H.: Hypoxidose. Klin Wchschr 1944, 23: 221-2.

Ruff S., Strughold H.: Grundriss der Luftfahrtmedizin (Handbook of aviation medicine). 2nd; J. A. Barth, Leipzig 1944.

Strughold H.: Physiologie der Stratosphaere (Physiology of the stratosphere). Med Zschr 1944, 1: 1.

Strughold H.: Physiologie des Hoehenfluges (Physiology of high altitude flight). Luftfahrtmed. Lehrbr. No. 1. LMFI of RLM, Berlin 1944.

1945

Strughold H.: Geschwindigkeiten im Luftkrieg und physiologische Latenzzeiten (Speed in air-war and physiological latent periods). Paper, 6 pages. AMRI of RLM, Berlin march 1945.

Autrum H. J., Strughold H.: Reaktionszeit und Lichtintensitaet des Reizes (reaction time and light intensity of the stimulus [paper, not published]).

Autrum H. J., Denzer H. W., Strughold H.: Berichte über Koerpertemperatur und Sauerstoffmangel (Reports on body temperature and oxygen deficiency. [paper not published]).

Strughold H.: Flackerlicht als Waffe (flickering light as a weapon. [not published]).

1948

Strughold H.: Die Bedeutung des Sauerstoffs fuer das Leben (The importance of oxygen for life). Schriften d. Univ. Heidelberg 1948, 3: 86-95.

1949

Strughold H.: The Human Time Factor in Flight. 1.: The Latent Period of Optical Perception and its Significance in High Speed Flying. J Aviat Med 1949, 20: 300-7.
Armstrong H. G., Haber H., Strughold H.: Aero Medical Problems of Space Travel. Panel Meeting, School of Aviation Medicine. J Aviat Med 1949, 20: 383-417.

1950

Strughold H.: Development of Aviation Medicine in Germany. In: German Aviation Medicine World War II, Vol. 1, p. 3-11; ed. by The Surgeon General, US Department of the Air Force; US Govt Print Off, Washington 1950.
Strughold H.: Development, Organization and Experiences of Aviation Medicine in Germany during World War II. In: German Aviation Medicine World War II, Vol. 1, p. 12-51; ed. by The Surgeon General, US Department of the Air Force; US Govt Print Off, Washington 1950.
Strughold H.: Intermittent Light. In: German Aviation Medicine World War II, Vol. 2, p. 972-4; ed. by The Surgeon General, US Department of the Air Force. US Govt Print Off, Washington 1950.
Strughold H.: The Mechanoreceptors of Skin and Muscles under Flying Conditions. In: German Aviation Medicine World War II, Vol. 2, p. 994-9; ed. by The Surgeon General, US Department of the Air Force. US Govt Print Off, Washington 1950.
Strughold H.: Possibility of Live under Extraterrestrial Conditions. Symposium of Space Medicine. University of Illinois Press, Chicago 1950.

1951

Strughold H.: The Human Time Factor in Flight. 2. Chains of Latencies in Vision. J Aviat Med 1951, 22: 100-8.
Strughold H., Haber H., Buettner K., Haber F.: Where Does Space Begin? Functional Concept of the Boundaries between Atmosphere and Space. J Aviat Med 1951, 22: 342-9, 357.
Strughold H.: Physiological Considerations on the Possibility of Life under Extraterrestrial Conditions. In: Marbarger J.P.: Space Medicine; The Human Factor in Flights beyond the Earth. P. 31-48. The University of Illinois Press, Urbana 1951.
Strughold H.: Life on Mars in View of Physiological Principles. Tech Data Dig 1951, 16: 15-9.
Strughold H.: Wie wird sich der menschliche Organismus im schwerefreien Raum verhalten? Ein Beitrag zum Thema (How will behave the human body in a gravity-free space)? Weltraumfahrt 1951, 2: 81-2.

1952

Strughold H.: Ecological Aspects of Planetary Atmospheres with Special Reference to Mars. J Aviat Med 1952, 23: 130-40.
Strughold H.: From Aviation Medicine to Space Medicine. J Aviat Med 1952, 23: 315-18, 329; also in USAF Air Univ Quart Rev 1958, 10: 7-16; also in: 86th Congress, 2nd Session, Space Research in the Life Science: An Inventory of Related Programs, Resources and Facilities, p. 229-38. Washington, US Govt Print Off 1960, Appendix 1.
Strughold H.: The Physiological Day-Night Cycle in Global Flights. J Aviat Med 1952, 23: 464-73.

Strughold H.: Basic Environmental Problems Relating Man and the Highest Regions of the Atmosphere as Seen by the Biologist. In: Physics and Medicine of the Upper Atmosphere: A Study of the Aeropause; ed. by White C. S. und Benson O. O., p. 23-34, Albuquerque (New Mexico) 1952.
Haber F., Strughold H.: Physik und Physiologie des Drucksturzes im Weltraum (Physics and physiology of rapid decompression in space). Weltraumfahrt 1952, 4: 118-20.

1953
Gerathewohl S. J., Strughold H.: Motoric Responses of the Eyes When Exposed to Light Flashes of High Intensities and Short Duration. J Aviat Med 1953, 24: 200-7.
Strughold H.: Comparative Ecological Study of the Chemistry of the Planetary Atmospheres. J Aviat Med 1953, 24: 393-9, 464.
Strughold H.: The Sensitivity of Cornea and Conjunctiva of the Human Eye and the Use of Contact Lenses. Amer J Ophtom 1953, 30: 625-30.
Strughold H.: The Green and Red Planet. A Physiological Study of the Possibility of Live on Mars. The University of New Mexico Press, Albuquerque 1953.
Strughold H.: Das Leben auf dem Mars (Life on Mars). Weltraumfahrt 1953, 4: 24-6.

1954
Gerathewohl S. J., Strughold H.: Time Consumption of Eye Movements and High-Speed Flying. J Aviat Med 1954, 25: 38-45.
Strughold H.: Hypoxia, Hypoxidosis, Hypoxidation, Hibernation, Apparent Death and Suspended Animation. J Aviat Med 1954, 25: 113-22.
Strughold H.: Living Room in Space. Instructors J 1954: 297-306.
Strughold H.: Atmospheric Space Equivalent. J Aviat Med 1954, 25: 420-4.
Kendricks E. J., Strughold H., Douglas Aircraft Company, Haber H., Gerathewohl S. J.: Medical Problems of Space Flight. Instructors J 1954.
Strughold H.: Space Equivalent Conditions Within the Earth´s Atmosphere. Physiological Aspects. Astronautica 1954, 1: 192-8.
Strughold H.: Die Empfindlichkeit der Horn- und Bindehaut des Auges und die Anwendung von Contact-Schalen (The sensitivity of the cornea and conjunctiva of the eye and the use of contact lenses). Optometrie. Zschr Optom Brillenanpass 1954: 7-12.

1955
Strughold H.: The Ecosphere of the Sun. J Aviat Med 1955, 26: 323-8.
Strughold H.: The Medical Problems of Space Flight. Internat Record Med 1955, 168: 570-5.
Strughold H.: Physiologic Day-Night Cycle after Long Distance Flights. Internat Record Med 1955, 168: 576-9.
Strughold H., Taylor W. F.: The Oculomotoric Pattern of Circular Eye Movements During Increasing Speed of Rotation. Amer Psychologist 1955, 10: 490-1.
Strughold H.: Space Equivalent Conditions Within the Earth´s Atmosphere (Physiological Aspects). Astronautica Acta 1955, 1: 32-40.
Strughold H.: Weltraumaequivalente Bedingungen innerhalb der Erdatmosphaere (Space equivalent conditions within the Earth's atmosphere). Weltraumfahrt 1955, 6: 2-5.

1956
Strughold H.: The U.S. Air Force Experimental Sealed Cabin. J Aviat Med 1956, 27: 50-2.
Strughold H.: A Simple Classification of the Present and Future Stages of Manned Flight. J Aviat Med 1956, 27: 328-31.
Strughold H.: The Oxygen Belt in the Planetary System. J Astronaut 1956, 3: 27-9.
Strughold H.: Medical Problems Involved in Orbital Space Flight. Jet Propulsion 1956, 26: 745-8, 756.
Strughold H.: The Ecosphere in the Solar Planetary System (Helio-Ecosphere). Proceedings of the 7th International Astronautical Congress, 277-88. Assoziazione Italiana Razzi, Rome 17th – 22nd Sept. 1956.
Haymaker W., Strughold H.: Atmospheric Hypoxidosis. In: Handbuch der Speziellen Pathologischen Anatomie und Histologie (Handbook of special pathologic anatomy and histology). Ed. by Scholz W., Vol. 13, 1. part, p. 1673-711. Springer, Berlin 1956.
Strughold H.: Man into Space. Engineering Aspects of Physiological Problems of Providing for Man in Space Harvard School of Public Health, Guggenheim Center for Aviation, Health and Safety, Boston 1956.
Strughold H.: Engineering for Physiological Requirements. Orbital and Satellite Vehicles, Vol. 2, Ch. 19, Special Summer Program, MIT, Cambridge (Massachusetts) 1956.
Strughold H.: Space Medicine and Allied Topics. The Artemis Press, London 1956.

1957
Gerathewohl S. J., Strughold H., Stallings H. D.: Sensomotor Performance During Weightlessness. Eye-Hand Coordination. J Aviat Med 1957, 28: 7-12.
Strughold H.: The Possibilities of an Inhabitable Extraterrestrial Environment Reachable from the Earth. J Aviat Med 1957, 28: 507-12.
Strughold H.: Mechanoreceptors, Gravireceptors. J Astronautics 1957, 4: 61-3.
Gerathewohl S. J., Strughold H., Taylor W. F.: The Oculomotoric Pattern of Circular Eye Movements During Increasing Speed of Rotation. J Exper Psychol 1957, 53: 249-56.
Strughold H.: Medicine at Work. Health in the Heavens, JAMA 1957, 164: 765-9.
Strughold H., Gerathewohl S. J.: Die medizinischen Probleme des Ueberschallfluges (Medical problems of supersonic flight). Inter Avia 1957, 12: 61-6.
Ruff S., Strughold H.: Grundriss der Luftfahrtmedizin (Handbook of aviation medicine). 3rd ed., J.A. Barth, Munich 1957.
Strughold H.: Space Medicine. In: The Space Encyclopedia. A Guide to Astronomy and Space Research. p. 229-34. London 1957.
Strughold H.: The Ecosphere in the Solar Planetary System (Helio-Ecosphere). Riv Med Aeronaut 1957, 20: 3-16; also in: Astronautica Acta 1957, 2.

1958
Strughold H.: Atmospheric Space Equivalent. J Aviat Med 1958, 29: 420-4.
Strughold H.: Basic Factors in Manned Space Operations. USAF Air Univ Quart Rev 1958, 10: 29-46.
Strughold H.: Guest Editorial: Space Medicine. New Physician 1958, 4: 2.
Kooistra J., Mitchell R., Strughold H.: The Behavior of Microorganism under Simulated Martian Environmental Conditions. Publ. of the Astronomical Soc. of the Pacific, Vol 70, No. 412.

Strughold H.: Staying Alive in Space. Air Force 1958, 41: 84-7.

Strughold H.: Interrelations of Space Medicine with other Fields of Science. Astronaut Engin Rev 1958, 17: 30-2, 37.

Strughold H.: General Review of Problems Common to the Field of Astronomy and Biology. Publications of the Astronomical Society of the Pacific 1958, 70: 43-50.

Strughold H.: Introduction. In: Vistas in Astronautics: Proceeding of the first Annual AFOSR Astronautics Symposium, p. 281-4. Pergamen Press, New York 1958.

Strughold H: Space Medicine and Astrobiology. Statement and Additional Materials Submitted by Hubertus Strughold 5th May 1958, p. 1215-60, 1542, 2486-2513. US Govt Print Off, Washington 1958.

Strughold H.: Geographie des Weltraumes: Spatiographie (Geography of space: Spatiography). Weltraumfahrt 1958, 8: 65-8.

Strughold H.: Der Mensch im Weltraum. Raumflugmedizin als Wegbereiter (Man in space. Space medicine as forerunner). Weltraumfahrt 1958, 8: 114-6; also in: Flug Revue 1958, 9: 12-4.

1959

Strughold H., Benson O. O.: Medical Progress: Space Medical Research. N Engl J Med 1959, 261: 494-502.

Strughold H.: Exotic Atmospheres on Earth. J Aviat Med 1959, 30: 311-4.

Strughold H.: The Evolution of Space Exploration. Air Force 1959, 42: 82.

Strughold H.: Space Medicine of the Next Decade as Viewed by a Physician and Physiologist. US Armed Forces Med J 4 1959: 397-405; also in: USAF Medical Service Digest 1959, 10: 16-20.

Strughold H.: From Aviation Medicine to Space Medicine. In: Man in Space. The United States Air Force Program for Developing the Spacecraft Crew. Ch.II, p. 7-18. Ed. by Gantz K. F., Duell, Sloan and Pearce, New York 1959.

Strughold H.: Basic Factors in Manned Space Operations. In: Man in Space. The United States Air Force Program for Developing the Spacecraft Crew. Ch. III, p. 19-41. Ed. by Gantz K. F., Duell, Sloan and Pearce, New York 1959.

Strughold H. (Ed.): Medical Aspects of Manned Flight. Space Technology. John Wiley & Sons, Inc., New York 1959.

Strughold H.: Definitions and Subdivisions of Space (Bioastronautical Aspect). Proceedings First Colloquium on the Law of Outer Space in the Chamber of the House of Parliament, p. 110-3. The Hague, at the IX Annual Congress of the International Astronautical Federation, 29. Aug. 1958. Springer, Wien 1959; also in: Compendium of Aerospace Medicine, ed. by Strughold H., Vol. 1., p. 17-22; USAF School of Aerospace Medicine, AMD (AFSC), Brooks AFB (Texas) 1977; also in: Bioastronautics 1959, 3 (8 p).

1960

Strughold H., Ritter O. L.: Solar Irradiance from Mercury to Pluto. J Aerospace Med 1960, 31: 127-30.

Strughold H., Ritter O. L.: Eye Hazards and Protection in Space. J Aerospace Med 1960, 31: 670-3.

Strughold H.: An Introduction to Astrobiology. Astronautics 1960: 20-1, 86-9.

Strughold H.: The Challenge of Medicine in the Space Age. Today´s Health 1960, 3: 36-40.

Strughold H.: Space Medicine and Astrobiology. Proc. 11th Int. Astronautical Congress 1960 in Stockholm, p. 671-87.

Strughold H., Ritter O.: The Gravitational Environment Space. In: Physics and Medicine of the Atmosphere and Space, p. 134-42; ed. by Benson O. O. and Strughold H., John Wiley & Sons, New York 1960.

Strughold H.: Interplanetary Space Flight from the Viewpoint of the Physician. In: Physics and Medicine of the Atmosphere and Space, p. 622-34; ed. by Benson O. O. and Strughold H., John Wiley & Sons, New York 1960.

Strughold H.: The Human Eye in Space (Physiologic Aspect). Proceedings of the Xth International Astronautical Congress, London 1959. p. 715-22. Springer, Wien 1960; also in: Astronautica Acta 1960, 5.

1961

Strughold H.: Orbital Characteristics of Earth and Moon Satellites As a Basis for Space Medical Studies. J Aerospace Med 1961, 32: 422-4.

Strughold H.: Sensory-Physiological Aspects of the Space Flight Situation. In: Psychophysiological Aspects of Space Flight; p. 57-65; ed.by Flaherty B. E.; Columbia University Press, New York 1961.

Strughold H.: Space Energies. Summation. In: Medical and Biological Aspects of the Energies of Space; p. 463-70; ed. by Campbell P., Columbia University Press, New York 1961.

Strughold H.: Space Medicine. In: Aerospace Medicine; p. 595-615; ed. by Armstrong H., Williams & Wilkins, Baltimore 1961.

Strughold H.: Planetary Atmospheres. In: Aerospace Medicine; p. 616-20; ed. by Armstrong H., Wiliam & Wilkins, Baltimore 1961.

1962

Strughold H., Ritter O. L.: Oxygen Production During the Evolution of the Earth´s Atmosphere. J Aerospace Med 1962, 33: 275-8.

Strughold H.: The Principle of the „Internal Atmosphere": Geobiological and Astrobiological Aspects. J Aerospace Med 1962, 33: 851-4.

Strughold H.: How Bioastronautics looks at the Moon. J Mississippi State Med Assoc 1962, 3: 397-403.

Strughold H.: Day-Night Cycling in Atmospheric Flight, Space Flight and other Celestial Bodies. Ann NY Acad Sci 1962, 98: 1109-15.

Strughold H., Ritter O.: Planetary Gravispheres. Astronautics 1962, 7: 26-7, 38.

Strughold H.: The Conditions Facing Life on Mars. Space Science 1962, 11: 2-7, 11.

Strughold H.: The Role of Medicine in the Space Age. USAF JAG Bulletin 1962.

1963

Strughold H.: Space Medicine Beyond the Moon. Texas State J Med 1963, 59: 1166-72.

Ritter O. L., Strughold H.: Seeing Planets from Space. Astronautics and Aerospace Engineering 1963, 7: 82-7.

Strughold H.: The Ecological Profile of Mars: Bioastronautical Aspect. In: Exploration of Mars; Proceedings of the American Astronautical Society Symposium on Mars. Denver (Colorado) 6.-7. June 1963; p. 30-44. North Hollywood Western Periodicals Co., 1963.

1964

Strughold H.: Air and Space Travel. The Torch 1964, 37: 4-8.

Strughold H.: Discussion. Rezension des Beitrages „Adaptations at Birth: Some Analogies to Space Travel." von M. E. Avery, M. D.. J Am Med Wom Assoc 1964, 19: 124-5.

Strughold H.: Acknowledgements by H. Strugold. In: Adam M-1. A Novel by William C. Anderson. Crown Publ., New York 1964.

Strughold H.: Ist Mars mit Eis bedeck (Is Mars covered with ice)?. Int Sci Tech 1964: 11-2.

Strughold H.: From Outer Space-Advances for Medicine, Ch. 12, In: Lillian Levy (ed.), Space, its Impact on Man and Society, New York, W.W. Norton & Co., Inc.

1965

Strughold H.: The Physiological Clock in Aeronautics and Astronautics. Ann N Y Acad Sci 1965, 134: 413-22.

Strughold H.: A Subsurface Marine Biospehre on Mars? Astronautics and Aeronautics 1965, 7: 82-6.

Strughold H.: Foreword. In: Campbell P. A.: Earthman, Spaceman, Universal Man? Pageant Press, New York 1965.

Bedwell T. C., Strughold H. (Ed.): Bioastronautics and the Exploration of Space. The Proceedings of the Third International Symposium on Bioastronautics and the Exploration of Space, 16th – 18th Nov. 1964. Springfield 1965.

Strughold H.: Foreword. In: Nowitzky A.M. : Spacecraft Sterilization Techniques and Equipment. Johnson Publishing Co., Boulder (Colorado) 1965.

1966

Strughold H.: A New Look at the Mars. Spaceflight 1966, 8: 302-6, 340; also in: TRW Space Log 1965/6: 2-13.

Strughold H.: Epilogue: Jules Verne, Physiologist. In: Dr. Ox´s Experiment. The Macmillan Company, 4. ed, p. 81-7, New York 1966.

Strughold H.: Martian Environmental Medicine. AIAA/AAS Stepping Stones to Mars Meeting. P. 553-7, Baltimore 1966; also in: Compendium of Aerospace Medicine. Vol. 2., p. 101-11; ed. by Strughold H.; School of Aerospace Medicine, Aerospace Medical Division (AFSC), Brooks AFB (Texas) 1979.

Strughold H.: Cycle Physiologique. Article for Encyclopedie de Léspace, France. Jour Et Nuit 1966.

1967

Strughold H., Ritter O. L.: Characteristics of Parking Orbits in Circummaritian Space. J Aerospace Med 1967, 38: 127-8.

Strughold H.: Synopsis of Martian Life Theories. Adv Space Sci Tech 1967, 9: 105-22.

Strughold H.: Lunar Medicine. Life Sciences Research and Lunar Medicine, p. 112-21; ed. by Malina F. J., Pergamon Press, New York 1967.

Strughold H.: Raumfahrtmedizinische Probleme auf dem Flugwege zum Mars (Space medical problems on the way to Mars). Astronautik 1967, 4: 22-5.

1968

Strughold H.: The Clock Inside your Body - In the Perspective of Modern Technology. Nadus J 1968, 4: 5-14.

Strughold H.: The Physiological Clock Across Time Zones and Beyond. Air Univ Rev 1968, 19: 28-33.
Strughold H.: Mars. Biological Aspect. Prepared vor publication in New Horizons, 1968, 32 pages.
Strughold H.: Planetary Environmental Medicine (Mars). In: Proceedings of the Fourth International Symposium on Bioastronautics and the Exploration of Space; p. 493-509. Ed. by Roadman C. H., Strughold H., Mitchell R. B. 1968.

1969
Strughold H.: Basic Biomedical Concept in the Jet and Space Age. Appl Mech Rev 1969, 22: 1339-42.

1971
Strughold H.: The Earth´s Environment and Aviation. In: Aerospace Medicine. Ch. 2, p. 22-34. Ed. by Randel H. W., The Williams & Wilkins Company, Baltimore 1971.
Strughold H.: Space Environment and Space Environment. In: Aerospace Medicine. Ch. 3., p. 35-46. Ed. by Randel H. W. The Williams & Wilkins Company, Baltimore 1971.
Strughold H.: Circadian Rhythms: Aerospace Medical Aspects. In: Aerospace Medicine. Ch. 4, p. 47-55. Ed. by Randel H. W., The Williams & Wilkins Company, Baltimore 1971.
Strughold H.: Rhythmostasis - A Fundamental Life Characteristics Aerospace Medical Aspect. Riv Med Aeron Sp 1971, 34: 168-75.
Strughold H.: Your Body Clock. Its Significance for the Jet-Traveller. Scribner, New York 1971.

1974
Strughold H.: Cycloecology in Space on the Moon and Beyond. In: Chronobiology; 417-23. Ed. by Schevin L. E. et al., Tgaku Shoin, Tokio 1974.
Strughold H.: The Rhythmostat in the Human Body (In the Jet and Space Age). Compendium of Aerospace Medicine. Vol. 1., p. 131-8; ed. by Strughold H.; SAM, Brooks AFB, Texas 1977
Strughold H.: The Metrification of America. Aeromedic 1974, 1: 7-8.

1975
Strughold H., Hale H. B.: Biological and Physiological Rhythms. In: Foundations of Space Biology and Medicine, Vol. II, Book 2, Ch.13, p. 535-48. National Aeronautics and Space Administration, Washington (D. C.) 1975.
Strughold H.: Gifts from the Sun. The Torch. Kutztown Publishing Co., Kutztown (Pennsylvania) 1975: 36-40.

1976
Strughold H.: The Gravitational Situation in Space. Ed. by Benson O. O. Jr., Strughold H.; Chapter IX; in: Physics and Medicine of the Atmosphere and Space.

1977
Strughold H.: (Ed.) Compendium of Aerospace Medicine. Vol. 1.; USAF School of Aerospace Medicine, AMD (AFSC), Brooks AFB (Texas) 1977.

1979
Strughold H.: (Ed.) Compendium of Aerospace Medicine. Vol. 2; USAF School of Aerospace Medicine, AMD (AFSC), Brooks AFB (Texas) 1979.

List of speaches, presentations and lectures of Hubertus Strughold 1946 – 1979

Papers archived at the Aerospace Medical Library at Brooks AFB, Texas in the midnineties

1946
Strughold H.: Die Bedeutung des Sauerstoffs für das Leben (The importance of oxygen for life). Presentation, 12 p., Heidelberg 8 th Dec. 1946.
Strughold H.: Warmgerichte auf Breigrundlage sind am besten (Hot mash dishes are best). Introduction, 1 p. Heidelberg 1946/7

1948
Strughold H.: Medical Aspects of Space Travel. Panel Discussion, 11 p. SAM, Randolph AFB (Texas) April 1948.
Strughold H.: Presentation, no topic mentioned. Congress for experimental medicine. Galveston (Texas) 8 th May 1948.

1949
Strughold H.: No topic mentioned. Physiology Congress in Detroit (Michigan) Apr. 1949.
Strughold H., Haber H.: Some Medical Problems Associated with Potential Flight Beyond the Stratosphere. Paper, 10 p. Presented at the annual meeting of the Aero Medical Association, New York (New York) 30 th Aug. 1949.

1950
Strughold H.: Physiological Considerations of Life on Mars. Presentation prepared for the 2nd aerospace medicsl symposium at the University of Chicago (Illinois) 3 rd March 1950.
Strughold H.: Intracellular Air Contents in Animal Hairs. Paper, 4 p. USAF SAM, Department of Space Medicine, USAF SAM, Randolph AFB (Texas) Sept. 1950.
Strughold H: Summation. Paper, 8 p. USAF SAM, Randolph AFB (Texas) Jan. 1950.

1951
Strughold H.: Investigations on the Usefulness of Contact Lenses in Flight. Paper, 7 p. Randolph AFB (Texas) May 1951.
Strughold H.: Suggestions Concerning the Proposed Program for the „Symposium on the Upper Atmosphere". Paper, 2 + 16 p. Statement for commander of USAF SAM, Randolph AFB (Texas) 5 th June 1951.

1952
Strughold H.: Physiological Day-Night-Cycle, Earth Rotation, and High Flying Speed. Paper, 12 p. Presented at the Airline Medical Directors Meeting, USAF SAM, Randolph AFB (Texas) 23 rd Feb. 1952.
Strughold H.: From Aviation Medicine to Space Medicine. Paper, 6 p. Presented at the annual meeting of the Space Medical Association of Aero Medical Association. Washington (D. C.) 17 th-19 th March 1952. Also in: Compendium of Aerospace Medicine. Vol. 1; ed. by Strughold H.; USAF SAM, Brooks AFB (Texas) 1977: 13-16.

Strughold H.: The Atmospheres of Earth and Mars Viewed in the Light of Recent Physiological Concepts. Paper, 9 p. USAF SAM, Randolph AFB (Texas) 8th July 1952.
Strughold H.: Internal Atmosphere. Paper, 10 p. USAF SAM, Randolph AFB (Texas) Aug. 1952. Also in: Compendium of Aerospace Medicine. Vol. 2; ed. by Strughold H.; SAM, Aerospace Medical Division (AFSC), Brooks AFB (Texas) 1979: 135-41.
Strughold H.: Space Medicine. Speech at the Society of the Sigma XI, University of Texas, Austin (Texas) 9th Dec. 1952.

1953

Strughold H.: Planetary Atmospheres as Seen by the Biologist. Paper, 14 p. Presentation at the Metereological Society of San Antonio (Texas) 27th Feb. 1953.
Strughold H.: Report at the Meeting of the Space Biology Committee, Holloman AFB (New Mexico) 2rd-3rd March 1953.
Strughold H.: Sealed Cabin - Physiological Requirements. Paper, 4 p. Department of Space Medicine, USAF SAM, Randolph AFB (Texas) 3rd April 1953.
Strughold H.: Medical Problems of Flight Outside the Atmosphere. Luncheon speech at the Menger Hotel in front of the „American Legion Post No. 10" (Business and Professional Men). Paper, 8 p. San Antonio (Texas) 15th July 1953; in similar form hold at the Air Force Historians Luncheon, Lackland AFB (Texas) 21rd Oct. 1953 as wall as at the Military Accountants and Statisticians, Brooke Army Medical Center 24th Nov. 1953.
Strughold H.: Various lectures at the Surgeons Refresher Course (23rd July 1953), San Marcos Kiwanis Club (13th Aug. 1953), San Antonio Kiwanis Club (20th Aug. 1953).
Strughold H.: Can Air Enter the Veins from the Arterial System? Paper, 7 p. USAF SAM, Randolph AFB (Texas) 11th Sept. 1953.
Strughold H.: The Evolution of the Earth´s Atmosphere. Lecture, 15 p. USAF SAM, Randolph AFB (Texas) 29th Sept. 1953.
Strughold H.: Some Thoughts about the Stars at Christmas. Luncheomn speech at the Military Civilian Club of San Antonio, San Antonio (Texas) 7th Dec. 1953. In: Compendium of Aerospace Medicine. Vol. 2; ed. by Strughold H.; School of Aerospace Medicine, Aerospace Medical Division (AFSC), Brooks AFB (Texas) 1979: 197-200.

1954

Strughold H.: Bullets from Space. Paper, 10 p. Lecture for National Sojourners Chapters No. 17 US Army am Menger Hotel, San Antonio (Texas) 17th Feb. 1954.
Sweeney H. M., Strughold H.: The Current Picture of Space Flight. Paper, 2 p. USAF SAM, Randolph AFB (Texas) 16th March 1954.
Strughold H.: Principles of Space Medicine. Paper, 20 p. Lecture for Primary Course, AME Class, USAF SAM, Randolph AFB (Texas) 28th Apr. 1954.
Strughold H.: Historic Background. Paper, 6 p. Speech on 21th May 1954.
Strughold H.: A Current Picture of Space Medicine. Paper, 18 p. Speech for Reserve officers at Webb AFB, Big Springs (Texas) 16th July 1954.
Strughold H.: Space Equivalent Conditions Within the Earth´s Atmosphere (Physiological Aspects). Presented at the 5th IAF-congress in Innsbruck, (Austria) 6th Aug. 1954.

Strughold H.: A Hermetic Cabin in Space. Paper, 12 p. Presentation at the Meeting of the San Antonio Group of the American Society of Mechanical Engineers, Witte Museum Art Gallery, San Antonio (Texas) 12 th Oct. 1954.
Strughold H.: General and Medical Observations During a Recent European Trip. 3 p. Presentation for USAF SAM Staff, Stafford Hall, Randolph AFB (Texas) 3 rd Dec. 1954.

1955
Strughold H.: Sealed Cabin Craft - A Revolutionizing Step in the Development of Flight. Paper, 7 p. Luncheon speech at Brooks Field Reserve Officers Club, Brooks AFB (Texas) 10 th March 1955.
Strughold H.: A Simple Classification of the Present and Future Status of Manned Flight. Speech at the Annual meeting of Space Medicine Association, Washington (D. C.) 21 th March 1955.
Strughold H.: The US Air Force Experimental Sealed Cabin. Speech at the Annual meeting of Space Medicine Association, Washington (D. C.) 21 th March 1955.
Strughold H., Gerathewohl S. J., Stallings H. D.: Sensomotoric Adaptations During Weightlessness. Presentation at the Space Medicine Session, Annual meeting of the Aero Medical Association, Drake Hotel, Chicago (Illinois) 16 th April 1955.
Strughold H.: Gravi-Receptors. Presentation at Space Medicine Session, Annual meeting of the Aero Medical Association, Drake Hotel, Chicago (Illinois) 16 th April 1955.
Strughold H.: The Medical Problems of Space Flight. Paper, 12 p. Speech at the First International Symposium on Health and Travel, Starlight Roof, Waldorf-Astoria Hotel, New York (New York) 23 rd June 1955.
Strughold H.: Medical Problems above 40,000 Feet. Paper, 3 p. Seminar FSRC, USAF SAM, Randolph AFB (Texas) 13 th Sept. 1955.
Strughold H.: Space Medicine. Paper, 23 p. Speech at Annual Banquet of Texas State Aviation Association, Plaza Hotel 5 th Nov. 1955. Same presentation at Flying Safety Meeting, Kelly AFB, San Antonio (Texas) 13 rd Oct. 1955.
Strughold H.: Medical Problems Involved in Orbital Space Flight. Paper, 16 p. Prepared for presentation at Space Medicine Session of American Rocket Society Annual Meeting at the Diamond Jubilee Annual Meeting of The American Society of Mechanical Engineers at Congress-Hotel in Chicago (Illinois) 13 th-18 th Nov. 1955.
Strughold H.: Space Medicine - The Youngest Offspring of Aeskulapius. Luncheon speech at Meeting of the Texas Academy of Internal Medicine, 10 th Dec. 1955.
In: Compendium of Aerospace Medicine. Vol. 2; ed. by Strughold H.; USAF SAM, Aerospace Medical Division (AFSC), Brooks AFB (Texas) 1979: 21-30.

1956
Strughold H.: New Events Along the Vertical Frontier. Paper, 18 p. Speech at Symposium Dinner, San Antonio (Texas) 19 th Jan. 1956.
Strughold H.: Space Medicine in the Next 20 Years. Paper, 11 p. Adress at banket in honor of Asst. Secy. Defense (Health & Medical) Dr. Frank B. Berry, The Health and Advisory Committee, and Medical Sciences Panel, National Research Council, Washington (D. C.) 10 th Feb. 1956.
Strughold H.: The Human Factor Involved in Flights to be Anticipated Within the next 20 Years. Paper, 12 p. USAF SAM, Randolph AFB (Texas) 7 th March 1956.

204

Strughold H.: Space Medicine. Paper, 13 p. Speech at Sigma XI Annual Initiation Banquet, Houston (Texas) 25th May 1956.
Strughold H.: Medical Support of Space Flight. Paper, 14 p. Presented at Human Factors Technical Symposium, Congress Hotel, Chicago (Illinois) 5th· 6th June 1956.
Strughold H.: Graduation Adress. Paper, 12 p. Prepared for presentation for Jet Pilot Class 56-C of the 3560th Pilot Training Wing an der Webb AFB (Texas) 28th July 1956.
Strughold H.: Man Into Space. Engineering Aspects of the Physiological Problems of Providing for Man in Space. Paper, 31 p. Based on tape recording of Lecture at the Summer Session in Orbital and Satellite Vehicles, M.I.T. 17th Aug. 1956.
Strughold H.: Space Medicine as an Environment for Manned Flight, Human Engineering of the Space Cabin and the Status of Weightlessness. Speech at the Engineering Society of Detroit and Joint Meeting with the Detroit Section of American Rocket Society, Detroit (Michigan) 19th Sept. 1956.
Strughold H.: The Ecosphere in the Solar Planetary System (The Life Zone or Ecosphere in Our Solar Planetary System). Presentation prepared for 7. IAF-Meeting in Rome (Italy) 17th- 22th Sept. 1956.
Strughold H.: Medical Problems in Space Operations. Paper, 7 p. Speech at the Meeting of Excelsior Society, on request of (Asst.) Secretary of Defense Dr. F.B. Berry, Ojai Inn, Ojai (California) 5rd Oct. 1956.
Strughold H.: Mechanoreceptors, Gravireceptors. Paper, 7 p. Presented at 3rd Annual meeting of American Astronautical Society, New York (N. Y.) 7th Dec. 1956.
Strughold H.: Man at the Threshold of Space Flight. Lecture for F.S.R.C. 1956.

1957
Strughold H.: Introduction. Human Factors Panel. Paper. In: Summary Session Astronautics Symposium, San Diego (California) 18th- 20th Feb. 1957: 42-51.
Strughold H.: Teaching and Research in Space Medicine. Paper, 12 p. Briefing for MEND, USAF SAM, Randolph AFB (Texas) 28th March 1957.
Strughold H.: What are the Possibilities of an Inhabitable Extra-Terrestrial Environment Reachable from the Earth? Presentation at Scientific Meeting of AMA, Denver (Colorado) 8th May 1957.
Strughold H.: Specifications for a Simulated Space Surrounded Space Cabin Simulator for School of Aviation Medicine. Paper, 3 p. With andwritten corrections. USAF SAM, Randolph Field (Texas) 22th May 1957.
Strughold H.: General Review of Problems Common to the Field of Astronomy and Biology. Symposium of the International Mars Committee, Lowell Observatory Flagstaff (Arizona) 18th June 1957.
Strughold H.: Memorandum for Major General Benson, Commander SAM. Paper, 3 p. USAF SAM, Randolph Field (Texas) 5th July 1957.
Strughold H.: The Life Zone or Ecosphere in our Solar Planetary System. Presentation at International Astronautical Congress, Rome (Italy) Oct. 1957.
Strughold H.: Space Medicine. Paper, 4 p. SAM USAF, Randolph AFB (Texas) 29th Nov. 1957.
Strughold H.: My European Trip to the International Astronautical Federation Congress in Barcelona 1957. Presentation, 14 p. Partly with handwritten supplements and corrections. USAF SAM, Randolph AFB (Texas) 1957.

1958

Strughold H.: Interrelations of Space Medicine with other Fields of Science.
Paper, 13 p. Presented at the Annual meeting of the Institute of Aeronautical
Sciences, New York, (New York) 28th Jan. 1958.

Strughold H.: Presentation with not topic mentioned at the 3rd Jet Age Conference of
the Air Force Association in Washington (D. C.) 26th - 28th Feb. 1958.

Strughold H.: Space Medical and Astrobiological Research (Bioastronautics).
Paper, 6 p. SAM USAF, Randolph AFB (Texas) Feb. 1958.

Strughold H.: Symposium on Simulated Atmospheres and Foreign Environments
in Space Operations. Paper, 7p. Presented at the 29th Annual meeting of AMA in
Washington (D. C.) 24th March 1958.

Strughold H.: Space Medicine - Man in the Space Environment. Paper, 27 p.
Presented at UCLA Courses in Space Technology, Los Angeles, San Diego,
San Francisco (California) 14th - 18th Apr. 1958.

Strughold H.: Space Medicine and Astrobiology. Paper, 5 p. Report to be submitted to
House Select Committee on Astronautics and Space Exploration, Room 214,
New House Office Building, Washington (D. C.) 5th May 1958.

Strughold H.: Astrobiology. Paper, 13 p. Presented at the Symposium on Possible
Uses of Earth Satellites in Life Science Experiments, Washington (D. C.) 14th - 17th
May 1958.

Strughold H.: Prospects and Limitation of Human Space Flight. Paper, 6 p.
Presented at the Symposium der Aviation Writers Association Meeting, Carswell AFB
(Texas) 29th May 1958.

Strughold H.: Definitions and Subdivisions of Space (Bioastronautical Aspect).
Discussion Remark at the Colloquium on „The Law of Outer Space" in the Chamber
of the House of Parliament, The Hague, at the Annual Congress of the IAF,
29th Aug. 1958.

Strughold H.: Biophysics of the Environment of Space. Paper, 16 p. Speech at the
Society of Exploration Geophysicists, Municipal Auditorium, San Antonio (Texas)
13rd Oct. 1958.

Strughold H.: Summation. Presented at the Symposium on Space Medicine, Joint
Meeting of the School of Aviation Medicine and the Bexar County Medical Society,
RAFB Officers Club, Randolph AFB (Texas) 28th Oct. 1958.

Strughold H. und Ritter O.: Gravitational Environment of Space. Speech,
10th Nov. 1958.

Strughold H.: Spatiography (Astronautical Aspect). Paper, 6 p. USAF SAM,
Brooks AFB, (Texas) 1958.

1959

Strughold H.: Space Medicine Talk. Speech at the Chamber of Commerce,
Fredericksburg (Texas) 15th Jan. 1959.

Strughold H.: Outline - Rocketry and Medical and Biological Sciences. Paper, 8 p.
Presented at the Symposium on Rocketry, New York University, School of Education,
24th Jan. 1959.

Strughold H., Simons D. G.: Results of Biomedical Explorations of Space to Date.
Paper, 11 p. Presentation at the Institute of Aeronautical Sciences, New York (New
York) 27th Jan. 1959.

Strughold H.: The Environment of Space (Bioastronautical Aspects). Paper, 23 p.
Lecture at the Flight Surgeon´s Refresher Course, Randolph AFB (Texas) Jan. 1959.

Strughold H.: Space Medicine of the Next Decade as Viewed by a Physician and Physiologist. Paper, 14 p. Presented at the 10. Anniversary Commemoration of the Founding of the Department of Space Medicine, USAF SAM, Randolph AFB (Texas) 9th Feb. 1959. Paper, 12 p. Also in: Compendium of Aerospace Medicine. Vol. 1; ed. by Strughold H.; USAF SAM, Brooks AFB (Texas) 1977: 23-8.

Strughold H.: Briefing for Gen. Briggs and Air Academy Staff. Paper, 10 p. Air Academy 23. March 1959.

Strughold H.: Medical Aspects of Space Flight. Paper, 10 p. Presented at the Space Age Forum of the Southwest, Dallas (Texas) 14th Apr. 1959.

Strughold H.: Advances in Astrobiology. Paper, 18 p. Presented at the Lunar and Planetary Exploration Colloquium, Santa Monica (California) 25th Apr. 1959.

Strughold H.: Future Space Flight (Medical Aspects). Paper, 21 p. Presented at the 77. Annual meeting of the New Mexico Medical Society, Las Cruces (Texas) 7th May 1959.

Strughold H.: Impact of Space Medicine on Future Medicine. Presented at the 68th Annual meeting of the Arizona Medical Association, Chandler (Arizona) 2nd May 1959. In: Compendium of Aerospace Medicine. Vol. 2; ed. by Strughold H.; USAF SAM, Aerospace Medical Division (AFSC), Brooks AFB (Texas) 1979: 31-3. In similar form: Paper, 16. p. Presented at the Meeting of the Houston Surgical Society, Houston (Texas) 15th May 1959.

Strughold H.: The Role of Medicine in the Space Age. Paper, 18 p. Presented at the Combined Meeting of the Nevada State Medical and Reno Surgical Societies, Reno, Nevada 21nd Aug. 1959. Also in: Excerpt, p. 26-8. Speech at the Clinical Meeting of the American Medical Association in Dallas (Texas) no date.

Strughold H.: The Human Eye in Space (Physiologic Aspects). Paper, 20 p.; 2nd Paper 4 p. Draft for presentation at the International Astronautical Congress in London (England) 31th Aug. - 5th Sept. 1959.

Strughold H.: Anatomy of Space (Physiological Aspect). 13 p. Presented at the Meeting of the American Society of Anesthesiologists, Inc., Bal Harbour (Florida) 5th - 9th Oct. 1959. In: Compendium of Aerospace Medicine. Vol. 2; ed. by Strughold H.; USAF SAM, Aerospace Medical Division (AFSC), Brooks AFB (Texas) 1979: 35-40.

Strughold H.: Future Plans in Space Medical Research. Paper, 5 p. Briefing for the Committee on Science and Astronautics, AMC, Brooks AFB (Texas) 17th Nov. 1959. In: Compendium of Aerospace Medicine. Vol. 2; ed. by Strughold H.; USAF SAM, Aerospace Medical Division (AFSC), Brooks AFB (Texas) 1979: 41-3.

Strughold H.: Lectures on Space Medicine, Air University, USAF SAM, Randolph and Brooks AFB (Texas) 1959: I: The Role of Medicine in the Space Age (Medicine in the Third Dimension); II: Space Equivalent Conditions Within the Earth´s Atmosphere; III: Environmental Ecology of the Solar System: 1. Spatiography; IV: Environmental Ecology of the Solar System: 2) Planetography; V: Classification of Space Operations and Their Medical Characteristics; VI: The Space Cabin, Medical Aspect; VII: The Exotic Psychophysiological World of Weightlessness; VIII: The Astronaut´s Visual World in Space; IX: A World Without Day and Night; X: Moon, Venus, and Mars as Astronautical Targets.

Strughold H.: Ophtalmologische Gesichtspunkte des Raumfluges (Ophtalmologic impcts on space flight). Presentation at 10th IAF-Congress in London (England) 1959.

1960
Strughold H.: Biophysics of the Space Environment. Paper, 33 p. Lectures in
Aerospace Medicine, USAF Aerospace Medical Centre, Brooks AFB (Texas)
11th Jan. 1960.
Strughold H.: Planetary Ecology (Celestial Bodies/Astrobiology). Paper, 28 p.
Lectures in Aerospace Medicine, USAF Aerospace Medical Centre. Brooks AFB
(Texas) 11th Jan 1960. In similar form: Paper, 21 p. Presented at the Meeting of
Astrophysical Society, Trinity University, San Antonio (Texas) 14th March 1960.
Also a substantially unchanched paper (19 p.) for briefing of Command and Staff
of School, Maxwell AFB (Alabama) 26th May 1960. Also in similar form: Paper, 24 p.
Prepared for Publikation im Journal of Astronautics.
Strughold H.: Summation. Paper, 8 p. Lectures of Aerospace Medicine. USAF
Aerospace Medical Centre, Brooks AFB (Texas) 15th Jan. 1960.
Strughold H.: Medical Problems of Man in Space. Paper, 18 p. Presented at the Law-
Science Week, Hotel Shamrock, Houston (Texas) 17th Feb. 1960.
Strughold H.: Remarks Regarding Extraterrestrial Life. Paper, 1 p. USAF AMC,
Brooks AFB (Texas) Feb. 1960.
Strughold H.: New Medical Horizons in the Space Age. Paper, 14 p. Presented at the
Chicagoland Health Fair, Chicago (Illinois) 18th March 1960.
Strughold H.: Aero Association of Space Medicine with Preventive Medicine. Paper,
3 p. Briefing for General Benson. USAF SAM, Brooks AFB (Texas) Feb. 1960.
Strughold H.: The Spaceflight Situation (Sensory-Physiological Aspect). Paper, 17 p.
Presented at the Psycho-physiological Aspects of Spaceflight Symposium, USAF
AMC, Brooks AFB (Texas) 26th - 27th May 1960. Also in: Compendium of Aerospace
Medicine. Vol. 2; ed. by Strughold H.; USAF SAM, Aerospace Medical Division
(AFSC), Brooks AFB (Texas) 1979: 75-82.
Strughold H.: Space Medicine and Astrobiology. Paper, 40 p.. Presented at the 11.
International Astronautical Congress, Stockholm (Schweden) 15th - 20th Aug. 1960.
Also in: Compendium of Aerospace Medicine. Vol. 2; ed. by Strughold H.; SAM,
Aerospace Medical Division (AFSC), Brooks AFB (Texas) 1979: 45-61.
Strughold H.: The Photic Environment in Space and on the Neighbouring Celestial
Bodies: Biological Aspect. Presented at the 2nd International Symposium on
Submarine and Space Medicine, Karolinska Institute, Stockholm (Schweden)
18th - 19th Aug. 1960. In: Compendium of Aerospace Medicine. Vol. 2; ed. by
Strughold H.; School of Aerospace Medicine, Aerospace Medical Division (AFSC),
Brooks AFB (Texas) 1979: 63-74.
Strughold H.: The Gravitational „Territories" of the Celestial Bodies of the Solar
System. Paper, 5 p. Presented at the Space Law Colloquium as part of the 11.
International Astronomical Congress, Stockholm (Schweden) 15th - 20th Aug. 1960.
Strughold H.: Space Medicine Briefing. Paper, 10 p. Presented for the Group for the
Advancement of Psychiatry, Aerospace Medical Centre, Brooks AFB (Texas)
21th - 22nd Sept. 1960.
Strughold H.: Space Energies: Summation. Presented at the Energies of Space
Symposium, AMC, Brooks AFB (Texas) 24th - 26th Oct. 1960. In: Compendium of
Aerospace Medicine. Vol. 2; ed. by Strughold H.; School of Aerospace Medicine,
Aerospace Medical Division (AFSC), Brooks AFB (Texas) 1979: 83-8.
Strughold H.: Advanced Studies. Paper, 7 p. Briefing for Daddario, member of the
Congress, USAF AMC, Brooks AFB (Texas) 2nd Dec. 1960.

1961

Strughold H.: Biophysics of the Space Environment. Paper, 34 p. Lectures in
Aerospace Medicine, USAF AMC, Brooks AFB (Texas) 16th- 20th Jan. 1961.
Strughold H.: Sense and Nonsense of Manned Space Flight: An Optimistic-Realistic
Approach. Presentation at the banquet of the ATC Information Conference at
Randolph AFB (Texas) 23rd Jan. 1961. In: Compendium of Aerospace Medicine. Vol.
2; ed. by Strughold H.; School of Aerospace Medicine, Aerospace Medical Division
(AFSC), Brooks AFB (Texas) 1979: 89-95.
Strughold H.: The Planets Around Us (Medicobiological Aspect). Paper, 36 p.
Presented at the War College, Air University, Maxwell AFB (Alabama) 22nd March
1961. In similar form: The Planets Around Us: The Astro-Biological Aspect. Paper,
35 p. First lecture, Visiting Lecturers´ Program of the Faculty Council, Wright-
Patterson AFB (Ohio) 28th March 1961.
Strughold H.: Extraterrestrial Environments. Paper, 67 p. Presented at the Institute
of Technology, Air University, Wright-Patterson AFB (Ohio) 27th- 28th March 1961.
Strughold H.: Recent Space Developments on the International Scene Oxygen
Production during the Evolution of the Earth´s Atmosphere). Paper, 12 p. Presented
at the Fellows Meeting in Chicago (Illinois) 24th Apr. 1961.
Strughold H.: Impact of Space Medicine on Medicine in General. 22 p. Presented at
the Mayo Clinic, Rochester (Minnesota) 10th May 1961.
Strughold H.: New Scientific Horizonts in the Space Age. 13 p. Presented at the
official opening of the Roger Bacon Science Center, Winona (Minnesota)
11th May 1961.
Strughold H.: The Evolution of the Planetary Atmospheres. Paper. Presented at the
American Astronautical Society Meeting, Grand Prarie (Texas) 17th May 1961.
Strughold H.: Temporal Coordination of Day-Night-Cycle after Intercontinental
Flight. Paper, 8 p. Presentation prepared for the Symposium on Circadian
Systems, University of Minnesota Medical School, Minneapolis (Minnesota)
4th- 7th June 1961.
Strughold H.: The Visual Panorama in Space on the Moon and the Neighbouring
Planets. Paper, 17 p. Presented at the Meeting of the wives of the Reserve Officers
Units, Navarro Room, St. Anthony Hotel (Texas) 22nd June 1961.
Strughold H.: Presentation, no topic mentioned. 12th IAF-Kongress in Washington
(D. C.) 2nd- 7th Oct. 1961; Co-Chairman at the Bioastronautics-Round-Table (Men
under Space Flight Stress).
Strughold H.: The Changing Visual Scenery from Aeronautics to Astronautics. Paper,
17 p. Presented at the Dining-In (U2-Pilots), Laughlin AFB (Texas)
22nd Sept. 1961. In: Compendium of Aerospace Medicine. Vol. 1; ed. by Strughold
H.; USAF SAM, Brooks AFB (Texas) 1977: 29-36.
Strughold H.: The Human Eye in the Visual Environment on the Moon. Discussion
Remark prepared for the Meeting of the LIL Committee of the International
Academy of Astronautics, Washington D.C., 2nd- 5th Oct. 1961. In: Compendium of
Aerospace Medicine. Vol. 2; ed. by Strughold H.; School of Aerospace Medicine,
Aerospace Medical Division (AFSC), Brooks AFB (Texas) 1979: 97-9.
Strughold H.: Crossing the Threshold of Space. The Role of Medicine. Paper, 8 p.
Presented at the ATC Commanders´ Call, Randolph AFB (Texas) 9th Oct 1961.
In more extensively paper with 26 p. Presented on 19th Oct. 1961.

Strughold H.: Day-Night Cycles in Atmospheric Flight, Space Flight, and other Celestial Bodies. Paper, 13 p. Presentation at the Conference on Rhythmic Functions in the Living System, The New York Academy of Sciences, New York, (N. Y.) 8th - 11th Nov. 1961.
Strughold H.: The Ecological Profile of Mars (and its Medico-Biological Implications). Paper, 15 p. Presentation prepared for the 128th Meeting of the American Association for the Advancement of Science (AAAS), Denver (Colorado) 26th - 30th Dec. 1961.
Strughold H.: Comments. Paper, 6 p. Concerning the Russian Cosmic Medical Doctor V. G. Yazdovsky during his Attendance of the Annual Meeting of the IAF in Washington (D. C.) 2nd - 7th Oct. 1961.

1962
Strughold H.: The Ecologic Profile of the Moon. Lectures of Aerospace Medicine, p. 347-67, USAF AMC, Brooks AFB (Texas) 8th - 12th Jan. 1962.
Strughold H.: Ecology of Planets (Astrobiology). Paper, 26 p. Lectures in Aerospace Medicine, AMC, Brooks AFB (Texas) 11th Jan. 1960.
Strughold H.: The Physical Environmental Profiles of the Planets and Their Medico-Biological Implications. Lecture I - 24 p. Lecture II - 18 p. Prepared for the War College, Maxwell AFB (Alabama) 1th Feb. 1962.
Strughold H.: Biophysical and Biomedical Profiles on Other Planets and the Moon. Lecture at the War College, Maxwell AFB (Alabama) 1th Feb. 1962.
Strughold H.: Space Medicine. Presentation at the Annual meeting of the Iowa Medical Society at the Veteran Memorial Audititorium, Des Moines (Iowa) 15th May 1962.
Strughold H.: The Human Elements in Astronautics. 9 p. Article to be published in the Los Angeles Times, San Antonio (Texas) May 1962.
Strughold H.: Planetary Ecology (Mars and Venus). Lecture, Medical Support for Space Flight. USAF AMC (AFSC), USAF SAM, Brooks AFB (Texas) 5th June 1962.
Strughold H.: From Aeronautics to Astronautics. Lecture, Medical Support for Space Flight. USAF AMC (AFSC), USAF SAM, Brooks AFB (Texas) 5th June 1962.
Strughold H.: Meteorites, Dust, and Gaseous Matter. Lecture, Medical Support for Space Flight. USAF AMC (AFSC), USAF SAM, Brooks AFB (Texas) 6th June 1962.
Strughold H.: Solar Electromagnetic Radiation. Vorlesung, Medical Support for Space Flight. USAF AMC (AFSC), USAF SAM, Brooks AFB (Texas) 6th June 1962.
Strughold H.: Atmospheric Physics. Lecture at the Bioastronautics for Space Research Pilots Course. USAF SAM, Brooks AFB (Texas) 9th July 1962.
Strughold H.: The Role of Medicine in the Space Age. Paper, 12 p. Presented at the American Bar Association in San Francisco (California) on 4th Aug. 1962.
Strughold H.: Space: The International Scene. Paper, 14 p. Presented at the meeting of the San Antonio Section of the Aerospace Medical Division, Officers Open Mess, Brooks AFB (Texas) 12th Sept. 1962.
Strughold H.: Ecophysiological Profile Tables of Space, Moon, Mars and Earth. Paper, 12 p. Presentation prepared for the International Symposium on Basic Environmental Problems of Man in Space in Paris (France) 29th Oct.- 2nd Nov. 1962. Paper in: Compendium of Aerospace Medicine. Vol. 1; ed. by Strughold H.; USAF SAM, Brooks AFB (Texas) 1977: 37-42.
Strughold H.: The Face of Mars (Medical Biological Aspect). Paper, 12 p. Presented at the Meeting of the South Texas Geological Society, San Antonio (Texas) 13th Nov. 1962.

Strughold H.: The Visual Panorama in Space, on the Moon and the Neighbouring
Planets. Paper, 14 p. Presented at the Girl Friday Luncheon at Lackland AFB (Texas)
19 th Dec. 1962.
Strughold H.: Space Medicine. Paper, 21 p. Prepared for publication in the „The
Book of Health". The Medical Arts Publishing Foundation; Houston (Texas) 1962.

1963
Strughold H.: Guest lecture at the 28. Annual banquet, Lockhart Chamber of
Commerce (Texas) 10 th Jan. 1963.
Strughold H.: Space Medical Problems Beyond the Moon. 23 p. Presented at the
27th Anniversary Meeting of the International Medical Assembly of Southwest
Texas, Granada Hotel, San Antonio (Texas) 30 th Jan. 1963; in similar form:
Human Problems in Exploration Beyond the Moon. Paper, 19 p. incomplete.
Strughold H.: The Ecological Profile of Mars: Bioastronautical Aspects. Paper, 23 p.
Lectures in Aerospace Medicine. USAF SAM, Brooks AFB (Texas) 8 th Feb. 1963. In
similar form: Presented at the American Astronautical Society Symposium on the
Exploration of Mars, Denver (Colorado) 6 th - 7 th June 1963. In: Compendium of
Aerospace Medicine. Vol. 1; ed. by Strughold H.; USAF SAM, Brooks AFB (Texas)
1977: 43-52.
Strughold H.: The Physiological Clock in Aeronautics and Astronautics. Lectures in
Aerospace Medicine, p. 389-400. USAF AMD. Brooks AFB (Texas)
4 th - 8 th Feb. 1963.
Strughold H.: New Scientific Horizons in Medicine and Biology in the Space Age.
Paper, 18 p. Presented at the Aerospace Educational Workshop, AFCAP, Austin
(Texas) 1 th March 1963.
Strughold H.: Space Visual Phenomena and Adaptation. Paper, 13 p. Presented at
the MEND Bioastronautical Symposium, Air Force Missile Test Centre (AFMC),
Patrick AFB (Florida) 18 th - 19 th Apr. 1963.
Strughold H.: Mars as an Astronautical Target. Presented at the Dining-In,
ACO School, Lackland AFB (Texas) 17 th June 1963.
Strughold H.: Biophysics of the Environment of Mars. Paper, 3 p. Presented at the
Advanced Placement Physics Program Conference of the Educational Testing
Service, Trinity University, San Antonio (Texas) 21 th June 1963.
Strughold H.: Basic Medical Research in the Adaptation of Man and Machine in
Aviation and Space Travel. Guest speech at the First Symposium oft he German
Soviety für Aviation and Space Medicine (Deutschen Gesellschaft für Luft- und
Raumfahrtmedizin - DGLRM), Physiological Institute oft he Munich University
(Germany) 8 rd - 9 th Oct. 1963.
Strughold H.: The Mission of Space Medicine. Paper, 10 p. Prepared for the
Grolier´s encyclopedia (Year Book 1963).

1964
Strughold H.: The Solved and the Unsolved Problems. Paper, 11 p. Lectures
of Aerospace Medicine, USAF Aerospace Medical Centre. Brooks AFB (Texas)
3 rd -7 th Feb. 1964.
Strughold H.: A Comparison of US and USSR Bioastronautics. Presentation at the
35. Annual meeting of AsMA in Miami Beach (Florida) 11 th May 1964.

Strughold H.: No title mentioned. Presentation at the 3rd Int. Symposium on Bioastronautics and the Exploration of Space, San Antonio (Texas) Nov. 16th -18th 1964.
Strughold H.: Life in a Theoretical Zone Below the Surface of Mars. Paper, 1964. In: Compendium of Aerospace Medicine. Vol. 2; ed. by Strughold H.; School of Aerospace Medicine, Aerospace Medical Division (AFSC), Brooks AFB (Texas) 1979: 143-51.
Strughold H.: Space Medicine: Manned Space Flight. Paper, 7 p. Prepared for publication in the American Annual 1964.

1965
Strughold H.: A Deep Look at Mars (The Martian Biosphere). Paper, 18 p. Presented at the Meeting of the Southwest Section of the American Institute of Aeronautics and Astronautics, Randolph AFB Officers´ Club (Texas) 18th March 1965.
Strughold H.: Solved and Unsolved Problems. Speech for Medical Students of the Tuft´s Univ. of the State Univ. of New York (New York) 15th June 1965.
Strughold H.: Space Medicine Looks at Mars. Paper, 17 p. Presented at the Meeting of the Aviation Writers Association, Gramercy Inn, Washington (D. C.) 12th July 1965.
Strughold H.: Lectures of Aerospace Medicine, USAF SAM (Texas) 22nd July 1965.
Strughold H.: A New Look at Mars Since Mariner IV. Medical Biological Aspect. Speech at the Dining-In, Ellington AFB (Texas) 10th Oct. 1965. In same form: Paper, 14 p. Presented at the Luncheon Meeting des San Antonio Optimist Club, Gunter Hotel, San Antonio (Texas) 19th Oct. 1965.
Strughold H.: The Metric System - Revolution or Evolution. Paper, 5 p. Panel Diskussion at the October meeting of the San Antonio Subsection of American Society of Mechanical Engineers, San Antonio (Texas) 26nd Oct. 1965.
Strughold H.: Pioneer Developments in Space Medicine. Lecture for class 65-B: 13 p. Bioastronautics for Space Research Pilots. USAF SAM, Brooks AFB, Texas 29th Nov. 1965.
Strughold H.: The Physiological Clock in Aeronautics and Astronautics. Paper presented at the Conference on Civilian & Militarian Uses of Aerospace).

1966
Strughold H.: A New Look at Mars - Medico-Biological Aspect. Paper, 15 p. Speech at the French Club, Witte Museum, San Antonio (Texas) 28nd Feb. 1966. In similar form: Lecture for Aerospace Medicine Residency Class 66 A, 18 p. USAF SAM, AMD Brooks AFB (Texas) 10th June 1966.
Strughold H.: Martian Environmental Medicine. Paper, 19 p. Presented at the Symposium „Stepping Stones to Mars" jointly conducted by the American Institute of Aeronautics and the American Astronautical Society, Baltimore 28th - 30th March 1966.
Strughold H.: General Bioastronautic Aspects of the Solar Planetary System. Paper, 11 p. Lecture for the Aerospace Medicine Residency Class 66 A. USAF SAM, AMD Brooks AFB (Texas) 10th June 1966.
Strughold H.: A New Look at Mars: Biological Aspect. Lecture, Bioastronautics for Space Research Pilots, Class 66 B, Brooks AFB (Texas) 5th Aug. 1966.
In: Compendium of Aerospace Medicine. Vol. 2; ed. by Strughold H.; USAF SAM, AMD (AFSC), Brooks AFB (Texas) 1979: 125-33.

Strughold H.: Space Medical Problems en Route to Mars (Raummedizinische Probleme auf dem Flugwege zum Mars). 15 p. Presentation, read at the 15th Internat. Rocket- and Space Travel Symposium (Raketen- und Raumflug-Jahressymposium) of the Hermann Oberth Society, Bremen (Germany) 22nd-25th Sept. 1966.

Strughold H.: Lunar Medicine. Paper, 22 p. Presented at the Second Lunar International Laboratory Symposium (LIL), Organized by the International Academy of Astronautics in Madrid (Spain) 13rd Oct. 1966. In: Compendium of Aerospace Medicine. Vol. 1; ed. by Strughold H.; School of Aerospace Medicine, Brooks AFB (Texas) 1977: 53-62.

Strughold H.: Basic Physiological Concepts for Bioengineering. Paper, 10 p. Presented at the Univ. of Texas Bioengineering Seminar, Austin (Texas) 3th Nov. 1966. Also in: Compendium of Aerospace Medicine. Vol. 1; ed. by Strughold H.; School of Aerospace Medicine, Brooks AFB (Texas) 1977: 63-73.

Strughold H.: The Physiological Clock in Air and Space Travel. Paper, 13 p. Lecture for Medicine Residency Class 67 A, SAM USAF, Brooks AFB (Texas) 7th Dec. 1966.

Strughold H.: Sensory Physiological Control of Body Balance and Movement on Earth, Mars, Moon and in Space. Paper, 8 p. Brooks AFB (Texas) 1966.

Strughold H.: A Martian Biosphere? Report-No. AAS 66-339, USAF SAM, Brooks AFB (Texas) 1966.

1967
Strughold H.: Lex Cosmica. Col Rule´s Lecture. Paper, 16 p. Lectures in Aerospace Medicine, Brooks AFB (Texas) 7th Feb. 1967.

Strughold H.: Solved and Unsolved Space Medical Problems International Status 1966-67. Paper, 27 p. Lectures of Aerospace Medicine. USAF AMC, Brooks AFB (Texas) 6th-9th Feb. 1967.

Strughold H.: Locomotion on the Moon. Paper, 4 p. Presented at the Third Texas and Southwestern Astronomers Neighbourhood Meeting, The University of Texas, Austin (Texas) 3rd March 1967.

Strughold H.: Recent Astronomical Discoveries and the Martian Life Theory. Paper, 6 p. Presented at the Third Texas and Southwestern Astronomers Neighbourhood Meeting, The University of Texas, Austin (Texas) 4th March 1967. In: Compendium of Aerospace Medicine. Vol. 1; ed. by Strughold H.; USAF SAM, Brooks AFB (Texas) 1977: 75-8.

Strughold H.: Solved and Unsolved Problems in Aerospace Medicine - International Status, 1967. 27 p. Presented on the occasion oft he visit of Lt. General Richard L. Bohannon, Surgeon General, USAF, with his distinguished guests the Allied Air Surgeons General, Brooks AFB (Texas) 6th Apr. 1967. In: Compendium of Aerospace Medicine. Vol. 1; ed. by Strughold H.; USAF SAM, Brooks AFB (Texas) 1977: 79-91.

Strughold H.: Biological "Fuel Cells" (From the Electric Fish to Man). In: Compendium of Aerospace Medicine. Vol. 1; ed. by Strughold H.; SAM, Brooks AFB (Texas) 1977: 93-100. Also in: Proceedings of 13th Annual Meeting of American Astronautical Society (AAS 67-121), 6 p. Statler Hilton Hotel, Dallas (Texas) 1st- 3rd May 1967.

Strughold H.: Gravisphere, Gravipause: Astronautical Aspect. For Presentation at the American Astronautical Society Conference on Use of Space Systems for Planetary Geology and Geographics. Boston (Mass.) 25th- 27th May 1967. In: Compendium of

Aerospace Medicine. Vol. 2; ed. by Strughold H.; School of Aerospace Medicine, Aerospace Medical Division (AFSC), Brooks AFB (Texas) 1979: 171-4.
Strughold H.: Hemis-Fair 1968 in the Space Age. Paper, 7 p. Presented at San Antonio Council of Presidents Annual Awards Banquet, St. Anthony Hotel, San Antonio (Texas) 5th June 1967. Also in: Space Age; Congress. Rec. - House, H 8033-4, Washington (D. C.) 26th June 1967.
Strughold H.: Life on Mars in View of Recent Discoveries of Earth-Based and Space-Bound Astronomy. Prented at the Meeting of the Armed Forces Management Association, Randolph AFB (Texas) 22nd June 1967. In: Compendium of Aerospace Medicine. Vol. 2; ed. by Strughold H.; USAF SAM, AMD (AFSC), Brooks AFB (Texas) 1979: 175-80.
Strughold H.: Pioneer Developments in Space Medicine. Paper, 21 p. Lecture for the „Bioastronautics for Aerospace Research Pilots", Class 67-A, Brooks AFB (Texas) 10th July 1967.
Strughold H.: General Bioastronautics of Our Planetary System. Paper, 17 p. Lecture for „Aerospace Medicine Residents - Class 68 A", Brooks AFB (Texas) 24th July 1967.
Strughold H.: The Influence of Solar Electromagnetic Radiation Upon the Planetary Environments (Helio-Ecosphere). Paper, 7 p. Lecture for the „Aerospace Medicine Residents – Class 68 A", Brooks AFB (Texas) 25th July 1967.
Strughold H.: The Sleep and Wakefulness Cycle in the Perspective of Air- and Space Travel. Paper, 26 p. Lecture for the „Aerospace Medicine Residents, Class 68A", SAM USAF, Brooks AFB (Texas) 11th Aug. 1967.
Strughold H.: Martian Station. Re-tiped to indicate changes, USAF SAM, Brooks AFB (Texas) 17th Aug. 1967.
Strughold H.: The Secretaries´ Language and Art in the Space Age. Paper, 12 p. Presented at the Luncheon of the AMS Secretaries, Brooks AFB (Texas) 27th Sept. 1967. Also in: Compendium of Aerospace Medicine. Vol. 1; ed. by Strughold H.; USAF SAM, Brooks AFB (Texas) 1977: 101-6.
Strughold H.: Physics and Chemistry of the Earth´s Atmosphere. Paper, 22 p. Lecture for the „Aerospace Medical Primary Class - 67C", USAF SAM, Brooks AFB (Texas) 9th Oct. 1967.
Strughold H.: The Spectrum of Space Medical Problems Solved and Unsolved, Status 1967. Paper, 15 p. Presented at the Kimbrough Urological Seminar, Brooks AFB (Texas) 30th Oct. 1967.
Strughold H.: The Era before Manned Space Flight. Paper, 23 p. Lecture for the „Aerospace Medicine Primary Class 67-C", Brooks AFB (Texas) 7th Dec. 1967.
Strughold H.: The Atmospheres of Earth and Mars in the Light of Recent Physiological Concepts. Paper No. 67-52, 10 p. American Rocket Society 1967.

1968
Strughold H.: Unorthodoxies and Controversies in Planetary and Space Science. Paper, 15 p. Presented at the Banquet of 6th Working Group on Extraterrestrial Resources, San Antonio (Texas) 19th Feb. 1968. Also in similar form (15 p.) at the AFSC Information Officer´s Luncheon, Officers Club, Brooks AFB (Texas) 30. Apr. 1968. In: Compendium of Aerospace Medicine. Vol. 1; ed. by Strughold H.; USAF SAM, Brooks AFB (Texas) 1977: 107-13.
Strughold H.: Life on Mars in View of Recent Discoveries of Earth-Based and Space-Bound Astronomy. 13 p. Luncheon speech at Christian Laymen, NCO Club, Brooks AFB (Texas) 29th May 1968.

Strughold H.: Planetary Environmental Medicine (Mars). Fourth International Symposium on Bioastronautics and the Exploration of Space, The Convention Centre, San Antonio (Texas) (The Hemis Fair City) 27th June 1968.

Strughold H.: Aerospace Age Impact Upon Administration. Paper, 12 p. Presented at the Meeting of the San Antonio Chapter of the Society for Personnel Administration, Officers´ Club, Brooks AFB (Texas) 21st July 1968.

Strughold H.: Bioelectro Energetics. Fuel Cell Aspects. Paper, 14 p. Prepared for presentation at the AGARD Bionics Symposium in Brussels (Belgiun) 18th - 20th Sept. 1968. Also in: Principles and Practise of Bionics. AGARD CP 44, Brussels 1968. Also in: Compendium of Aerospace Medicine. Vol. 2; ed. by Strughold H.; SAM, Aerospace Medical Division (AFSC), Brooks AFB (Texas) 1979: 117.

Strughold H.: On the Road to „Metrication". Paper, 8 p. Presented at the San Antonio Zero Defects Area Council Luncheon, Brooks AFB Officers Club (Texas) 24th Sept. 1968. Also in: Compendium of Aerospace Medicine. Vol. 1; ed. by Strughold H.; USAF SAM, Brooks AFB (Texas) 1977: 115-8.

Strughold H.: The Physiological Clock Across Time Zones and Beyond. Paper, 23 p. Presented at the Third Civil Aviation Medical Association (CAMA) Symposium on Modern Concepts in Civil Aviation Medicine. USAF SAM, Brooks AFB (Texas) 27th Sept. 1968.

Strughold H.: The Anatomy of Sleep. Paper, 24 p. Presentation at the Luncheon Meeting of the Officers´ Wives Club, Brooks AFB (Texas) 15th Oct. 1968.

Strughold H.: Panel Discussion: Where do we go from here? The Proceedings of the Fourth International Symposium on Bioastronautics and the Exploration of Space, p. 595-608.

Strughold H.: Pioneer Developments in Space Medicine or Bioastronautics. Paper, 22 p. Lecture for the Bioastronautics for Aerospace Research Pilots, Brooks AFB (Texas) 1968. Similar lecture (9 p.) for the „Bioastronautics for Aerospace Research Pilots", Brooks AFB (Texas) 1970. Also in: Compendium of Aerospace Medicine. Vol. 1; ed. by Strughold H.; USAF SAM, Brooks AFB (Texas) 1977: 1198.

1969
Strughold H.: Biomedical Benefits from Space. Paper, 13 p. Luncheon speech at the Exchange Club of San Antonio (Texas) 21th May 1969.

1970
Strughold H.: The Seventies - The Decade of Global Metrication. Paper, 10 p. Presented for USAF Security Services, Kelly AFB (Texas) Feb. 1970. In similar form: 10 p. Presented at the Meeting of the Civilian Engineers in San Antonio (Texas) 8th Jan. 1973.

Strughold H.: Pioneer Developments in Space Medicine or Bioastronautics. Paper, 9 p. Lecture for the Bioastronautics for Aerospace Research Pilots, Brooks AFB (Texas) 1970.

1971
Strughold H.: Cycloecology in Space on Moon and Beyond. In: Space Biology and Medicine; 417-23. Congress of the Society for the Study of Biological Rhythms, Little Rock (Arkansas) 8th - 10th Nov. 1971.

Strughold H.: The Biological Clock or The Circadian Rhythm in the Jet and Space Age. Paper, 26 p. Prepared for presentation, USAF SAM, Brooks AFB (Texas) 1971.
Strughold H.: Presentation, no title at the Annual Meeting der Space Medicine Branch der AsMA in Houston (Texas) 1971.

1973
Strughold H.: The Sleep and Activity Cycle in the Mars International Laboratory (MIL).Prepared for presentation at MIL Panel Meeting at the Congress of the International Academy of Astronautics in Baku (USSR)
7th-13th Oct. 1973. In: Compendium of Aerospace Medicine. Vol. 1; ed. by Strughold H.; USAF SAM, Brooks AFB (Texas) 1977: 129-30.

1974
Strughold H.: Space Science for Poetry. Paper, 11 p. San Antonio (Texas) 4th Oct. 1974.
Strughold H.: The Rhythmostat in the Human Body (In the Jet and Space Age). Paper, 14 p. Presentation at the Southwest Research Institute, 24th Oct. 1974.

1975
Strughold H.: The Sun: The Fountain of Energy for Life. Paper, 16 p. Presented at the Torch Club of San Antonio (Texas) 10th March 1975.
Strughold H.: Semantics for Poetry in the Space Age. Paper, 11 p. Presented at the Poetry Seminar in San Antonio (Texas) 3rd Oct. 1975. In: Compendium of Aerospace Medicine. Vol. 1; ed. by Strughold H.; USAF SAM, Brooks AFB (Texas) 1977: 139-44.

1976
Strughold H.: The Two Hundred Year Jubilee of the Discovery of Oxygen. Remarks following a Lecture at the USAF School of Aviation Medicine 1976. In: Compendium of Aerospace Medicine. Vol. 2; ed. by Strughold H.; USAF SAM, Aerospace Medical Division (AFSC), Brooks AFB (Texas) 1979: 191-2.

1977
Strughold H.: Gifts from the Sun. Paper, 13 p. Presented at the „Daughters of the American Revolution". San Antonio de Bexar Chapter (Texas) 6th Jan. 1977.
Strughold H.: Speech on the occasion of the inauguration of the Strughold Aeromedical Library. In: Compendium of Aerospace Medicine. Vol. 1; ed. by Strughold H.; USAF SAM, Brooks AFB (Texas) 19th Jan. 1977: 11-2.
Strughold H.: The Sun: The Fountain of Energy for Life. Paper, 9 p. Presented at the San Antonio Astronomical Association, San Antonio (Texas) 18th Feb. 1977.
In similar form: Presented at the Commencement Ceremony at St. Mary´s University in May 1977. Also in: Compendium of Aerospace Medicine. Vol. 1; ed. by Strughold H.; School of Aerospace Medicine, Brooks AFB (Texas) 1977: 145-53.
Strughold H.: Impact of the Celestial Bodies on the Human Mind (Stars, Planets, the Moon, Comets, UFOs), draft: Impact of the Starry Sky on the Human Mind. Paper, 8 p. Presented at the San Antonio Astronomical Association (Texas) 9th Dec. 1977.
In similar form: Presented at the Optimist Club, San Antonio (Texas) 19th July 1978. In: Compendium of Aerospace Medicine. Vol. 2; ed. by Strughold H.; USAF SAM, Aerospace Medical Division (AFSC), Brooks AFB (Texas) 1979: 193-6.

Strughold H.: The Historical Impact of the Star-Covered Sky Upon the Human Mind. Paper, 8 p. Presented at the San Antonio Astronomical Association (Texas) 9th Dec. 1977.

Strughold H.: Biographie. In: Compendium of Aerospace Medicine. Vol. 1; ed. by Strughold H.; School of Aerospace Medicine, Brooks AFB (Texas) 1977: 7-10.

1978

Strughold H.: Speech on the occasion of the induction into the International Space Hall of Fame, Alamogordo (New Mexico) 6th Oct. 1978. In: Compendium of Aerospace Medicine. Vol. 2; ed. by Strughold H.; USAF SAM, AMD (AFSC), Brooks AFB (Texas) 1979: 11-2.

1979

Strughold H.: Lyndon B. Johnson, The Promoter of Space Exploration. Personal Memoirs. In: Compendium of Aerospace Medicine. Vol. 2; ed. by Strughold H.; USAF SAM, Aerospace Medical Division (AFSC), Brooks AFB (Texas) 1979: 13-8.

Strughold H.: Meeting Walt Disney in the Early Space Age. In: Compendium of Aerospace Medicine. Vol. 2; ed. by Strughold H.; USAF SAM, Aerospace Medical Division (AFSC), Brooks AFB (Texas) 1979: 19.

Strughold H.: At the Threshold of the Cosmozoicum. In: Compendium of Aerospace Medicine. Vol. 2; ed. by Strughold H.; USAF SAM, Aerospace Medical Division (AFSC), Brooks AFB (Texas) 1979: 113-6.

Strughold H.: Cosmic Sleep. In: Compendium of Aerospace Medicine. Vol. 2; ed. by Strughold H.; USAF SAM, Aerospace Medical Division (AFSC), Brooks AFB (Texas) 1979: 119-24.

Strughold H.: The Life Zone in the Planetary System. In: Compendium of Aerospace Medicine. Vol. 2; ed. by Strughold H.; USAF SAM, Aerospace Medical Division (AFSC), Brooks AFB (Texas) 1979: 153-60.

Strughold H.: Mechanoreceptors, Gravireceptors, Acceleroreceptors. In: Compendium of Aerospace Medicine. Vol. 2; ed. by Strughold H.; USAF SAM, Aerospace Medical Division (AFSC), Brooks AFB (Texas) 1979: 161-4.

Strughold H.: Out of Space - Advances for Medicine. In: Compendium of Aerospace Medicine. Vol. 2; ed. by Strughold H.; USAF SAM, Aerospace Medical Division (AFSC), Brooks AFB (Texas) 1979: 181-9.

Strughold H.: Mars - The Roman God of War and of Agriculture. In Compendium of Aerospace Medicine. Vol. 2; ed. by Strughold H.; USAF SAM, Aerospace Medical Division (AFSC), Brooks AFB (Texas) 1979: 201.

Strughold H.: Solar Energy Dictionary. In: Compendium of Aerospace Medicine. Vol. 2; ed. by Strughold H.; USAF SAM, Aerospace Medical Division (AFSC), Brooks AFB (Texas) 1979: 203-10.

Oral history taken by author with:

- Alcott, Edward B., Ph.D., Historian, Dept. AF, HQ Human Systems Centre, Brooks AFB (Texas), 6th Feb. and 22nd Aug. 1997.
- Boubel, Tamara, San Antonio (Texas) 30th Nov., 1th-7th Aug. 1996, 2nd Dec. 1997, 17th May 1998.
- Bretschneider, Kai-Thorsten, Dr., Klausdorf/Schwentine (Germany) 26th Aug. 1996.
- Bussche H. van den, Prof. Dr. med., Univ. Hamburg (Germany) 28th Jan.1999.
- Daumann F.-J., Dr. med., General M.C. ret., past President of DGLRM, Head of GAFIAM (GeAF Institute of Aviation Medicine – FlMedInstLw), Fuerstenfeldbruck (Germany) 30th Dec. 1996 and 19th Feb. 1998.
- Doerner, K., Prof. Dr. Dr., Westf. Clinik for Psychology, Psychosomatic and Neurology, Guetersloh (Germany) 6th March 1996.
- Draeger J., Prof. Dr., Clinic of Opthalmology of the Univ. Hospital Eppendorf, Hamburg (Germany) 17th Dec. 1998.
- Dressen, Public prosecutor (Staatsanwalt), Central Office of the State Judicial Administration (Zentrale Stelle der Landesjustizverwaltungen; (110 AR 813/96)), Ludwigsburg (Germany) 18th July 1996.
- Fichtner, G., Prof. Dr., Head of Inst. of Medical History of Univ. Tuebingen (Germany) 14th Feb. 1996.
- Frank, P., Dr., Secretary of DGLRM, Fuerstenfeldbruck (Germany) 22nd Apr. 1996, 18th Apr. 1998.
- Freeman, Marsha, 21st Century Science and Technology, Washington (D. C.) 3rd Feb. 1997.
- Friedrich, Office man (Archivamtmann), State archive (Staatsarchiv) Nürnberg (Germany) 30th July 1996.
- Fuchs, Heinz S., Prof. Dr., Gen. GeAF M.C. ret., Bonn (Germany) 29th May 1995 and letter correspondences until publication in Private archive of Dr. Harsch.
- Gibson, Air Commodore, England, 11th Jan. 1999.
- Goerke, Heinz, Prof. Dr. med. Dr. h. c. mult., Munich (Germany) 3rd Feb. 1998.
- Griesbaum, Joachim, Chief University Archives at Albert-Ludwigs-University Freiburg, 18th July, 1996.
- Graul E. H., Prof. Dr., Marburg (Germany) 17th Dec. 1998.
- Gunga, H. C., Dr., Physiolog. Inst., FU Berlin(Germany) 26th Sept. 1995, 31st Oct. 1996, 20th Nov. 1997.
- Haenel, Dr., Univ.-Archives of Goettingen, 16th July, 1996.
- Hanschke, Wolfgang, Lt.Col. GeAF, Brooks AFB (Texas) 26th Apr. 1996.
- Hoelscher, Paulamaria, Dr. med., Ludwigshafen (Germany) 1st Dec. 1997.
- Hollmann, Wildor, Prof. Dr. med. Dr. h.c., German Sports University Cologne (Deutsche Sporthochschule Koeln), 3nd Apr. 1996 and 11th Jan. 1999.
- Karlheim, Hubert, Dr. med. et phil., relative, Stadthagen, May 11th 1996.
- Kessler, Dr., Scientific employee, Rupert Karls Univ. Heidelberg 15th July 1996.
- Kilwing, Elli, born Karlheim, friend from Westtuennen, June 1st 1996.
- Kirsch, Karl, Professor Dr. med., Free University Berlin, 16th May 1997, 6th Jan. 1999 and 26. Jan. 2013.

- Klueting, E., Dr., Managing director, Westphalian Homeland Association (Heimatbund), Muenster (Germany) 22nd Aug. 1997.
- Koester, Margot, Dipl.-Chem., Head Poggendorff editorial stuff, Sachsony Acad. of Sciences, Leipzig (Germany) 19th June and 1st Oct. 1996.
- Kolander, Hilde, born Lorenz, Hespecke, 5th and 19th Nov. 1996.
- Kuehn, Gerhard, Sauerland working group on family research, Sundern (Germany) 12th Nov. 1996.
- Lauschner, E. A., Prof. Dr. med. (1911-96), Gen. GeAF M.C. ret. Emmering, 25th June 1992.
- Linne, Karsten, Hamburg Foundation for Social history of the 20th century, Hamburg (Germany) 29th May and 5th June 1996.
- Longe, Patrick D., SSgt, USAF, 311 HSW Historian, Brooks AFB (Texas) 30th Nov. 1998.
- Lorenz, National Archives Department Potsdam (Germany) 22. Aug. 1996
- Luelf, Alfons, native researcher, Westtuennen, 26th Feb., 4th and 7th May and 27th June 1996.
- Mai, Paul, Dr., CV-Archives, Regensburg, March 12th 1996.
- Menard, D., USAF Museum, Wright Patterson AFB (Ohio) 8th July and 12th Aug. 1996.
- Modler, Raimo, Großalsleben (Germany) 4th Feb. 1996.
- Mohler, Stanley R., M.D., Professor and Vice Chair, Director Aerospace Medicine, Wright State University, Dayton (Ohio), 16th July 1996 und 21th Jan. 1998.
- Mueller, Bruno H. C., Prof. Dortmund (Germany) 18th May 1996.
- Muellmann, Adalbert, Dr., Sauerland Homeland Society 30th July 1996.
- Mutke G., Space Gynecologist and Me-262-pilot, Munich 1999
- Oberdorf, Guenter, Iserlohn, 1st June, 1996.
- Oberdorf, Ida, relative from Rhynern, 27th February 1996
- Peter, Juergen, Dr., Hanau (Germany) 18th Feb. 1998.
- Rayman, Russel B., M.D., Executive Director, Aerospace Medical Association, Alexandria (Virginia), 5th Aug. 1996.
- Scarpa, Philip J., National Aeronautics and Space Administration, Kennedy Space Center (Florida) 24th July 2000.
- Starkey, Don J., Director, Space Center Division, NM Office of Cultural Affairs, Alamogordo (New Mexico) 15th Dec. 1998.
- Steinberg, Elan, Executive Director, World Jewish Congress, New York (New York) 7th July 1996.
- Strughold, Mary, wife, Mico (Texas) 3rd August 1996.
- Ueter, Ferdinande, relative, born Strughold (1928-1998), from Rheda-Wiedenbrueck 13th Sept. and 1st October 1997
- Voss, H., Hamm 18th July 1996.
- Thomas M., head of the home town and history association in Siegen 2nd May 1996.
- Weber, Ulrich, Hamm (Germany) 25th March 1996.
- Weisser U., Prof. Dr. med., Univ. Hamburg (Germany) 27th Jan. 1999.
- Welsch, Dr. med., Head II. Department of GAFIAM (Flight Physiology), Koenigsbrueck (Germany) 11th Sept. 1998.
- Zhang Ru Cun, Dr. med., Institute for Manual Medicine and Traditional Chinese Medicine, Bad Oeynhausen (Germany) 5th Feb. and 9th March 1996.
- Zhang, Tsu Te, Dr. med. (1911-96), Luzhou, Sichuan Provinz (PR China) 24th July 1996.

219

Literature

Albring W.: Gorodomlia. German Rocketry Pioneers in Russia (Deutsche Raketenforscher in Russland). Luchterhand Literaturverlag, Hamburg 1991.

Alexander L. The treatment of shock from prolonged exposure in cold especially in winter. Washington DC. Office of Publication Board, Department of Commerce, Report #250. 1946.

Armstrong H. G.: The Origin of Aerospace Medicine. US Armed Forces Med J 1959, 10: 389-92.

Ashman C., Wagman R. J.: The Nazi-Hunters. The shocking true Story of the Continuing Search for Nazi Criminals. Pharos Books, New York, 1988.

Autrum H. My Life (Mein Leben). Springer, Berlin 1996.

Baerwolf A: For many weeks in Space? (Wochenlang im All? Gespräch mit Professor Strughold). Welt am Sonntag newspaper, 29th Aug. 1965.

Baerwolf A.: Burnout. Rendezvous with the moon (Brennschluss - Rendezvous mit dem Mond). Ullstein, Berlin 1969.

Baerwolf A.: Sitting beside the chair. Interview with H. Strughold on the occasion of his 80th birthday (Neben den Stuhl gesetzt: Der Raumfahrtmediziner Hubertus Strughold wird 80 Jahre alt). Welt newspaper, 14th June, 1978.

Baerwolf A.: The secret factory: Americas victory in a technological war (Die Geheimfabrik. Amerikas Sieg im Technologischen Krieg). Herbig, Muenchen 1994.

Baerwolf A.: The Mars-Factory (Die Marsfabrik. Aufbruch zum roten Planeten). Herbig, Muenchen 1995.

Beamish R. J.: The story of Lindbergh. The lone Eagle. The International Press, 1927.

Beckh H v.: The Space Medicine Branch of the Aerospace Medical Association. Aviat Space Environ Med 1979, 50: 513-6.

Beddies T. Kinder-"Euthansie" in Berlin-Brandenburg (Children-Euthanasia in Berlin-Brandenburg), in: Beddies T. and Huebner K. (Ed.). Documents regarding Psychiatrie in Nazi Germany (Dokumente zur Psychiastrie im Nationalsozialismus). Berlin 2003: 219-48.

Benford R. J.: Report from Heidelberg. The Story of the Army Air Forces Aero Medical Center in Germany 1945-1947. Heidelberg 1947.

Benford RJ. "German Aviation Medicine during World War II". Superintendent of Documents, U. S. Government Printing Office, Washington, D.C. 1948.

Benford R. J.: Doctors in the Sky. The Story of the Aero Medical Association. Charles C. Thomas. Springfield 1955.

Berger R, Nazi Science - The Dachau Hypothermia Experimants. NEJM 322:1435-1440. 1990.

Berry C. A.: The Beginnings of Space Medicine. Aviat Space Environ Med 1986, 57 : A58-63.

Benz W.: S. Rascher – A Career (Dr. med. Sigmund Rascher - Eine Karriere. In: Dachauer Hefte. Studien und Dokumente zur Geschichte der nationalsozialistischen Konzentrationslager) Issue 4, p. 190-214. Ed. by Benz W., Distel B., Dachau 1988.

Benzenhoefer U.: Medical crimes against Humanity (Aerztliche Verbrechen gegen die Menschlichkeit: Vor 50 Jahren wurde der Nürnberger Aerzteprozeß eroeffnet). Niedersaechsisches Aerztebl 1996, 10: 13-5.

Benzinger T. Aero Medical Department of the Testing Station Rechlin, 1934 - 1944 (Medizinische Abteilung der Erprobungsstelle der Luftwaffe Rechlin). ATI No. 58275. AAF Aero Medical Center, Heidelberg 1946.

Blumenthal R. "The Mixed Reasons for News, U.S. Nazi-Hunt" New York Times, 11/28/1976, page 185.

Bower T. "The Paperclip Conspiracy, The Hunt for Nazi Scientists". Publisher: Little, Brown. 1987.

Bower T.: From Dachau to the Moon. How nazi Scientists become the Fathers of US-Space Program (Von Dachau zum Mond. Wie Nazi-Forscher zu den Vaetern der US-Weltraumfahrt wurden.) Die Zeit No. 20, 8.th May 1987.

Bower T.: Conspiracy Paperclip (Verschwoerung Paperclip. NS-Wissenschaftler im Dienste der Siegermaechte.) List, Munich 1988.

Braun W. v.: The Development of Rocketry in Germany (Das deutsche Raketenwesen. In: Clarke A.C. [Ed.]: Wege in den Weltraum. Die Pioniere berichten). P. 52-82. Econ Verlag, Duesseldorf-Wien 1969.

Bretschneider K.-T.: Friedrich Hermann Rein. Scientist in Germany and Physiologist in Goettingen (Wissenschaftler in Deutschland und Physiologe in Göttingen in den Jahren 1932-1952). Medical thesis, Goettingen 1997.

Buechner, F.: Plans and Coincidence. Remembering my Life as a University Teacher. (Plaene und Fuegungen. Lebenserinnerungen eines deutschen Hochschullehrers.) Munich, Berlin 1965.

Campbell P. A.: The Present Space Medicine Effort at the School of Aviation Medicine. US Armed Forces Med J 1959, 10: 392-7.

Clamann H. G. Report on Rapid Decompression Experiments (Vorlaeufiger Bericht ueber Drucksturzversuche. Einschl. Schreiben an S. Ruff, Berlin-Adlershof, 6th Sept. 1939. In: Archive of USAF School of Aerospace Medicine, Brooks AFB, Texas.

DeHart R. L.: Aerospace Medicine in Perspectives: The Modern Perspectives. In: Fundamentals of Aerospace Medicine, Ed. by DeHart, p. 26-40. Lea & Febiger, Philadelphia 1985.

Deutsch E.: The Nuremburg Code (Der Nuernberger Kodex. Das Strafverfahren gegen Mediziner, die zehn Prinzipien von Nuernberg und die bleibende Bedeutung des Nuernberger Kodex). In: Troehler U. and Reiter-Theil S. (ed.) Ethics and Medicine (Ethik und Medizin. Was leistet die Kodifizierung von Ethik)? p. 103-14. Wallstein-Verlag, Goettingen 1997.

Doerner K., Ebbinghaus A., Linne K. (Ed.). The Nuremberg Doctor Trials 1946/1947 (Der Nuernberger Aerzteprozess 1946/47). Mikrofiche-Edition. KG Sauer, Munich 2000.

Ebert C.: Personal biographies of lectureres of the Medical Faculty in Wuerzburg (Die Personalbiographien der Ordinarien und Extraordinarien der Anatomie mit Histologie und Embryologie, der Physiologie und der Physiologischen Chemie an der Medizinischen Fakultät der Julius-Maximilians-Universitaet Wuerzburg). Medical theses, Erlangen-Nuremberg 1971.

Eckart WU. Medicine during the Nazi Dictatorship. Ideology, practice, consequences (Medizin in der NS-Doktatur. Ideologie, Praxis, Folgen). Boehlau, Weimar 2012.

Engle E., Lott A. S.: Man in Flight - Biomedical Achievements in Aerospace. Leeward Publ., Annapolis 1979.

Faust H.: Why to the moon? (Warum Flug zum Mond?) Handelsblatt 1965, 119: 17.

Feiden M. K. German Space Doctor considers that manned satellites are possible (Deutscher Weltraummediziner hält bemannte Satelliten für moeglich). Essener Daily (Tageblatt), 15th Oct. 1957.

Fischer A. C.: Aviation Medicine on the Threshold of Space. National Geographic 1955, CVIII: 240-78.

Freeman M.: The Story of the German Space Pioneers (Hin zu neuen Welten. Die Geschichte der deutschen Raumfahrtpioniere.) Boettiger, Wiesbaden 1995.

Fuchs H. S.: Hubertus Strughold – Father of Space Medicine (In memoriam Hubertus Strughold, des „Vaters der Raumfahrtmedizin"). Wehrmed. Mschr. 1986, 3: 128-30.

Fuchs H. S.: From Aviation to Space Medicine. In Memoriam Hubertus Strughold – „Father of Space Medicine". Von der Luft- zur Raumfahrtmedizin. In Memoriam Hubertus Strughold - „Vater der Raumfahrtmedizin". Astronautik 1987, 1: 5-7.

Fuchs H. S.: Hubertus Strughold (Kurzbiographien aus der Luft- und Raumfahrt). Luft- und Raumfahrt 1987, 4: 2p.

Fuchs H. S.: Obituary (Nachruf H. Strughold). DGLRM Mitt. 1988, 1: 8-12.

Gartmann, H.: Artificial Satellites (Künstliche Satelliten). Die Kosmos-Bibliothek, Vol. 218. Franckh´sche Verlagsbuchhandlung, Stuttgart 1958.

Gartmann, H.: Dreamer, Researcher, Designer (Traeumer, Forscher, Konstrukteure. Die Abenteuer der Weltraumfahrt). Econ-Publ., Duesseldorf 1958.

Gauer O., Haber H.: Man under Gravity-Free Conditions. In: German Aviation Medicine World War II; Ch. VI, p. 641-4. Ed. by The Surgeon General, US Department of the Air Force, U.S. Govt. Print. Office, Washington 1950.

Gauer O., Opitz E., Palme F., Strughold H. Parachute Jump and Time Reserve in High Altitudes (Fallschirmabsprung und Zeitreserve in großen Hoehen). Luftfahrtmed 1942, 6: 340-55.

Gerst T.: Reorganization and Consolidation of Medical self-administration (Neuaufbau und Konsolidierung: Aerztliche Selbstverwaltung und Interessen-vertretung in den drei Westzonen und der Bundesrepublik Deutschland 1945-1995. In: Geschichte der deutschen Aerzteschaft); p. 195-242. Ed. by Juette R.; Deutscher Aerzte-Verlag, Cologne 1997.

Glasgow T. A.: „Father of Space Medicine. ´Halley´s comet launched his career. Aerospace Historian 1970, 17: 6-9.

Goyer R.: 50 Years of the USAF. Flying 1997, 70: 100-2.

Graul E. H.: Space Medicine (Weltraummedizin. Der Mensch in der Zerreissprobe). Ullstein, Frankfurt-Berlin 1970.

Grosse-Brockhoff F.: Pathologic Physiology and Therapy of Hypothermia. German Aviation Medicine World War II, Bd. II, S. 828 ff., Washington 1950.

Grosse-Brockhoff F.: Cold damage (Kaelteschaeden). In: Handbook of Internal Medicine, 4. ed., part VI/2, p. 46 f. Berlin 1954.

Harsch V.: German Acceleration Research from the Very Beginnings. Aviat Space Environ Med 2000a, 71(8): 854-6.

Harsch V. German Acceleration Research from the Very Beginnings. Aviat Space Environ Med 2000b, 8: 854-6.

Harsch V.: 40 years of German Sociatey for Aviation and Space Medicine (Die Deutsche Gesellschaft fuer Luft- und Raumfahrtmedizin e.V. (DGLRM) 1961-2001). Norderstedt 2001.

Harsch V.: Hamburg Aviation Medical Institute (Das Institut für Luftfahrtmedizin in Hamburg-Eppendorf (1927-1945)). Rethra Publ., Neubrandenburg 2003.

Harsch V. "Life, Work and Times of Hubertus Strughold, 1898-1986." (Leben, Werk und Zeit des Physiologen Hubertus Strughold, 1898-1986). Rethra Verlag. Neubrandenburg 2004.

Harsch V. Theodor Benzinger, German Pioneer in High Altitude Physiology Research and Altitude Protection. Aviat Space Environ Med 2007, 9: 906-8.

Harsch V., Wirth D. (Ed.) 60 Years Aerospace Medicine in Germany after WWII (60 Jahre Luft- und Raumfahrtmedizin in Deutschland nach 1945). Rethra-Verlag, Neubrandneburg 2008

Henke J., Oldenhage K.: OMGUS-Handbook. (Die amerikanische Militaerregierung in Deutschland 1945-1949). Ed. by C. Weisz. Oldenbourg Publ., Munich 1994.

Hense W.: The sky comes cloeser (Der Sternenhimmel ist uns naeher gerueckt. Professor Dr. Strughold machte Urlaub im Sauerland. Interview mit Raumflugmediziner). Newspaper article, 1957.

Hippke E.: Opening adress at the first aeromedical meeting in Berlin 1937 (Eroeffnungsansprache auf der ersten deutschen Tagung für luftfahrtmedizinische Forschung in Berlin, 25. - 28. Oktober 1937). Luftfahrtmed 1938, 2: 149-57.

Hippke E.: Personalia (Personalien: Oberstarzt a. D. Professor Dr. Heinz von Diringshofen). Wehrmed Mschr 1967: 311-2.

Hoffmann D. (Ed.): Operation Epsilon. The Farm-Hall-Protocols (Die Farm-Hall-Protokolle oder Die Angst der Alliierten vor der deutschen Atombombe). Rowohlt Publ., Berlin 1993.

Hunt L.: Secret Agenda. The United States Government, Nazi Scientists, and Project Paperclip, 1945 to 1990. St. Martin´s Press, New York 1991.

Jungk R.: The Space Professor (Der Weltraumprofessor). Newspaperarticle, no date.

Justice B.: Russia Hunted for Space Medicine Ace: US Got Him. Star Telegram, 3rd Oct. 1961.

Kanovitch B.: Medical experiments in concentration camps in Nazi Germany. (Die Medizinischen Experimente in den Konzentrationslagern des Nationalsozialismus. In: Ethik und Medizin. Was leistet die Kodifizierung von Ethik?). Ed. by Troehler U. and Reiter-Theil S.; p. 89-101. Wallstein-Verlag, Goettingen 1997.

Kirsch K., Winau R.: The Early Days of Space Medicine in Germany. Aviat Space Environ Med 1986, 57: 633-5.

Klee E.: Auschwitz (Auschwitz, die NS-Medizin und ihre Opfer). S. Fischer Publ., Frankfurt a. M. 1997.

Koch G. Human Genetics in my Time (Humangenetik und Neuro-Psychiatrie in meiner Zeit (1932-1978). Jahre der Entscheidung). Verlag Palm & Enke, Erlangen und Jena. 1993.

Kogon E.: The SS-State and its Concentration Camps (Der SS-Staat. Das System der deutschen Konzentrationslager). 31st ed., Wilhelm Heyne Verlag, Munich 1995.

Kornbluh M. Bulletin of the Atomic Scientists. 1992. 48: 42-43.

Kornmueller A. E., Palme F., Strughold H.: Ueber Veraenderungen der Gehirnaktionsstroeme im akuten Sauerstoffmangel (EEG-changes due to acute lack of oxygen). Luftfahrtmed 1941, 5: 161-83.

Kudlien F.: Doctors in Nazi-times (Aerzte im Nationalsozialismus). Kiepenhauer & Witsch 1995

Kurowski F.: Allie´s hunt for German Scientists (Alliierte Jagd auf deutsche Wissenschaftler. Das Unternehmen Paperclip.) Kristall bei Langen-Mueller, Munich 1982.

Lasby C. G.: Project Paperclip: German Scientists and the Cold War. Atheneum, New York 1975.

Lauschner E. A.: The Beginnings of Aviation Medicine in Germany. Aviat Space Environ Med 1984, 55: 355-7.

Levitt I. M.: Space Travel today and tomorrow (Weltraumfahrt heute und morgen). Deutsche Buchgemeinschaft, Berlin 1961.

Link M. M., Colemann H. A.: Medical Support of the Army Air Forces in World War II. Office of the Surgeon General, USAF, Washington, 1955.

Lytle S.: Space Doctor. While NASA was thinking about Earth Orbits, he was planning for Mars. 1985: 48-50.

Mackowski MP. "Testing the limits: aviation medicine and the origins of manned space flight". College Station, TX. University of Texas A and M Press. 2006.

Magnus K.: Rocket-Slaves. German Scientists behind the red barbed wire (Raketensklaven. Deutsche Forscher hinter rotem Stacheldraht). DVA, Stuttgart 1993.

Marbarger J. P.: Space Medicine. The Human Factor in Flights Beyond the Earth. Ed., University of Illinois Press, Urbana 1951.

Marbarger J. P.: A Snapshot of the Early History of the Space Medicine Branch. Paper, 8 p. Presented at the Annual Meeting der AsMA in Miami, Florida 1992.

Maser W.: Nuremberg Tribunal of the Winners (Nürnberg: Tribunal der Sieger). Droste, Duesseldorf 1988.

Matschke R. G.: See Survival (Ueberleben auf See. Medizinische Aspekte der Schiffbruechigen in historischen Darstellungen). Med. thesis, Duesseldorf 1975.

McGinnis P. J.: The Re-Emergency of Space Medicine as a Distinct Discipline. Aviat Space Environ Med 1998, 69: 1107-11.

Military Medical Ethics, Volume 2. Washington D.C. U.S. Department of Defense, Office of the Surgeon General, US Army, Borden Institute. 2003.

Mitscherlich A.: Inhuman medicine (Unmenschliche Wissenschaft). Goettinger Universitaetszeitung 1946, 17/18: 6-7.

Mitscherlich A., Mielke F.: Medicine without Humanity (Medizin ohne Menschlichkeit - Dokumente des Nürnberger Ärzteprozesses). Fischer Publ., Frankfurt a. M. 1989.

Moritz E. (Ed.): Current Biography Yearbook 1966. Hubertus Strughold, p. 394-6. Wilson Company, New York 1967.

Nadas A.: Obituaries: Hubertus Strughold. JAMA 1987, 258: 312.

o. Verf. (no author): Centre Personnel Activities make National TV Program. Astromedic 23 rd Nov. 1961.

Noell W. Special physiology of the brain during Anoxia. In : German Aviation Medicine Worls War II. Prepared under the auspices of the Surgeon General, U.S. Air Force. U.S. Government Printing Office, Washington D.C. 1950: 286-300.

Noell W. The human EEG during anoxia. In : German Aviation Medicine World War II. Prepared under the auspices of the Surgeon General, U.S. Air Force. U.S. Government Printing Office, Washington D.C. 1950: 301-3.

Nuremburg Trials Document. Document #437. Affadavit of Dr. Sigmund Ruff. October 25, 1946.

Nuremburg Trials Document. Document #451. Cross Examination of Dr. Wolfgang Lutz. December 12, 1946. Pages 266-274.

Office of History: A Short History of Air University. HQ Air University, Maxwell AFB (Alabama) 31 th Dec. 1995.

224

Peter J.: The Nurenberg Trials (Der Nuernberger Aerzteprozess: im Spiegel seiner Aufarbeitung anhand der drei Dokumentensammlungen von Alexander Mitscherlich und Fred Mielke). Lit Verlag, Hamburg 1994.

Piccard A.: Above the clouds, below the waves (Ueber den Wolken, unter den Wellen). Brockhaus, Wiesbaden 1954.

Poggendorf-Redaktion - Editorial Office: Strughold, Hubertus, Physiol. Saechsische Akademie der Wissenschaften. Vol. VII., 1971.

Poeppinghege R.: Rejection to the Republic (Absage an die Republik. Das politische Verhalten der Westfälischen Wilhelms-Universität Münster 1918-1935). Agenda, Muenster 1994.

Pueschel E.: The distress organization of the German Luftwaffe (Die Seenot-verbaende der deutschen Luftwaffe und ihr Sanitätsdienst 1939-1945). Droste Publ., Duesseldorf 1978.

Radinger W., Schick W.: Secret Projects of Messerschmitt (Messerschmitt Geheimprojekte). Aviatic, Planegg 1991.

Reimer T.: Development of Aviation Medicine in Germany (Die Entwicklung der Flugmedizin in Deutschland). Medical theses, Cologne 1979.

Rein F.H. Science and Inhumanity (Wissenschaft und Unmenschlichkeit). Goettinger Universitaetszeitung 1947, 2 (14): 3-5.

Roadman C. H.: Aerospace Medicine. Air Univ Rev 1968, 19: 2 f.

Roadman C. H.: Welcome to the Fourth International Symposium on Bioastronautics and the Exploration of Space. In: Fourth International Symposium on Bioastronautics and the Exploration of Space. Ed. by Roadman C. H., Strughold H., Mitchell R. B.; p. Xi-XIV., Springfield 1968.

Romberg H. W. Der Fallschirmabsprung aus großen Hoehen. Luftwissen 8 (1941) 10: 310-4.

Roth K. H.: Deadly Hights – The Hypoxia-experiments in the concentration camp Dachau and their relevance for the aeromedical Research in the 3 rd Reich (Tödliche Höhen: Die Unterdruckkammer-Experimente im Konzentrationslager-Dachau und ihre Bedeutung für die luftfahrtmedizinische Forschung des „Dritten Reiches". In: Vernichten und Heilen. Der Nürnberger Ärzteprozeß und seine Folgen). p 93-109. Ed. by Ebblinghaus A., Dörner K. Aufbau-Publ., Berlin 2001.

Ruhenstroth-Bauer G and Nachtsheim H. Die Bedeutung des Sauerstoffmangels für die Auslösung des epileptischen Anfalls (The significance of oxagen deficiency as trigger for an seizure). Klin Wschr 23 (1944) 18-20.

Ruhenstroth-Bauer. Reader Letter „Experiments with Children". Weekly newspaper Die Zeit 2000 No. 8. From www.zeit.de: 2000 No. 8.

Ruff S. Rescue Possibilities from High Altitude Flights (Ueber Rettungsmoeglich-keiten beim Flug in grossen Hoehen). Presentation at the 9th Scientific Members Meeting of the German Academy of Aviation Research on 6th November 1942. Pages 3-18 (found at University Library Hannover (ZS 4730 g (1057).

Ruff S., Strughold H. Outlines of Aviation Medicine (Grundriss der Luftfahrtmedizin). 2nd edition. Johann Ambrosius Barth, Leipzig 1944.

Schafer G. E.: US Air Force School of Aerospace Medicine Celebrates 50th Anniversary. Aerospace Med 1968, 39: 328-31.

Scherff K.: Airlift to Berlin (Luftbrücke Berlin). Motor Buch Publ., Stuttgart 1998.

Schott H.: Chronic of Medicine (Die Chronik der Medizin). Chronik Verlag, Dortmund 1993.

Schmul HW. The Kaiser Wilhelm Institute for Anthropology, Human Heredity and Eugenics, 1027-1945. Crossing Boundries. (Grenzüberschreitungen. Das Kaiser-Wilhelm-Institut für Anthropologie, menschliche Erblehre und Eugenik 1927-1945) Springer. 2008. Wallstein, Goettingen 2005.

Schmidt U. Justice at nuremburg, leo alexander and the nazi doctors trial. New York, NY. Palgrave Macmillian. 2004.

Schwabe K.: German University Teaschers and Hitlers War (Deutsche Hochschullehrer und Hitlers Krieg (1936-1940). In: Die Deutschen Eliten und der Weg in den Zweiten Weltkrieg). Broszat M., Schwabe K. (Ed.); Beck´sche Verlagsbuchhandlung, Munich 1989: 291-333.

Schwerin von A. Experimentalization of Humans (Experimentalisierung des Menschen. Der Genetiker Hans Nachtsheim und die vergleichende Erbpathologie 1920-1945). Wallstein Verlag, Goettingen. 2004.

Schwerdtfeger, Luft U.: Medical Assistance to britisch and american Pilots. Aeromedical Report 26/44. HQ Luftwaffe´s Medicval Corps (Ed.) 1944.

Siegmund W.: The Grammar school Hammonense 1657-1957 (Das Gymnasium Hammonense 1657-1957. Entnommen der Festschrift zum 300-jaehrigen Jubiläum von 1957, S. 31-156. In: 325 Jahre Gymnasium Hammonense). Edited by the society of the friends of the grammar school Hammonense, Griebsch Priting Company, Hamm 1982.

Sonnenborn R. A.: Manned spaceflight isn´t a big deal anymore (Flug eines bemannten Raumschiffs zur Zeit kein grosses Problem mehr. Interview mit Professor Dr. Dr. Strughold vom Luft- und Raumfahrtmedizinischen Zentrum in Texas.) Westf. Anzeiger 5 th Sept. 1960.

Strughold H.: Long Trip to Mars now to Strennous for Man. Science News Letter 6 th Febr. 1960.

Strughold H.: Celsius overtaking Fahrenheit in U.S.. S. 1 E, San Antonio Express 13 th Sept. 1979.

Strughold H.: Deep Manned Space Probes. Los Angeles Times 17 th June 1962.

Strughold H.: 15 Years of Space Medicine. Astro Medic 1964, 3.

Strughold H.: In: The New Space Age. A Guide to Astronomy and Space Exploration. Dutton, New York 1969.

Stuhlinger E., Ordway F. I.: Wernher von Braun (Aufbruch in den Weltraum. Die Biographie). Bechtle Verlag, Esslingen-Munich 1992.

Taddey G (Ed.): Lexikon of German History. Kroener, Stuttgart 1979.

Taylor T.: The Nuremburg Trials (Die Nürnberger Prozesse. Hintergruende, Analysen und Erkenntnisse aus heutiger Sicht.) Wilhelm Heyne Verlag, Munich 1996.

The National Association of Doctors in the U.S.: Dr. Hubertus Strughold, M.D., Ph.D. „Father of Space Medicine". In: The Nadus Journal 1968, 4: 4-5.

Thomas S.: Hubertus Strughold. The Father of Space Medicine whose Dramatic Advanced Planning Envompasses the Universe. In: Men of Space, Vol. 4, p. 233-72. Chilton Company - Book Div., Philadelphia 1962.

Unger F.: The Physiological Institute at the Military Medical Academy in Berlin (Das Institut für Allgemeine und Wehrphysiologie an der Militärärztlichen Akademie in Berlin (1937-1945)). Medical theses, Hannover 1991.

USAF: German Aviation Medicine World War II, 2 Vol., Washington D.C. 1950
USAF: Brooks AFB 75th Anniversary Celebration. Brooks AFB (Texas) 7 th-13 th Nov. 1992.

Ward J. E.: The remarkable Herr Professor (Dr. Hubertus Strughold). Speed Age
Sept. 1959: 42-3, 56.

Weindling P. Genetics and Human Experimentation in Germany, 1940-1950
(Genetik und Menschenversuche in Deutschland, 1940-1950). In: Schmuhl H.W.
(Ed.). Rassenforschung am Kaiser-Wilhelm-Instituten vor und nach 1933. Wallstein,
Goettingen 2003: 245-74.

Weindling PJ. Nazi medicine and the nuremburg trials. NewYork, NY. Palgrave
Macmillan. 2004.

Weiss H.: A Westphalian becomes a Space Pioneer. (Ein Westfale als Weltraum-
pionier. Prof. Dr. Strughold für kurze Zeit in der Heimat.) Westfalenpost
30 th Sept. 1954.

Milliams D. C.: The History and Mystery of the Menger Hotel. Republic of Texas
Press, Plano, Texas 2000.

Zimmermann W.: Interview from Space (Interview aus dem „Weltraum" - Rhynern
und Westtuennen auf Besuchsliste.) Westfälischer Anzeiger, 17 th Oct. 1957.

Zuntz N.: Physiology and Hygiene in Aviation (Zur Physiologie und Hygiene der
Luftfahrt. In: Luftfahrt und Wissenschaft; Ed. Sticker J.), Vol. 3. Verlag von Julius
Springer Publ., Berlin 1912

Register of Figures, Tasbles and Documents

Figures

Tables

Documents

Index

Notes:

The Authors

Dr. Mark Campbell is a board certified general surgeon and a Fellow of the American College of Surgery, the Aerospace Medicine Association, and the Texas Surgical Society. He currently is in general surgery private practice in Paris, Texas. He has been a member of the Space Medicine Association and The Aerospace Medical Association (AsMA) since 1988. Dr. Campbell has been a private pilot since 1984 and received his Air Force Flight Surgery wings in 1994. He was a NASA Flight Surgeon from 1994 to1995 and was deployed to Star City, Russia to support the Shuttle-Mir program. He has authored or co-authored 34 published papers concerning surgical care during space flight and surgical techniques in weightlessness and is the author of a chapter on "Surgical Care in Space" in the recently published textbook, "Principles of Clinical Medicine for Space Flight ". He was on the Aviation Space and Environmental Medicine journal advisory board from 2006-2009 and edited the journal section, "Classics in Space Medicine". He was the President of the Space Medicine Association from 2007-2008 and is currently Vice-President of the Aerospace Medical Association. He is currently also the chairman of the AsMA Commercial Space Flight Working Group, which produced a position paper on "Medical Issues for Suborbital Commercial Space Flight Crewmembers" and is on the FAA Commercial Space Transportation Advisory Committee. He is the Historian for the Space Medicine Association.

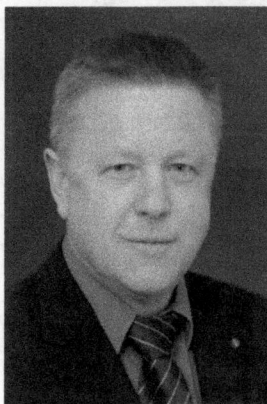

Dr. Viktor Harsch is an aerospace medicine specialist in Neubrandenburg (ETNU), Germany. He has been a flight surgeon for the Luftwaffe since 1999. He was deployed as AirMedEvac-specialist to Bosnia-Herzegowina, Georgia, Uzbekistan, and Afghanistan. He is currently in private family medicine practice concentrating on occupational health and travel medicine. He received AME training at CAMI in Oklahoma in 1996 and advanced aerospace medicine training at Brooks AFB in Texas in 2002. He finished his medical thesis on aviation history in Goettingen in 1996. He is a private pilot and has published over 12 articles and portions of 8 books related to aerospace medicine history. He is a member of the German Society for Aviation and Space Medicine (DGLRM) and the Aerospace Medical Association (AsMA). He is a Fellow of the Aerospace Medical Association and the International Academy of Aviation and Space Medicine. He is the Historian of the German Society of Aviation and Space Medicine.

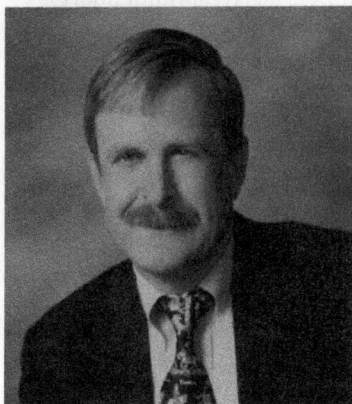

Mark Campbell   **Viktor Harsch**

RETHRA VERLAG
- NEUBRANDENBURG -
RETHRA PUBLISHING

www.rethra-publishing.de

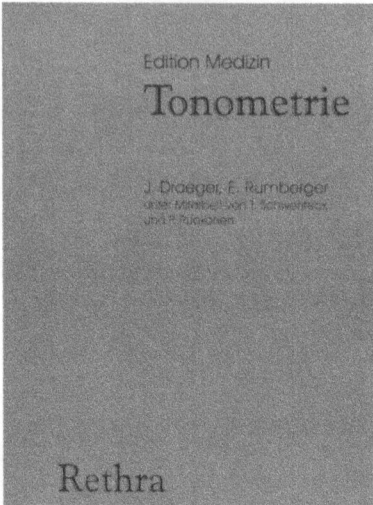

Draeger J., Rumberger E. (2008):
Tonometry.
162 pages, 88 figures, 23.80 €
ISBN: 9783937394176

Contributors:

Draeger J. (ed.), Rumberger E. (ed.),
Ruokonen P., Schwenteck T.

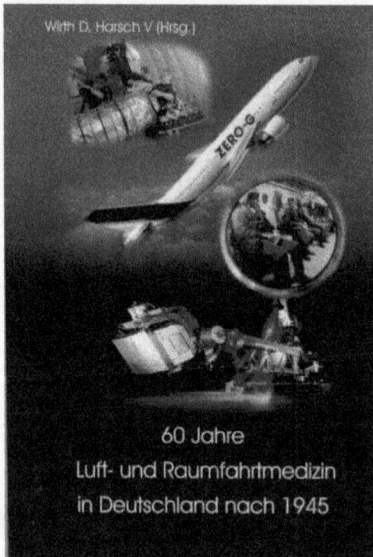

Wirth D. and Harsch V. (2008):
60 years of Aviation and Space Medicine in Germany after 1945.
Rethra Verlag, Neubrandenburg.
252 pages, 78 figures, 29.80 €
ISBN: 9783937394107

Contributors:

Gerzer R., Gunga H.C., Haehn P., Harsch V. (ed.), Hendrik A., Kimmich K., Kirsch K., Klein K.E., Knueppel J., Kressin J., Milfeit R., Pongratz H., Ruyters G., Stueben U., Ulmer H.V., Welsch H., Wirth D. (ed.), Wurster J.

www.ingramcontent.com/pod-product-compliance
Lightning Source LLC
Chambersburg PA
CBHW020833210326
41598CB00019B/1886